Food Cults

Rowman & Littlefield Studies in Food and Gastronomy

Food studies is a vibrant and thriving field encompassing not only cooking and eating habits but also issues such as health, sustainability, food safety, and animal rights. Scholars in disciplines as diverse as history, anthropology, sociology, literature, and the arts focus on food. The mission of **Rowman & Littlefield Studies in Food and Gastronomy** is to publish the best in food scholarship, harnessing the energy, ideas, and creativity of a wide array of food writers today. This broad line of food-related titles will range from food history, interdisciplinary food studies monographs, general interest series, and popular trade titles to textbooks for students and budding chefs, scholarly cookbooks, and reference works.

Titles in the Series

Appetites and Aspirations in Vietnam: Food and Drink in the Long Nineteenth Century, by Erica J. Peters
Three World Cuisines: Italian, Mexican, Chinese, by Ken Albala
Food and Social Media: You Are What You Tweet, by Signe Rousseau
Food and the Novel in Nineteenth-Century America, by Mark McWilliams
Man Bites Dog: Hot Dog Culture in America, by Bruce Kraig and Patty Carroll
A Year in Food and Beer: Recipes and Beer Pairings for Every Season, by Emily Baime and Darin Michaels
Celebraciones Mexicanas: History, Traditions, and Recipes, by Andrea Lawson Gray and Adriana Almazán Lahl
The Food Section: Newspaper Women and the Culinary Community, by Kimberly Wilmot Voss
Small Batch: Pickles, Cheese, Chocolate, Spirits, and the Return of Artisanal Foods, by Suzanne Cope
Food History Almanac: Over 1,300 Years of World Culinary History, Culture, and Social Influence, by Janet Clarkson
Cooking and Eating in Renaissance Italy: From Kitchen to Table, by Katherine A. McIver
Eating Together: Food, Space, and Identity in Malaysia and Singapore, by Jean Duruz and Gaik Cheng Khoo
Nazi Hunger Politics: A History of Food in the Third Reich, by Gesine Gerhard
The Carrot Purple and Other Curious Stories of the Food We Eat, by Joel S. Denker
Food in the Gilded Age: What Ordinary Americans Ate, by Robert Dirks
Food Cults: How Fads, Dogma, and Doctrine Influence Diet, edited by Kima Cargill

Food Cults

How Fads, Dogma, and Doctrine Influence Diet

Edited by Kima Cargill

ROWMAN & LITTLEFIELD
Lanham • Boulder • New York • London

Published by Rowman & Littlefield
A wholly owned subsidiary of The Rowman & Littlefield Publishing Group, Inc.
4501 Forbes Boulevard, Suite 200, Lanham, Maryland 20706
www.rowman.com

Unit A, Whitacre Mews, 26-34 Stannary Street, London SE11 4AB

British Library Cataloguing in Publication Information Available

Library of Congress Cataloging-in-Publication Data

Names: Cargill, Kima, author.
Title: Food cults : how fads, dogma, and doctrine influence diet / edited by Kima Cargill.
Description: Lanham : Rowman & Littlefield, [2017] | Series: Rowman & Littlefield studies in food and gastronomy | Includes bibliographical references and index.
Identifiers: LCCN 2016027109 (print) | LCCN 2016046779 (ebook) | ISBN 9781442251311 (cloth : alk. paper) | ISBN 9781442251328 (electronic)
Subjects: LCSH: Food habits—Social aspects. | Food preferences—Social aspects. | Nutrition—Social aspects. | Diet—Social aspects.
Classification: LCC GT2855 .F658 2016 (print) | LCC GT2855 (ebook) | DDC 394.1/2—dc23
LC record available at https://lccn.loc.gov/2016027109

™ The paper used in this publication meets the minimum requirements of American National Standard for Information Sciences Permanence of Paper for Printed Library Materials, ANSI/NISO Z39.48-1992.

Printed in the United States of America

Contents

Introduction

What do we mean when we call any group a cult? Defining that term is a slippery proposition; the word is provocative—even pejorative, according to some.[1] Does it necessarily refer to a religious group? A group with a charismatic leader? Or something darker and more sinister?

Most people associate the term *cult* with religion. Indeed, the term originated in the early seventeenth century from the Latin *cultus*, meaning "to worship." Early sociologists in the United States and Germany introduced this term as a sociological classification to distinguish different types of religious behavior.[2] Outside of the social sciences, the term was also used in the 1930s medical literature in the United States to describe faith-healing practices, first linking cults with healing and the body. The term came to emphasize the deviant nature of a religious group,[3] which was often characterized by tension with and disenfranchisement from mainstream culture.[4] Certainly many groups called cults have been on the fringes of society due to their unorthodox beliefs, but it is also true that some of them eventually became mainstream (see Christianity). In fact, Saul Levine, a psychiatrist who works with the concerned families of cult members, humorously defines cults as any group to which relatives are opposed, citing Catholics, Mormons, Orthodox Jews, born-again Christians, and the company IBM as examples of groups he has heard referred to as cults.[5]

Recently scholars have attempted to neutralize the connotation of the word *cult*, arguing that membership is often part of a larger quest for spirituality and community.[6] Psychiatrist Marc Galanter argues that cults are better thought of as a type of charismatic group characterized by a consensual belief system, a high level of social cohesiveness, and a charismatic leader,[7] while other scholars have further expanded the term to include political groups.[8]

Cults cut across religion, psychotherapy, self-help, politics, and business trainings;[9] yet little attention has been paid to the ways that nutritional and dietary ideologies inspire similar fervor among adherents. In addition, such "food cults" are very often led by a guru or charismatic leader promising longevity, fertility, and vitality, just as we see in other kinds of cults. Note that food cults differ from communities defined by a regional cuisine in that they are chosen as an ideology, as opposed to groups defined by cuisine that emerges naturally from ecological restraints and dietary opportunities.[10] Membership in a food cult often becomes a central organizer of one's identity, revolving around a group dogma or ideology, often providing a conversion experience, a charismatic leader, and a community of "worship" (either in person or, increasingly, online). Documenting these extreme beliefs and practices allows us to see the ways in which food serves as a nexus for religious beliefs, pseudoscience, sexuality, death anxiety, preoccupation with the body, asceticism, and hedonism, to name a few.

Outside of academic discussions, we can also see where the term *cult* is increasingly used in popular culture to refer to the near-religious devotion for certain consumer brands (e.g., Cult of Mac), as well as a way to describe powerful trends that straddle health, fitness, and spirituality (e.g., the cult of Bikram yoga). The *Oxford English Dictionary*[11] embraces this broader usage, defining *cult* as

1. A particular form or system of religious worship or veneration, esp. as expressed in ceremony or ritual directed towards a specified figure or object.
2. A relatively small group of people having (esp. religious) beliefs or practices regarded by others as strange or sinister, or as exercising excessive control over members.
3. A collective obsession with or intense admiration for a particular person, thing, or idea.

Thus we should also consider food cults through the lens of popular culture, allowing us to see how dietary ideologies mediate identity within the context of a consumer economy. In fact, anthropologist Marvin Harris suggested that "in market economies such as the United States, good to eat may mean good to sell,"[12] highlighting how our food preferences, beliefs, and choices are often shaped by supply-side forces. To that end, many of the contributors to this volume explore how contemporary Western dietary trends emerge simply because they are sold to us as products with countless promises.

Ultimately I embrace the broadest definition of *cult* because it allows the widest intellectual berth in exploring the mechanisms of group and individual identity, the distortion of nutritional science, the ways in which food behaviors express our anxieties, and how dietary practices organize us psychologically. While there are a variety of scholarly accounts of various food communities across disciplines, there is no single collection that pulls together these works or anchors these communities in a theory of why we gravitate toward them and the social and psychological functions they serve.

This volume documents and investigates domestic and international, contemporary and historic food communities characterized by extreme nutritional beliefs or viewed as "fringe" movements by mainstream culture. For example, raw foodists claim that a strictly raw food diet promotes "a sense of well-being, better physical functioning, less bodily pain, more vitality, and improved emotional and social performance."[13] Yet scientific studies of raw food diets have shown that its adherents experience constant hunger, failure to menstruate, decreased libido, and dramatic reductions in reproductive functioning. It is difficult to believe that ravenous, infertile people feel good. From an evolutionary perspective, we should feel worse, not better, when our reproductive functioning is imperiled. In other words, a raw food diet is not adaptive for human beings, so how do we make sense of subjective reports of improved vitality from raw foodists?

One possibility is that raw foodists' claims of improved well-being are valid in spite of decreased reproductive functioning—in other words, the diet may have a paradoxical effect that science cannot yet explain. Another possibility, however, is that the subjective sense of improved well-being is strictly psychological. If the second hypothesis is true, how, then, might we explain this phenomenon? Chapter 1 of this volume uses psychoanalytic and existential theories to explain why a raw food diet and so many others appeal to our deepest unconscious wishes, so much so that we are often blind to the false promises thus offered. In chapter 2, Leighann R. Chaffee and Corey L. Cook use theories from cognitive psychology to explain the mechanisms of pseudoscientific thinking and how we are often duped into belief systems by clever gurus and marketers who use the same psychological tactics that circus performers, magicians, and psychics have utilized for centuries.

While the first two chapters of this volume provide psychological models for understanding food cults, the next set of chapters broadens the focus to interdisciplinary case studies of specific historical and contemporary food cults and communities. We might imagine that dietary trends and nutrition are unique to contemporary culture, but Paul A. Brazinski reminds us that such practices existed in biblical times, prompting the questions: Is there something innate in humankind that draws us toward dietary rituals or cults? Or do contemporary food cults simply originate in early religious rituals, now secularized and urbanized for many of us?

Several chapters explore how food cults provide a framework for "healthism," often characterized by purification and cleansing rituals. Samuel Veissière and Liona Gibbs-Bravo, for example, enter the world of juicing culture, finding themselves unable to resist the seductive (and expensive) promises of moral and nutritional superiority. Meanwhile, Tina Sikka examines "superfoods," arguing that superfood companies construct an image of progressive pro-health products in order to mask an underlying reliance on neoliberal business practices and gendered stereotypes. In contrast to these superfood companies, other corporations use discursive practices appealing to the "glutton" in order to maximize profits, argues Carlnita P. Greene, who uses Olive Garden as a case study for the cult of gluttony.

Several other contributors explore the dynamics of extreme nutritional ideologies, such as paleo/primal/caveman diets versus vegetarianism, veganism, and fruitarian diets. Lenore Bell makes a compelling case in arguing that the paleo diet, combined with the CrossFit exercise program, emerged after 9/11 in New York as a means to calm anxieties surrounding future terrorist attacks. Amanda Maxfield and Andrea Rissing analyze online discourses by primal dieters versus those of fruitarians, finding that, in spite of their ostensibly oppositional dietary approaches, the two groups are actually quite similar in their logics, tactics, and motivations. Michele Scott, meanwhile, returns us to the theme of neoliberalism as it mediates dietary practices and identity, comparing the paleo diet to the elective restrictive diet.

Just as one cannot live on bread alone, no volume on dietary ideologies would be complete without discussing gluten-free diets. L. Sasha Gora examines the revival of sourdough baking in Europe and North America in contrast to the development of gluten-free lifestyles, arguing that these polarizing practices mediate anxiety surrounding food, culture, and choice. Jennifer Martin, meanwhile, explores the tensions between "card-carrying" members of the gluten-free cult—that is, sufferers of celiac disease—and the newly arrived gluten-free "hobbyists" who bring additional market demand for gluten-free menus and products but run the risk of undermining the credibility of the movement.

Finally, several contributors focus on specific ethnic groups and their food practices. Preety Gadhoke and Barrett P. Brenton, for example, argue that foodways and related belief systems among Native Americans in North America are products of traumatic loss and social devastations. Moving to the other side of the globe, De-Valera Botchway and Charles Prempeh examine marijuana ingestion for nutrition among ghetto Muslim youth in Ghana. Meanwhile, Liora Gvion and Irit Sharir conclude the volume with their chapter on the formation of maternal identity via food practices in Israel.

Bon appétit!

NOTES

1. Paul J. Olson, "The Public Perception of 'Cults' and 'New Religious Movements,'" *Journal for the Scientific Study of Religion* 45, no. 1 (2006): 97–106.
2. L. von Wiese and H. P. Becker, *Systematic Sociology: On the Basis of the Beziehungslehre and Gebildelehre of Leopold Von Wiese* (Hoboken: J. Wiley & Sons, 1932); Ernst Troeltsch, *The Social Teaching of the Christian Churches* (New York, 1931), *II779* (1912).
3. C. Bader and A. Demaris, "A Test of the Stark-Bainbridge Theory of Affiliation with Religious Cults and Sects," *Journal for the Scientific Study of Religion* 35, no. 3 (September 1996): 285–303.
4. J. T. Richardson, "Definitions of Cult: From Sociological-Technical to Popular-Negative," *Review of Religious Research* 34, no. 4 (June 1993): 348–56.
5. Saul Levine, "Life in the Cults," in *Cults and New Religious Movements*, edited by Marc Galanter, 95–108 (Washington, DC: American Psychiatric Association, 1989).
6. Bader and Demaris, "A Test of the Stark-Bainbridge Theory."
7. Marc Galanter, ed., *Cults and New Religious Movements: A Report of the American Psychiatric Association* (Washington, DC: American Psychiatric Association, 1989).
8. D. Tourish and T. Wohlforth, *On the Edge: Political Cults Right and Left* (New York: M. E. Sharpe, 2000).
9. Tourish and Wohlforth, *On the Edge*, 3.
10. M. Harris, *Good to Eat: Riddles of Food and Culture* (New York: Simon and Schuster, 1985).
11. OED Online, "Cults," http://www.oed.com/view/Entry/45709?rskey=7CMReS&result=1#eid.
12. Harris, *Good to Eat.*
13. Richard W. Wrangham, *Catching Fire: How Cooking Made Us Human* (New York: Basic Books, 2009).

BIBLIOGRAPHY

Bader, C., and A. Demaris. "A Test of the Stark-Bainbridge Theory of Affiliation with Religious Cults and Sects." *Journal for the Scientific Study of Religion* 35, no. 3 (September 1996): 285–303.

Galanter, Marc, ed. *Cults and New Religious Movements: A Report of the American Psychiatric Association.* Washington, DC: American Psychiatric Association, 1989.

Harris, M. *Good to Eat: Riddles of Food and Culture*. New York: Simon and Schuster, 1985.

Levine, Saul. "Life in the Cults." In *Cults and New Religious Movements*, edited by Marc Galanter, 95–108. Washington, DC: American Psychiatric Association, 1989.

OED Online. "Cults." http://www.oed.com/view/Entry/45709?rskey=7CMReS&result=1#eid.

Olson, Paul J. "The Public Perception of 'Cults' and 'New Religious Movements.'" *Journal for the Scientific Study of Religion* 45, no. 1 (2006): 97–106.

Richardson, J. T. "Definitions of Cult: From Sociological-Technical to Popular-Negative." *Review of Religious Research* 34, no. 4 (June 1993): 348–56.

Tourish, D., and T. Wohlforth. *On the Edge: Political Cults Right and Left*. New York: M. E. Sharpe, 2000.

Troeltsch, Ernst. *The Social Teaching of the Christian Churches*. New York, 1931. *II779* (1912).

von Wiese, L., and H. P. Becker. *Systematic Sociology: On the Basis of the Beziehungslehre and Gebildelehre of Leopold Von Wiese*. Hoboken: J. Wiley & Sons, 1932.

Wrangham, Richard W. *Catching Fire: How Cooking Made Us Human*. New York: Basic Books, 2009.

Chapter One

The Psychology of Food Cults

Kima Cargill

Most of the chapters in this volume describe the beliefs and practices of specific food cults. But before we learn about those specific communities we should first think broadly about why people are attracted to such groups at all. What are the psychological mechanisms involved in the joining of groups defined by extreme or fervent dietary ideologies? Of course, dietary practices and nutritional beliefs do not just serve physical health—they serve a great many psychological functions as well. Salubrious psychological effects can include a sense of agency and empowerment, as well as pride in self-care. Conversely, eating behavior and nutritional beliefs can be an expression or source of psychological distress.

In my clinical psychology practice I have seen many of the ways in which dietary practices and beliefs can mediate distress. For example, one of my former patients who was diagnosed with obsessive-compulsive disorder developed a great many rules about food that she eventually came to understand as an extension of her fears about infection and contamination. Similarly, it is common for patients with paranoid schizophrenia to believe that their food is poisoned, contaminated, or compromised—an extension of the characteristic paranoid and persecutory delusions. In addition, depressed individuals frequently lose their appetite as part of the neurovegetative and anhedonic symptoms of depression,[1] thereby experiencing food as tasteless, bleak, and unpalatable. In the same way that food fears and anxieties exist on this individual level, groups can experience a shared psychology surrounding food or drink. For example, adherents of urotherapy believe that drinking one's own urine increases longevity and fertility, along with curing a wide variety of common ailments.[2] Groups such as these, often considered cults, are frequently dismissed as extremists, especially when their nutritional dogma is not founded on science, but I believe there is much to learn by understanding their practices. Making meaning of such extreme or unusual behavior informs all psychological phenomena. To that end, the study of cults is nothing more than the study of idiosyncratic healing movements or cultures that hold potent appeal.[3] Doomsday cults, for example, might seem like deviant groups, but they circle around an obliterating question that we all spend considerable psychic energy managing: When and how will the world end? In other words, extremists sometimes serve as proxies for us in how they engage with the fears that we all face. Paradoxically, that may be the very reason why such groups become the object of scorn. By directing our derision at such "crackpots" we project, and therefore externalize, our deepest fears. In this chapter I explore these dynamics by focusing on three psychological functions of food cult membership:

1. the ways in which it offers a medium for group identity and cohesion
2. how it functions as secular religions in contemporary Western culture
3. how such groups offer a means to manage and contain some of our deepest existential anxieties

GROUP IDENTITY AND COHESION

First and foremost, participation in a cult of any sort provides belongingness—a sense of being part of something bigger and more meaningful than ourselves. Saul Levine, a leading expert on cult behavior, observed, "It may sound silly, but one cannot be a cult unto oneself. It takes numbers of people acting in a concerted, shared, cohesive effort to produce the phenomenal elevation of the group in importance and the subjugation of the self, which we see so regularly."[4] Consider that from a developmental psychology perspective, the individual's construction of identity and sense of security both originate socially—usually in the mother/infant dyad and later extending to the nuclear family, larger kinship networks, and clans or tribes. As we mature into adulthood, our relationships with new groups are developmentally anchored in these early experiences, and we are then tasked with balancing the sometimes competing demands of group versus individual identity. In *Group Psychology and Analysis of the Ego*, Sigmund Freud argued that there is a tension between individual and group identity, such that surrender to a collective entity is irrational in his view, and therefore doing so must involve some reward.[5] He hypothesized that the reward is a powerful sense of harmony if the group structure recalls familial patterns of comfort and security. Such submersion of ego into the group, he reasoned, provides a temporary release of control, ultimately resulting in idealization and love of the group. In a manner of speaking, the group absorbs the individual, calming and soothing anxiety through symbiosis. In fact, empirical evidence supports the notion that cult membership rewards the individual with improved psychological well-being, a finding that we shall return to later in this chapter.

Not only does group identification provide instinctive comfort and attachment, but it also serves to define individual identity by putting into relief the ways in which we are similar to and different from others. Psychologists Mihaly Csikszentmihalyi and Eugene Rochberg-Halton argued that individual identity is driven by two dynamic forces: *differentiation*, in which we seek separation from others by emphasizing our distinct individuality, and *similarity*, in which we express our integration and sameness with our social context.[6] We seem to need to experience ourselves as simultaneously similar to and different than others. Consider as an everyday example how bumper stickers serve the dual purposes of differentiation and similarity. They distinguish a car owner as unique, by being, say, a lover of ferrets or the Grateful Dead. At the same time, they call out to other like-minded members of those tribes, who might honk and wave to express solidarity. Similarly, participation in food cults, or any cults, stands to achieve the goals of differentiation and similarity. Being a raw foodist, for example, exists in sharp contrast to mainstream Western dietary practices; yet at the same time it provides a group of support and like-minded others.

Writing about the appeal of cults, psychiatrist Saul Levine noted that "the sense of belonging cannot be overemphasized. It creates an inner 'specialness' (some might call it 'preciousness'), and a united feeling of 'us (inside) against them (outside).'"[7] Note that with this comment Levine introduces a new idea—that cult membership provides not only belongingness but also a potential means of expressing antagonism. Indeed, such antagonism, or an "us against them" mentality, may be a universal human trait, existing across cultures, geographies, and epochs. But why? Why would we naturally (if that is indeed the case) seek to create and enforce antagonistic boundaries between groups? Is it simply human nature to dichotomize ourselves into opposing groups as a heuristic for understanding differences? Are men really from Mars and women really from Venus? Are cats better than dogs? Are there really two kinds of people in the world: those who think there are two kinds of people in the world and those who don't?

My mother once told me that in the small Oklahoma town where she grew up, all town life was strictly demarcated by membership in either the Methodist Church or the Church of Christ—two nearly indistinguishable sects of Protestantism when considered within the broader context of world religions. After Sunday church services each group repaired to separate cafeterias to eat. Members of each group were expected to exclusively socialize with, date, and marry members of their own group. Those who deviated from these norms were subject to ostracism and strict social punishment. Given the very minor theological differences between these two religions, we might imagine that strict adherence to these boundaries was driven less by meaningful doctrinal differences than by the need for a convenient social heuristic in the construction of in-groups and out-groups—what Freud referred to as the "narcissism of minor differences."[8]

In explaining such antagonistic behavior, political psychoanalyst Vamik Volkan has argued that humans have an "inescapable need" for enemies and allies.[9] The cornerstone of his theory is that this psychological need is the foundation for the development of ethnic and national identity, as well as a means to regulate ourselves when under threat. He says that we engage in regressive behavior when within the safety of our groups, developing shibboleths and imbuing objects with mystical value as talismans against out-groups. National flags, mascots, and even architectural features, for example, are the kinds of symbols that come to define specific groups and become charged with meaning. In fact, he believes that most multigenerational ethnic conflicts originate in this phenomenon, citing Serbs versus Croatians, Palestinians versus Israelis, and Turks versus Greeks.[10] But what if we are not born into such tribalism? What if we were born into relatively peaceful, safe, and uncontested territory? What if, like many people in the contemporary United States, we don't have strong ethnic or regional identities or a clear sense of how we fit into a meaningful clan? How, then, do we satisfy the "inescapable need" for enemies and allies? I submit that it is these conditions that drive us to seek out dogmatic groups based on voluntary membership. Indeed, cult researchers Dennis Tourish and Tim Wolford argued that an essential behavior of contemporary cults is the creation of a "grandfalloon"—an irredeemable out-group that serves to cement group loyalty and solidarity.[11] Cult membership, in other words, provides a surrogate mechanism for satisfying the inescapable need for enemies and allies.

Consider someone who strongly identifies with a paleo diet, who then by necessity distinguishes themselves from starch eaters—those poor folks who are victim to agriculture's ills. In fact, arguments over this narcissism of small differences comprise much of the content in online discussion forums for paleo, primal, caveman, and Neolithic diets. For example, one commenter writes, "Paleo puts the Paleolithic Era on a pedestal and says that this is the ideal model for how a human should eat. Primal is more vague and doesn't get very specific about which era was the best or not, just that our modern lifestyle doesn't work, so it's good to dial things back to a more primitive time."[12] Other examples abound, showing how grandfalloons can be defined by dietary differences. For example, many ethnic slurs are based on dietary habits: Krauts for Germans; Rice Eater, Bug Eater, or Dog Eater for various Asian groups; Limey for Brits (which originated from British sailors eating and smelling like limes in order to ward off scurvy); and Curry-Muncher, used in Africa to refer to Indians. In fact, historically the foods that one group eats often become a salient marker for other groups that don't or won't eat that food. For example, many Hindu castes adhere to a strict vegetarian diet and believe that Indian Muslims, who typically eat meat, are bloodthirsty and carnal. The dietary beliefs unify the in-group and delineate its members from the out-group.

In addition to providing this mechanism for group identity and cohesion, food cult membership offers additional comfort by way of organizing rituals and rules.

FOOD CULTS AS SECULAR RELIGIONS

Psychiatrists E. M. Pattison and Robert Ness argue that cults offer a form of communion, which they define as "an intimate psychosocial network characterized by a high level of psychic-emotional bonding and a shared set of belief, values, and behavioral orientations."[13] Yet communion is not just a social ritual but also a moral one. Historically, family, tribe, and religion filled humans' social and moral needs, but in the contemporary United States and much of the secular urban West, people are less likely than ever to live in close proximity to families or to participate in organized religion. Psychiatrist Marc Galanter argues that this is why cults emerge—that when there is a crisis in the culture and individuals become deprived of a meaningful orientation to their lives they seek out meaning through artificial or voluntary structures.[14] Similarly, Pattison and Ness argue that people gravitate to cults as a means to create smaller structures of meaning if the broader culture has become more abstract, impersonal, and utilitarian. They document the historical chronology of such structures of meaning, originating with villages or tribal settings defined by agricultural solidarity. These tribal structures later evolved into more complex feudal societies defined by merchant guilds and organized religions. That period was followed by the early stages of industrial society in which fraternal orders and labor unions emerged. Finally, in postmodern urbanized societies, they say that structures of meaning have become "all manner of flying saucer groups, self-help groups and health cults."[15] While this humorous characterization might sound like an indictment of postmodern urban culture, their ultimate conclusion is that cults are really nothing more than "culture writ small."[16]

In short, the loss of stabilizing structures in urban industrial environments makes life more ambiguous and difficult. People find it increasingly burdensome to constantly carve out a singular identity and have an unmet desire for community, rules, and a means to distinguish right from wrong. Accordingly, the Pew Research Center recently reported that 23 percent of Americans now identify as atheist or agnostic, up from 16 percent in 2007.[17] Among millennials, 70 percent claim no religious affiliation and say that religion is not important in their lives. This secularization has left many searching for the structure and identity that religion once provided. Even "atheist churches" have sprung up in some areas,[18] suggesting that religion, or at least church attendance, provides something important besides the belief in God. Food cults arguably replace what religion once did by prescribing organizing food rules and rituals. Like religion, they provide meaning in confusing situations, giving us moral guidelines and comfort. In urban, secular cultures and locations such as the United States, food cults are arguably more appealing than ever, both because they function as new religions and because of the unprecedented cultural premium placed on health, longevity, and the body. Several chapters in this volume explore this phenomenon by examining the beliefs and practices surrounding juicing, paleo lifestyles, superfoods, and fruitarianism.

While religion often provides comfort and community, it can also bring guilt, salvation, purification, judgment, and ritual. Food cults that function as new religions do not disappoint in this regard. They provide adherents with a vehicle for all of these phenomena and then some. For example, one of my patients, a lapsed Catholic, seemed to have transferred much of her religious thinking onto her diet. Themes of good and evil, temptation and sacrifice, temperance and salvation dominated her thoughts and language surrounding food. She voraciously read popular diet books, combed online forums, and visited various healers and nutritionists—the more extreme, the better. It seemed that she was seeking not just nutritional guidance but also a rigid framework involving deprivation and sacrifice. When she once described a trip to the grocery store I could almost imagine her walking through the aisles with a devil on one shoulder and an angel on the other. Not only had she replaced the moral framework of Catholicism with these rigid and elaborate dietary doctrines, but she had also replaced priest and confessional with psychologist and psychotherapy.

Historian Harvey Levenstein, in describing widespread food fears in America, argued that residual Puritanism and its tradition of self-denial made Americans especially vulnerable to nutritionists' cautions against pleasure and hedonism.[19] This guilt over self-indulgence, along with the belief that self-denial is the road to salvation, surely played a role in the appeal of restrictive or self-punishing food cults. For example, adherents of calorie-restricting longevity diets often practice a grueling 40 percent daily calorie reduction for years, believing that such restriction yields a longer life span and lower rates of cancer, diabetes, and other diseases, in spite of mixed scientific evidence in both humans and nonhumans.[20] Like so many religions, a great many extreme diet communities often feature fasting, asceticism, conversion, and renewal as their central tenets.

Another way in which cults of all types parallel religion is in the offering of a conversion experience to newcomers. Many later chapters in this volume discuss the centrality and importance of a conversion experience in the appeal of food cults. In chapter 5, for example, ethnographer Liona Gibbs-Bravo recounts how she was seduced into the world of juicing through a highly proscribed cleansing ritual:

> On the second night of my cleanse, I found myself sitting at a barbecue sipping my Mean Green juice while my friends ate their burgers, scrolling through Instagram to see what other juicers were up to. I felt a quiet satisfaction in knowing that by giving up that burger I was becoming a healthier, *better person*. This intense feeling of self-satisfaction and moral superiority in my deprivation in fact remained as a strong undercurrent throughout my cleanse process. When I was staring at the clock with my stomach growling waiting desperately for the time I could start my next juice, or having trouble falling asleep because I was so hungry, I felt I would be rewarded for this work by emerging as a cleaner, happier person.

Similarly, Leighann Chaffee and Corey Cook, in their chapter on pseudoscientific nutritional beliefs, observe that "many food cults gain popularity through books written by an author touting the transformative power of making a major dietary change (e.g., low-carb, paleo, and gluten-free diets all claim that restricting one or more ingredients results in weight loss, greater energy, and overall better health)." Like religious leaders, dietary gurus often assert their credibility and attract their following by describing their own conversion experience. The followers frequently deify the leaders of these extreme dietary movements—a hallmark of all cults. For example, Mark Sisson, leader of the currently popular primal diet, maintains a well-trafficked website called Mark's Daily Apple—the name of which itself is arguably an oblique reference to original sin. There he posts nutritional sermons combined with musings on the modern world and its temptations. Adherents write in with their stories of conversion and salvation, thanking Sisson for his guidance and example, often crediting him with saving their lives or showing them the right path. For example, an eighteen-year-old named Andrew writes in, "I would like to thank Mark Sisson and the Primal lifestyle for saving my life." He then goes on to recount a harrowing hiking trip in the desert in which he became separated and lost from his group. He credits the primal lifestyle with his ability to stay calm, accurately read his map, and relocate the hiking trail, concluding with "thank you Mark and the rest of the Primal Blueprint team for all you've done for me and so many others worldwide. In multiple senses I owe my life to your efforts."[21] Such accounts also indicate that membership in food cults serves as a means of calming our anxieties, the topic of the final section of this chapter.

FOOD CULTS, ANXIETY, AND THE RELIEF EFFECT

In 1936, *Fortune* magazine observed, "The willingness to eat not for pleasure but for health is doubtless due to a fundamental U.S. trait: the fear of being sickly. Perhaps in England, but certainly not in France or Spain or Germany or Russia, will you find people so anxious to believe that by eating a certain way they can achieve a life buoyant and vigorous. Here it is the gourmet who is the curiosity, the dietitian who is the prophet."[22] This passage suggests that certain cultures may be primed to experience more food anxiety than others. Such cultures are consequently likely to be more vulnerable to food fads, trends, and cults that promise structure and safety in the face of both ambiguous and ubiquitous threats to the self. Paleo and related diets, for example, were not the first dietary trends in the United States to idealize preindustrial or primitive diets. In fact, earlier fears over modern food processing led to natural food diets whose rhetoric bears uncanny resemblance to today's paleo/primal adherents. In the 1920s, one doctor promoted the diet of the "uncivilized" people of the remote Himalayan Hunza Valley in Kashmir, claiming that their unprocessed foods led to unusually fertile and long lives. By contrast, "civilized man, by desiccation, by heating, by freezing and thawing, by oxidation and decomposition, by milling and polishing, had eliminated the natural from his food and substituted the artificial, bringing on a host of health problems."[23] The so-called Hunza diet and the description of the Hunza people became a popular tale of Shangri-La, inspiring a best-selling book and Hollywood movie. Levenstein argues that such anxieties about food have surely existed since ancestral times but that industrialization and globalization have "ratcheted up" these fears by placing unprecedented distance between food sources and our tables. Such distance is threatening because food that is prepared out of our control could be contaminated, tainted, or poisoned. Eating food we did not grow or prepare ourselves is a leap of faith in food safety laws, regulation, and anonymous third parties. That leap of faith generates anxiety that we must manage and defend against. In addition to the reality that bad food can kill us, there are also a great many other elements of food and nutrition that affect our fertility, longevity, and general well-being. Food cults speak to these anxieties by providing systems of meaning and support that act as psychological talismans against existential threats.

Indeed, Galanter has found that many cult members experience enhanced well-being, which he terms the "relief effect."[24] His research with members of new religious movements shows that this therapeutic effect often comes with considerable sacrifice, but increased comfort and well-being is generated by the group closeness and conformity provided by cults. Building on Galanter's findings, psychologist Brock Kilbourne found that in order for a cult to provide this relief effect it must be structured with the following characteristics:

1. a special supportive, empathic, and confiding relationship between the adherent and the group
2. a setting imbued with powerful symbols of expertise, help, hope, and healing

3. a special rationale, ideology, or indisputable myth that explains normality and abnormality and renders sensible the individual's self-preoccupations and inexplicable feelings
4. a special set of rituals and practices that confirms the individual's assumptive world[25]

Consider how food cults provide such relief from anxieties that are specific to embodiment and the physical self. Anxieties over fertility, longevity, and mortality, for example, differ from social and interpersonal anxieties. Somatic and existential anxieties seek relief that is more specific to the body. Special diets and food cults offer just such specific relief—a nutritional doctrine that promises to heal, along with the interpersonal closeness and intimacy of group membership. I first began to take notice of food cults several years ago in my clinical work with patients suffering from infertility. The majority of these patients are affluent, professional women who have delayed motherhood for educational and professional reasons. A smaller number of these patients are women who have suffered from long-term reproductive or endocrinological health problems, complicating or preventing their attempts to conceive. Most of them have spent tens of thousands of dollars and many years on intrusive procedures such as intrauterine insemination (IUI) and in vitro fertilization (IVF). Generally speaking, these are not women who are willing to let go of the prospect of biological motherhood or move on to adoption or a life without children. Those groups typically do not make it as far as my office, as they are not experiencing clinically significant levels of distress.

In my work with these women, there is a nearly audible biological clock ticking in the room. It is this desperation that drives many of them to try nearly any promise of increased fertility, irrespective of scientific merit. Over time I discovered that many of my patients go to the same naturopathic dietitian, who presents herself as a specialist in fertility. While I have not met this practitioner personally, nor am I familiar with the rationale for her so-called fertility diet, I am quite skeptical of the approach. Many of my patients pay her large sums of money for Chinese herbs that they brew into teas. Many of them are also prescribed a diet of bone broth, ox-blood soup, eggs, and baby carrots to be ingested at certain times during their menstrual cycle and in certain ritualized ways. Certainly an individual's diet affects fertility and general well-being, but there is no scientific evidence that anything beyond generally good nutrition and folic acid have any effect on fertility.

Future research might demonstrate that specific foods, teas, or herbs increase fertility, although no such evidence currently exists. Any claims to that effect must be considered a combination of wishful thinking and good marketing. Much like the supplement industry preys on magical thinking and desperation among consumers, so too do the purveyors of many specialized diets. I have come to believe that the aforementioned dietitian has loosely formed a food cult because of the sense of solidarity and community offered by membership, the deification of the leader, and the relief effect provided by the sense that following this diet will result in increased fertility. Yet, like any other cult, these are likely hollow promises offered by a false prophet.

CONCLUSION

In short, membership in food cults serves the same psychological functions of cult membership of any kind. People are attracted to cohesive groups as a means of defining identity and delineating in-group and out-group membership. Cults often serve these needs while also providing a guiding doctrine and rituals for behavior—a religion of sorts. Taken together, these functions converge into a means of managing anxiety, providing a relief effect. With their focus on diet and nutrition, food cults provide all of these functions, along with the added attention to somatic concerns and the body—namely, many of our deeper existential anxieties center around fears of mortality, fertility, attractiveness, and disease. Food cults hold a natural appeal in that they often address these anxieties, promising a systematic method for using food to tame, control, and heal the body. While this chapter addresses the psychological appeal of food cults using an existential/psychoanalytic approach, the next chapter provides a complementary model resting on cognitive psychological theories. Chaffee and Cook review the literature on pseudoscientific thinking, applying those findings to specific examples of food cults and their claims.

NOTES

1. American Psychiatric Association, *Diagnostic and Statistical Manual of Mental Disorders*, 5th ed. (Arlington: American Psychiatric Publications Incorporated, 2013).

2. Michael Braumstein, "Urine Therapy: If Health Is What You Urine For, Try This . . ." http://www.heartlandhealing.com/pages/archive/urine_therapy/.

3. Marc Galanter, *Cults: Faith, Healing, and Coercion* (New York: Oxford University Press, 1999).

4. Saul Levine, "Life in the Cults," in *Cults and New Religious Movements*, edited by Marc Galanter, 95–108 (Washington, DC: American Psychiatric Association, 1989), 97.

5. Sigmund Freud, *Group Psychology and the Analysis of the Ego* (New York: Boni and Liveright, 1920).

6. Mihaly Csikszentmihalyi and Eugene Halton, *The Meaning of Things: Domestic Symbols and the Self* (Cambridge: Cambridge University Press, 1981), 38.

7. Levine, "Life in the Cults," 97.

8. Sigmund Freud, "The Taboo of Virginity (Contributions to the Psychology of Love III)(1918)," *Standard Edition* 11 (1917): 191–209.

9. Vamik D. Volkan, "The Need to Have Enemies and Allies: A Developmental Approach," *Political Psychology* (1985): 219–47.

10. Vamik D. Volkan, *Bloodlines: From Ethnic Pride to Ethnic Terrorism* (New York: Farrar, Straus and Giroux, 1997).

11. D. Tourish and T. Wohlforth, *On the Edge: Political Cults Right and Left* (New York: M. E. Sharpe, 2000), 6.

12. Paleogrubs, "Paleo vs. Primal: Which Way of Eating Is Best?" http://paleogrubs.com/paleo-vs-primal.

13. E. M. Pattison and Robert Ness, "New Religious Movements in Historical Perspective," in *Cults and New Religious Movements*, edited by Marc Galanter (Washington, DC: American Psychiatric Association, 1989), 45.

14. Marc Galanter, ed., *Cults and New Religious Movements: A Report of the American Psychiatric Association* (Washington, DC: American Psychiatric Association, 1989), 26.

15. Pattison and Ness, "New Religious Movements in Historical Perspective," 47.

16. Pattison and Ness, "New Religious Movements in Historical Perspective," 81.

17. Pew Research Center, "U.S. Public Becoming Less Religious," 2015. Published electronically November 3, http://www.pewforum.org/2015/11/03/u-s-public-becoming-less-religious/.

18. David Brooks, "Building Better Secularists," *New York Times*, February 3, 2015.

19. Harvey Levenstein, *Fear of Food: A History of Why We Worry about What We Eat* (Chicago: University of Chicago Press, 2012), 4.

20. Ricki J. Colman, Rozalyn M. Anderson, Sterling C. Johnson, Erik K. Kastman, Kristopher J. Kosmatka, T. Mark Beasley, David B. Allison, et al., "Caloric Restriction Delays Disease Onset and Mortality in Rhesus Monkeys," *Science* 325, no. 5937 (2009): 201–4; Leonie K. Heilbronn and Eric Ravussin, "Calorie Restriction and Aging: Review of the Literature and Implications for Studies in Humans," *American Journal of Clinical Nutrition* 78, no. 3 (September 1, 2003): 361–69; Julie A. Mattison, George S. Roth, T. Mark Beasley, Edward M. Tilmont, April M. Handy, Richard L. Herbert, Dan L. Longo, et al., "Impact of Caloric Restriction on Health and Survival in Rhesus Monkeys from the Nia Study," *Nature* 489, no. 7415 (2012): 318–21; Stephen R. Spindler, "Biological Effects of Calorie Restriction: Implications for Modification of Human Aging," in *The Future of Aging: Pathways to Human Life Extension*, edited by Gregory M. Fahy, Michael D. West, L. Stephen Coles, and Steven B. Harris (Dordrecht: Springer Netherlands, 2010), 367–438.

21. Mark Sisson, "Mark's Daily Apple," http://www.marksdailyapple.com/how-primal-literally-saved-my-life/#ixzz45o1w57QK.

22. "The Wonders of Diet," *Fortune*, 1936, 86 (as quoted in Levenstein, *Fear of Food*, vii).

23. Levenstein, *Fear of Food*, 109.

24. Galanter, *Cults and New Religious Movements*, 32.

25. Brock Kilbourne, "Psychotherapeutic Implications of New Religious Affiliation," in *Cults and New Religous Movements*, edited by Marc Galanter (Washington, DC: American Psychiatric Association, 1989), 132.

BIBLIOGRAPHY

American Psychiatric Association. *Diagnostic and Statistical Manual of Mental Disorders*, 5th ed. Arlington: American Psychiatric Publications Incorporated, 2013.

Braumstein, Michael. "Urine Therapy: If Health Is What You Urine For, Try This . . ." http://www.heartlandhealing.com/pages/archive/urine_therapy/.

Brooks, David. "Building Better Secularists." *New York Times*, February 3, 2015.

Colman, Ricki J., Rozalyn M. Anderson, Sterling C. Johnson, Erik K. Kastman, Kristopher J. Kosmatka, T. Mark Beasley, David B. Allison, et al. "Caloric Restriction Delays Disease Onset and Mortality in Rhesus Monkeys." *Science* 325, no. 5937 (2009): 201–4.

Csikszentmihalyi, Mihaly, and Eugene Halton. *The Meaning of Things: Domestic Symbols and the Self*. Cambridge: Cambridge University Press, 1981.

Freud, Sigmund. *Group Psychology and the Analysis of the Ego*. New York: Boni and Liveright, 1920.

———. "The Taboo of Virginity (Contributions to the Psychology of Love III)(1918)." *Standard Edition* 11 (1917): 191–209.

Galanter, Marc. *Cults: Faith, Healing, and Coercion*. New York: Oxford University Press, 1999.

———, ed. *Cults and New Religious Movements: A Report of the American Psychiatric Association*. Washington, DC: American Psychiatric Association, 1989.

Heilbronn, Leonie K., and Eric Ravussin. "Calorie Restriction and Aging: Review of the Literature and Implications for Studies in Humans." *American Journal of Clinical Nutrition* 78, no. 3 (September 1, 2003): 361–69.

Kilbourne, Brock. "Psychotherapeutic Implications of New Religous Affiliation." In *Cults and New Religous Movements*, edited by Marc Galanter, 127–46. Washington, DC: American Psychiatric Association, 1989.

Levenstein, Harvey. *Fear of Food: A History of Why We Worry about What We Eat*. Chicago: University of Chicago Press, 2012.

Levine, Saul. "Life in the Cults." In *Cults and New Religious Movements*, edited by Marc Galanter, 95–108. Washington, DC: American Psychiatric Association, 1989.

Mattison, Julie A., George S. Roth, T. Mark Beasley, Edward M. Tilmont, April M. Handy, Richard L. Herbert, Dan L. Longo, et al. "Impact of Caloric Restriction on Health and Survival in Rhesus Monkeys from the Nia Study." *Nature* 489, no. 7415 (2012): 318–21.

Paleogrubs. "Paleo vs. Primal: Which Way of Eating Is Best?" http://paleogrubs.com/paleo-vs-primal.

Pattison, E. M., and Robert Ness. "New Religous Movements in Historical Perspective." In *Cults and New Religious Movements*, edited by Marc Galanter, 43–84. Washington, DC: American Psychiatric Association, 1989.

Pew Research Center. "U.S. Public Becoming Less Religious." 2015. Published electronically November 3. http://www.pewforum.org/2015/11/03/u-s-public-becoming-less-religious/.

Sisson, Mark. "Mark's Daily Apple." http://www.marksdailyapple.com/how-primal-literally-saved-my-life/#ixzz45o1w57QK.

Spindler, Stephen R. "Biological Effects of Calorie Restriction: Implications for Modification of Human Aging." In *The Future of Aging: Pathways to Human Life Extension*, edited by

Gregory M. Fahy, Michael D. West, L. Stephen Coles, and Steven B. Harris, 367–438. Dordrecht: Springer Netherlands, 2010.

Tourish, D., and T. Wohlforth. *On the Edge: Political Cults Right and Left*. New York: M. E. Sharpe, 2000.

Volkan, Vamik D. *Bloodlines: From Ethnic Pride to Ethnic Terrorism*. New York: Farrar, Straus and Giroux, 1997.

———. "The Need to Have Enemies and Allies: A Developmental Approach." *Political Psychology* (1985): 219–47.

"The Wonders of Diet." *Fortune*, 1936, 86.

Chapter Two

The Allure of Food Cults

Balancing Pseudoscience and Healthy Skepticism

Leighann R. Chaffee and Corey L. Cook

"The antioxidants released from gogi berries go into your liver and trigger disease-fighting chemicals that *literally* dissolve cancer cells within your body."

Why do people "buy into" food cults and the latest diet craze? Proprietary and cult-following diets abound; yet the U.S. national health status indicates no significant evidence of their efficacy. From the early proprietary diets to pharmaceuticals later determined unsafe for consumers to present-day fad diets, their popularity indicates a human predisposition toward food cults. Consumers are incessantly bombarded with products, services, and diets to improve health, but the information overwhelms rather than advises. Further complicating matters, there is no clear distinction for the average consumer between scientific and pseudoscientific claims. Pseudoscience deliberately misleads, providing vague generalizations, influencing with vivid anecdotes, and lacking falsifiability.[1] This is especially problematic as the layperson often lacks the training or experience to distinguish pseudoscience from true scientific claims. The characteristics of pseudoscience are common ingredients in marketing and promotional materials. We aim to describe mechanisms by which pseudoscientific evidence misleads consumers and propagates food cult following, while providing contemporary examples of this phenomenon and suggestions for combating pseudoscientific claims about nutrition.

MECHANISMS OF PSEUDOSCIENCE

Practitioners of pseudoscience influence and manipulate others by employing a number of cognitive mechanisms that promote gut-level heuristics over rational judgments. Proponents of critical thinking, such as the Skeptics Society, identify characteristics common among pseudoscientific claims. Recognition of these claims can serve as warning signs that the information provided may be misleading or bogus. Researchers have also identified common influence tactics[2] used by salesmen, politicians, and various advertising campaigns. People promoting pseudoscientific claims in the context of diet and nutrition often use these same tactics. Additionally, participation in groups defined by nutritional dogma helps satisfy many of the inherent social desires faced by humans—a fact not lost on proponents of pseudoscience.

CHARACTERISTICS OF PSEUDOSCIENCE: DID YOU KNOW YOU CAN CHEAT DEATH WITH THE ANTIOXIDANT POWER OF POMEGRANATE JUICE?

Many of the characteristics of pseudoscience are easily evidenced by the claims made by food cults and their proponents. The most common trait of pseudoscientific claims, according to John Ruscio,[3] is the appearance of actual science, lending credibility to such claims. In the appearance of science, food cults often cite studies and statistics as support—this can take the form of graphs, percentages, and comparisons to other foods in commercials and other promotional sources. However, the studies cited may not have come from peer-reviewed sources (the gold standard in actual science), or the findings from these studies may be exaggerated or reported lacking important contextual factors. For example, studies showing a correlational link between a particular ingredient or substance and a negative effect such as obesity or increased cancer rate in laboratory animals are often used and exaggerated to demonstrate the evils of said substance or related substances. Likewise, studies demonstrating a correlational link between "good" substances are often exaggerated when they support ideas proposed by the food cult. In both cases, correlation is often equated with causation, and as any introductory statistics student can vouch, correlation does not imply causation. Food cults may also employ the use of buzzwords that sound credible and exaggerate the beneficial or detrimental properties of a particular food or dietary habits. Claims regarding toxins, antioxidants, and superfoods are abundant and often rife with qualifiers such as *natural* (versus *unnatural* or *modified*). For example, superfood crazes such as acai berries and kale are touted for their antioxidant count and detoxifying abilities. Although some of these terms have concrete scientific meaning, the average person is unlikely to know what that meaning is. Likewise, claims regarding the abilities of these foods (e.g., that kale can dissolve unhealthy foods in the body) are vague and unverified. The heuristic associations these words imply nonetheless affect people's perceptions and behaviors regarding these foods.

Another characteristic of pseudoscience endemic among food cults is reliance on anecdotes and personal testimony. Anecdotal information makes an ostensible connection between two things (e.g., a dietary change and weight loss), and then it jumps to conclusions regarding "A" causing "B." For example, according to Godairyfree.org, cutting all dairy from one's diet can "squash [*sic*] headaches, migraines, rashes, stuffy sinuses, chronic infections, arthritis pain, and even narcolepsy." Many food cults gain popularity through books written by an author touting the transformative power of making a major dietary change (e.g., low-carb, paleo, and gluten-free diets all claim that restricting one or more ingredients results in weight loss, greater energy, and overall better health). These instances, though not validated, are then sold as miracle cures that will work for virtually everyone. There are a number of substantiated problems with relying on anecdotal evidence. For one, anecdotal examples lack any form of control for isolated variables. Additionally, many dietary fads and food cults recommend a number of changes (e.g., drink plenty of water, exercise daily, and get plenty of sleep) along with cutting out most processed and fast foods. These changes alone are enough to produce substantial health benefits regardless of any other major dietary changes or specific restrictions and are strengthened by the placebo effects of expecting to feel better as a result of changes in diet. However, as skeptics are fond of pointing out, the plural of *anecdote* is not *data*, and large-scale, controlled testing needs to be conducted before one can make strong generalizations regarding the benefits or consequences of particular dietary habits.

Another problem with pseudoscientific claims made by food cults is that they are not falsifiable—which defies one of the fundamental tests of scientific inquiry. Actual food science is incredibly complex because many of the basic aspects of experimental research, such as the use of control groups and experimental control over potential influencing variables, simply cannot be employed. This is evidenced historically by examples such as the banana diet—the first widely adopted treatment of celiac disease.[4] In the early part of the twentieth century, children suffering from the then undiagnosed disease were prescribed a strict diet consisting of bananas and milk. While this was in fact a successful treatment of celiac disease (because of the lack of gluten in the diet), the inability to isolate variables led to widespread beliefs of the magical curative properties of bananas (which are still labeled a "superfood") and to widespread adoption of the "banana diet" for weight loss and a host of non-celiac-related ailments. While the benefits the children received were due to the cessation of gluten consumption, it is nearly impossible to "prove" that bananas alone were not the catalyst for these benefits, save for the use of long-term tightly controlled experimental studies. As the idiom states, "the absence of evidence is not the evidence of absence"—it is much more difficult to provide evidence of nonexistence than the converse.

INFLUENCE TACTICS

Social cognition researchers have identified a wide variety of ways that rational judgment is often displaced by the use of gut-level heuristic processing. Kahneman refers to these as "fast" and "slow" processing systems,[5] while other models use terms such as *automatic* versus *systematic* processing. In his research on influence, Cialdini identifies six common tactics employed by "influence practitioners." These tactics often work by bypassing the rational, systematic, and slow thinking level and accessing the automatic, unconscious, fast cognitive system. Such tactics include the endorsement of apparent authority figures such as celebrity doctors or well-liked celebrity figures, use of social validation statements regarding the popularity of a particular diet or behavior, and inducing cognitive dissonance in members regarding their eating behaviors by shaming those who break dietary rules.

The first of these tactics is reciprocity. Evidence suggests that reciprocity is likely the most commonly endorsed human value, and it underlies a number of religious and cultural beliefs, including the Golden Rule, karma, and an eye for an eye.[6] As such, people feel compelled to offer concessions to those who appear to have first provided some favor. The language of food cults is seeped with this persuasion tactic, often *offering* some purported life-changing information. By coloring the language of the dietary message as though it is a favor being done specially for the adherents, food cults compel their members to respond in kind and follow the dogmatic rules they prescribe. This is an especially powerful tool when employed by some charismatic leader who embodies traits associated with other reciprocity tactics—namely, *liking* and *authority*. People are much more likely to comply with the requests of people they like and who appear to be an authority on the respective domain or behavior. For example, many people turn to the celebrity Dr. Oz for dietary advice, including his "two-week rapid weight loss diet" and a list of foods that allow you to "eat your way to better genes." Food cult leaders often appear empathetic to the plights of their would-be adherents; they understand the afflictions (e.g., obesity, low self-esteem, joint pain, stomach problems, etc.) of their followers and offer a "solution" for their suffering. These leaders often embody authority because they, too, have a similar story of past afflictions and plight that they were only able to overcome through adoption of the food doctrine.

Interestingly, evidence also suggests that the more one sacrifices for something, the more strongly they will be committed to that particular behavior or thing. This is evidenced in real life by phenomena such as fraternity hazing and rites of passage, in which experiencing some humiliating event or psychological or physical abuse strengthens one's commitment to a group. This is due in part to another influence principle known as *commitment and consistency*. People have a deep-rooted desire to remain consistent with previously endorsed attitudes, in large part because of the negative emotions (i.e., dissonance) that occurs when one's attitudes and behaviors do not align. Because of this, food cults require gestures of commitment from members—they may have to deny themselves common and often delicious foods, purchase special food items and preparation tools, and request special menus or menu items when dining out. After all, as Jesuschristdiet.com informs us, sugar is a (literal) product of the devil. The more sacrifices required for a group based on dogma, the more dissonance its members will experience if they attempt to pull away from the group or defy its rules. Likewise, the more drastic the changes made by members of food cults, the more difficult it will often be for them psychologically to renounce their membership. Concerns about membership can be alleviated, however, by another principle—*social validation*. This principle helps people validate beliefs or behavior by seeing the examples of others. Although conformity is often viewed in negative terms, there are very strong social pressures to go along with the group, as the consequences of going against the group can be severe and include repercussions such as shaming and a loss of status and important social connections. The final principle identified by Cialdini is *scarcity*; things seem more attractive when their availability appears limited. For this reason, food cults often treat their members as part of an initiated enlightened caste of people who alone understand the true method of being healthy, happy, and prosperous.

It is also important to consider social and cognitive motivations for believing pseudoscientific claims behind many food cults. People can accomplish a number of social goals by participating in food cults. For example, people may gain a feeling of acceptance and belonging—a fundamental human need[7]—by being part of such groups, while others can gain social capital, status, and power by taking on a leadership or authoritative role within the group. Work by Christakis and Fowler[8] on obesity, for instance, indicates that health behaviors spread through social influence and that promotion of both poor and good health behaviors can spread throughout social networks. Nutritional pseudoscientific claims offer clean, definitive answers about what you should and should not eat, while the nature of actual health information is messy, complicated, and constantly changing in the face of new evidence. Motivation for definitive answers, coupled with the social pressures of belonging, are powerful tools for influencing behavior. The pressure created by the motivation to belong is difficult to overstate. Evidence suggests that for as long as *Homo sapiens* have been a species, we have relied on our social networks to help satisfy the most basic social and survival needs, including psychological support, self and kin protection, forming romantic and social relationships, successfully raising children, and (of course) getting enough food to be healthy and prosperous.[9] As such, ostracism and shunning from a group, which often results from not following group norms, can have potentially devastating effects, including anger, sadness, depression, and motivation to comply with those norms, therefore reaffirming the strength of the claims made by food cults.[10]

INFORMATION/MODERN ENVIRONMENT

An essential consideration of why people fall prey to bogus nutritional claims is the unique modern food environment. Consider the differences between the modern food environment and that of our hunter-gatherer ancestors. For a majority of their time on earth, hominids—the genus of bipedal primates that includes ancestral species such as *Homo erectus* as well as modern humans (*Homo sapiens*)—lived in a world of food scarcity rather than abundance. Our modern ancestors functioned as hunter-gatherers, or foragers, from 250,000 to roughly 8,000 years before the common era.[11]

These ancestors ate the foods available in their natural environment, and obtaining sufficient food was a significant challenge, requiring hours of work each day. Their cognitive resources were therefore employed to locate and acquire sufficient foods. Population densities were low, humans lived in small groups, and the advent of tools and harnessing of fire had great impact on the ability of foragers to obtain adequate energy and survive. Agrarian life emerged approximately eight thousand years ago, allowing humans to form villages and eventually large societies. Agriculture enabled population growth, but agriculturalists had to expend a great deal of energy to obtain adequate nutrition from the earth. Resources such as irrigation and land were commodities as villages and civilizations formed around sources of water.

Contrast these eras with our modern world, especially the past few decades. Our food environment is highly unique when compared with the rest of human history. The availability and convenience of high-energy, dense food, coupled with the abundance of food cues in the environment, are highly difficult to navigate. Food decision making is further complicated by the complexity of nutrition recommendations consumers receive, from proprietary to governmental policy, as these recommendations are convoluted and contradictory. As stated previously, we have a motivation for definitive answers, which are increasingly difficult to find when considering nutrition. Together, these aspects of the modern environment contribute to the human propensity to follow food cults and fad diets and to believe pseudoscientific nutritional claims.

First, the availability and convenience of high-calorie, palatable foods in the modern world complicate food decision making. Despite the fact that many developing nations are food insecure (with insufficient caloric energy available to sustain the population), adults in the industrialized world experience nutritional surplus and consume over 3,000 kcal per capita per day.[12] Contemporary humans live in a time of food abundance and variety, using cognitive resources to navigate the plethora of choices at the local convenience store. We are faced with more food and eating-related options on a daily basis than we faced historically and are thus forced to make more food-related decisions. Research by Schwartz[13] indicates a paradox of choice, such that we experience stress or diminished satisfaction with our choice as options increase. The norms and rules characteristic of food cults ease the stress and confusion created by our modern abundance of choice. The appeal of our ancestral, more "natural" environment is employed by many food cults (e.g., paleo, Jesus diet, and raw diet). The proponents of these diet cults reference the simpler times of paradise past and express a fear of modernity.[14]

An additional unique aspect of this modern food environment is the ubiquity of food cues; visual and informational food cues, including information relating to food, diets, and nutrition, are abundant. Take a moment to consider the images of food encountered daily—billboards, advertisements in print and online sources, commercials on television, and more. Environmental (visual) food stimuli are capable of influencing food consumption,[15] likely via the dopamine system.[16] For instance, Harris, Bargh, and Brownell[17] demonstrate that exposure to food advertisements increases consumption in elementary-school-aged children and adults, even for food products not advertised in the commercials. This phenomenon illustrates the priming effect, in which the dual-process cognitive system referred to earlier automatically processes information and thus influences behavior, such as increasing the consumption of food.

It is nearly impossible for modern humans to successfully navigate these ubiquitous food cues, and, as previously stated, exposure to visual food cues increases subsequent consumption. This is especially problematic given the obesity rate in developed nations, and many individuals engage in diets and food cults to lose weight. Unfortunately, these cues do not come in the form of advertisements alone; consider the multiple avenues by which the average individual encounters advice related to their food choices. On a daily basis, in addition to being bombarded by advertisements, we encounter online and print news media articles, read packaging claims on our products, have conversations with friends, receive health advice from an array of sources, receive emails with nutritional advice from our health insurance and personal gym, and attempt to heed nutritional recommendations put forth by the government. Regrettably, governmental nutrition recommendations in the United States further complicate food decision making. The United States Department of Agriculture (USDA) issues revised recommendations every five years. The purpose of these recommendations is to promote adequate nutrition, and, ideally, these recommendations should ease consumer navigation of the food environment. Historically, these USDA recommendations focused on the prevention of hunger and nutrient deficits, but the focus shifted to the prevention of chronic disease in the 1960s and 1970s with increased prevalence of heart disease after World War II.[18] Unfortunately, the process by which these recommendations are determined is highly complex; thus the resulting recommendations are complex. This complexity is derived from the USDA's conflict of interest in supporting agriculture and the food industry while simultaneously issuing nutrition recommendations. In an effort to avoid dichotomous labeling of some foods as "good" and others as "bad," the final recommendations include vague phrasing, such as in 2000 to "choose beverages and foods to moderate your intake of sugar."[19] The flip-flop on fats further exemplifies this complexity—in 2000, previous recommendations related to total fat were replaced with recommendations related to saturated and trans fats, and in 2010, the USDA introduced the term *SoFAS* for solid fats and added sugars.[20] These recommendations are grounded in empirical evidence for chronic disease risk, but they are confusing to the consumer who has absorbed decades of advice that all fats are to be avoided. This confusion is alleviated when the consumer turns to an authority figure, such as the promoter of a food or diet cult utilizing the principles of influence and pseudoscience to gain followers.

Governmental nutrition recommendations are not the only source of complex and often contradictory information. There are several modes by which nutritional information is transmitted to the public (for instance, government-published nutrition guidelines, dietary recommendations from health care practitioners, and proprietary fad diets). This abundant available information is commonly contradictory and ranges from accurate to moderately inaccurate to downright misleading or dangerous. For example, common high-end "healthy" grocery stores often stock books in print related to fad diets such as veganism, raw foodism, and gluten-free. These books rely on mechanisms of pseudoscience, anecdotal evidence, and influence tactics to promote their claims. These claims are even more pervasive on the Internet, where we are bombarded by lists such as eatthis.com's fifty-seven healthiest foods on the planet, twenty-three foods happy people eat, and five foods healthy people never eat at night.

How does the average consumer sort through this information? Rozin[21] argues that we have a lack of compensation for food advances, such as the availability and convenience of highly palatable foods and the ubiquity of food cues. For instance, we lack the ability to navigate scientific findings or nutritional information. In response to the information overload, we categorize foods as simply "good" or "bad." The inability to navigate this volume of information contributes to the susceptibility for food cult following. Levinovitz[22] argues that the moralization of "good" and "bad" dietary habits provided by the rules established within food cults simplifies the world by providing people with clear-cut, dogmatic answers—working in a manner similar to the rules set forth by religions. Food cults, communities, and proprietary diets therefore ease the stress of navigating the abundance of cues and conflicting information via rules and norms, and pseudoscience provides the simple nutritional answers that people desire.

Misinformation may be spread accidentally or through more deliberate intentions such as profit. In the contemporary world, these norms and rules are frequently spread via blogs and social media accounts. The hosts of these may have a range of health and nutritional expertise, with a variety of training. Much of the information shared is false and pseudoscientific in nature; yet it highly influences nutritional choices and the development of food-based communities. Social media facilitates the spread of information as users frequently comment or share their experiences, creating a sense of community or accountability and therefore satiating the need to belong.[23]

COMBATING PSEUDOSCIENCE

Is it possible to identify and resist these pseudoscientific claims? Unfortunately, the average person targeted by pseudoscientific claims does not possess the skills to distinguish between empirical and nonscientific evidence. An important first step is examining the claim to determine whether it is empirical or pseudoscientific in nature is by checking for the telltale signs of pseudoscience (e.g., reliance on anecdotal evidence, overgeneralization, statistics provided with little context). Additionally, recognizing the source of the information and the potential bias of the source is crucial. Sutherland, Spiegelhalter, and Burgman[24] suggest tips for interpreting scientific evidence, and they stress the potential for bias and the quality of research design. Consumers would additionally benefit from recognizing the motivations of those making nutritional claims, as the end goal for many pseudoscience practitioners is profit or influence, as well as a general understanding of the common influence tactics.[25] The pseudoscientific claim is vague by definition, thus making it difficult to evaluate the potential for bias or poor research design.

CONCLUSION

Food cults demonstrate the characteristics of pseudoscience by using anecdotes in place of evidence. Additionally, the social and cognitive mechanisms of pseudoscience, including endorsement by legitimate authority figures or celebrities, social validation, and cognitive dissonance, help explain the allure of food cults. Participation in food cults fulfills the fundamental human need to belong and may net social status, capital, or power through group membership. Although scientific thinking may be used to combat pseudoscience, it takes practice and effort, and food science is particularly complex. This problem is compounded by the current sheer abundance of both accurate and inaccurate information. The unique modern food environment, characterized by availability and convenience, with more visual food cues than the rest of human history and muddled by confusing and contradictory nutritional advice, is ripe for the promotion of food cults and fad diets. Unfortunately, most people do not have the skills necessary to navigate the wealth of information relating to diet and nutrition encountered on a daily basis, and food cults ease the stress created by copious dietary information through clear rules and regulations, while pseudoscience makes sweeping claims that essentially tell people what they want to hear. The information age further propagates food cults and groups through Internet presence via social media and blogs. Thus, pseudoscientific nutritional claims and promotion of food cults have a ubiquitous presence in the modern world, and these food cults are likely here to stay.

NOTES

1. C. James Goodwin and Kerri Goodwin, *Research in Psychology: Methods and Design* (Hoboken, NJ: Wiley & Sons, 2012).
2. Robert Cialdini, *Influence: The Psychology of Persuasion* (New York: Harper Business, 2006).
3. John Ruscio, *Critical Thinking in Psychology: Separating Sense from Nonsense* (Belmont, CA: Wadsworth, 2006).
4. Alan Levinovitz, *The Gluten Lie: And Other Myths about What You Eat* (New York: Regan Arts, 2015).
5. Daniel Kahneman, *Thinking, Fast and Slow* (New York: Farrar, Straus, and Giroux, 2012).
6. Michael Shermer, *The Science of Good and Evil: Why People Cheat, Gossip, Care, Share, and Follow the Golden Rule* (New York: Holt Paperbacks, 2005).
7. Roy Baumeister and Mark Leary, "The Need to Belong: Desire for Interpersonal Attachment as a Fundamental Human Motivation," *Psychological Bulletin* 117 (1995): 497–529.
8. Nicholas Christakis and James Fowler, "The Spread of Obesity in a Large Social Network over 32 Years," *New England Journal of Medicine* 357 (2007): 370–79.
9. Douglas T. Kenrick, Steven L. Neuberg, Vladas Griskevicius, D. Vaughn Becker, and Mark Schaller, "Goal-Driven Cognition and Functional Behavior: The Fundamental-Motives Framework," *Current Directions in Psychological Science 19* (2010): 63–67.

10. Kipling D. Williams and Steve A. Nida, "Ostracism: Consequences and Coping," *Current Directions in Psychological Science 20* (2011): 71–75.

11. David Christian, *This Fleeting World: A Short History of Humanity* (Great Barrington, MA: Berkshire Publishing Group, 2008), 11.

12. World Health Organization, "Global and Regional Food Consumption Patterns and Trends," *World Health Organization*, retrieved September 23, 2015, from http://www.who.int/nutrition/topics/3_foodconsumption/en/.

13. Barry Schwartz, "The Tyranny of Choice," *Scientific American*, 2004, retrieved from http://www.sciam.com.

14. See note 4 above.

15. Stanley Schachter, "Obesity and Eating: Internal and External Cues Differentially Affect the Eating Behavior of Obese and Normal Subjects," *Science* 161 (1968): 751–56.

16. Nora Volkow, Gene-Jack Wang, Joanna Fowler, Jean Logan, Millard Jayne, Dinko Franceschi, et al., "'Nonhedonic' Food Motivation in Humans Involves Dopamine in the Dorsal Striatum and Methylphenidate Amplifies This Effect," *Synapse* 44 (2002): 175–80.

17. Jennifer L. Harris, John A. Bargh, and Kelly D. Brownell, "Priming Effects of Television Food Advertising on Eating Behavior," *Health Psychology* 28 (2009): 404–13.

18. Marion Nestle, *Food Politics* (Los Angeles: University of California Press, 2013), 39.

19. Nestle, *Food Politics*, 44.

20. Nestle, *Food Politics*, 382.

21. Paul Rozin, "The Meaning of Food in Our Lives: A Cross-Cultural Perspective on Eating and Well-Being," *Journal of Nutrition Education and Behavior* 37 (2005): S107–S112.

22. See note 4 above.

23. Tang Yao, Qiuying Zheng, and Xiucheng Fan, "The Impact of Online Social Support on Patients' Quality of Life and the Moderating Role of Social Exclusion," *Journal of Service Research* 18 (2015): 369–83.

24. William Sutherland, David Spiegelhalter, and Mark Burgman, "Twenty Tips for Interpreting Scientific Claims," *Nature* 503 (2013): 335–37.

25. Robert Cialdini, *Influence: The Psychology of Persuasion* (New York: Harper Business, 2006).

BIBLIOGRAPHY

Baumeister, Roy F., and Mark R. Leary. "The Need to Belong: Desire for Interpersonal Attachment as a Fundamental Human Motivation." *Psychological Bulletin* 117 (1995): 497–529.

Christakis, Nicholas A., and James H. Fowler. "The Spread of Obesity in a Large Social Network over 32 Years." *New England Journal of Medicine* 357 (2007): 370–79.

Christian, David. *This Fleeting World: A Short History of Humanity*. Great Barrington, MA: Berkshire Publishing Group, 2008.

Cialdini, Robert B. *Influence: The Psychology of Persuasion*. New York: Harper Business, 2006.

Goodwin, C. James, and Kerri A. Goodwin. *Research in Psychology: Methods and Design*. 7th ed. Hoboken, NJ: Wiley & Sons, 2012.

Harris, Jennifer L., John A. Bargh, and Kelly D. Brownell. "Priming Effects of Television Food Advertising on Eating Behavior." *Health Psychology* 28 (2009): 404–13.

Kahneman, Daniel. *Thinking, Fast and Slow*. New York: Farrar, Straus, and Giroux, 2012.

Kenrick, Douglas T., Steven L. Neuberg, Vladas Griskevicius, D. Vaughn Becker, and Mark Schaller. "Goal-Driven Cognition and Functional Behavior: The Fundamental-Motives Framework." *Current Directions in Psychological Science* 19 (2010): 63–67.

Levinovitz, Alan. *The Gluten Lie: And Other Myths about What You Eat.* New York: Regan Arts, 2015.

Nestle, Marion. *Food Politics.* Los Angeles: University of California Press, 2013.

Rozin, Paul. "The Meaning of Food in Our Lives: A Cross-Cultural Perspective on Eating and Well-Being." *Journal of Nutrition Education Behavior* 37 (2005): S107–S112.

Ruscio, John. *Critical Thinking in Psychology: Separating Sense from Nonsense.* Belmont, CA: Wadsworth, 2006.

Schachter, Stanley. "Obesity and Eating: Internal and External Cues Differentially Affect the Eating Behavior of Obese and Normal Subjects." *Science* 161 (1968): 751–56.

Schwartz, Barry. "The Tyranny of Choice." *Scientific American* (2004). Retrieved from www.sciam.com.

Shermer, Michael. *The Science of Good and Evil: Why People Cheat, Gossip, Care, Share, and Follow the Golden Rule.* New York: Holt Paperbacks, 2005.

Sutherland, William J., David Spiegelhalter, and Mark A. Burgman. "Twenty Tips for Interpreting Scientific Claims." *Nature* 503 (2013): 335–37.

Volkow, Nora D., Gene-Jack Wang, Joanna S. Fowler, Jean Logan, Millard Jayne, Dinko Franceschi, et al. "'Nonhedonic' Food Motivation in Humans Involves Dopamine in the Dorsal Striatum and Methylphenidate Amplifies This Effect." *Synapse* 44 (2002): 175–80.

Williams, Kipling D., and Steve A. Nida. "Ostracism: Consequences and Coping." *Current Directions in Psychological Science* 20 (2011): 71–75.

World Health Organization. "Global and Regional Food Consumption Patterns and Trends." *World Health Organization.* Retrieved September 23, 2015, from http://www.who.int/nutrition/topics/3_foodconsumption/en/.

Yao, Tang, Qiuying Zheng, and Xiucheng Fan. "The Impact of Online Social Support on Patients' Quality of Life and the Moderating Role of Social Exclusion." *Journal of Service Research* 18 (2015): 369–83.

Chapter Three

Food Practices in Early Christianity

Paul A. Brazinski

Christian food practices greatly influence global diets and consumerism every year. For example, sales for McDonald's famous "Filet-o-Fish" peak on Fridays during Lent due to Catholic practices; even Chick-fil-A, the notorious chicken biscuit restaurant, sells fish sandwiches during this period to accommodate their fasting Christian customers who cannot eat meat except fish on these days. These food practices, especially fasting and imitating Jesus, have a long tradition in the history of Christianity.

Food has played an important role in the development of Christianity.[1] Several different food practices and cults originated and evolved throughout the history of Christianity. Some of these practices, such as the worship of the Eucharist, are well represented in scholarship.[2] However, the history of food cults in Christianity beyond the Eucharist is little researched. These habits helped shape the identity of early Christianity, especially those practices that contrast against the "other" vis-à-vis heretical groups.[3] This chapter aims to fill this lacuna by surveying early Christian food practices—namely, their origin and evolution over the first five centuries. In fact, Christianity arguably used their food traditions and practices to differentiate themselves from the "other" against heretical sects and other religions, such that food cults and practices were a central feature of early Christianity.

FOOD CULTS IN THE NEW TESTAMENT AND THE AGE OF APOLOGISTS (c. AD 33–220)

Christianity assimilated several of its early food habits from Judaism. Thus, a précis of Jewish traditions will help flesh out where Christian practices started and how they evolved to differentiate themselves from the "other," meaning early Judaism. Early Judaism turned to the Hebrew Bible for its food rules, most of which come from Leviticus and Deuteronomy.[4] These religious dietary laws are included in the *Kashrut*, which is the system of formulated rules of behavior in Judaism, while the food one may consume according to these regulations is called *kosher*.[5] The *Kashrut* provides a list of prohibited foods, which are typically justified with health or philosophical explanations.[6] For example, Deuteronomy 14:21 and Exodus 23:19 state that mixtures of meat and milk are prohibited. This practice is justified in that a mother should not cook a kid in her own milk. Other passages, such as Leviticus 11:3–8 and Deuteronomy 14:3–21, prohibit the consumption of certain animals, such as those with cloven hooves, fish without scales, amphibians, and reptiles.[7] Moreover, Judaism emphasizes a weekly meal called the Shabbat, which several scholars refer to vis-à-vis the Last Supper. Yet, although several early Christians would assimilate many of these customs, the emergence of Orthodoxy would start to reject several of these early Jewish practices for new Christian ones to differentiate their identity.

For example, the *Kashrut* has an emphasis on eating purified food in a sanitary area with clean individuals. Yet Jesus shared his table with social outcasts, such as prostitutes and sinners, which was taboo at the time (Matthew 9:10).[8] Moreover, Jesus in Acts 10:15 tells Peter, "Rise, Peter; kill, and eat." His command here was to eat anything from the earth, since everything that God created was good and already cleansed. Jesus also declared all foods clean in Mark 7:19.[9] It is important that this command was given to Peter, who would serve as the first bishop of Rome. This was yet another departure from kosher customs. Yet not every early Christian followed these new standards.

Paul the Apostle, in his Letter to the Galatians, speaks of his difficulty in keeping the Christian identity separate amid such intermingling with Judaism.[10] As Bauer and others like Ehrman have argued, the church is not a monolithic structure; there was much diversity in standards, practices, and principles in the early church to create its current identity.[11] Indeed, in a metaphor Bauer often cites, there were several horses in the race to be called mainstream Christianity; yet only the one named "Catholicism" won amid other heretical and nonmainstream movements. One of these versions of Christianity was the Judaizers.[12] These people called themselves Christians in Paul's time; however, they continued to follow several Jewish traditions.[13] One of the main issues that Paul mentions in the Letter to the Galatians concerning the Judaizers, along with circumcision, is food practices.[14] And this was not an isolated issue among the early leaders of Christianity. Indeed, even Peter was an early Judaizer until the council at Jerusalem, which pushed for a non-Jewish form of Christianity. Thus, Paul combated Jewish customs, such as kosher practices and circumcision, in forming the identity of early Christianity.

In doing so, Paul provides several statements about proper Christian food practices.[15] For example, in Romans 14:14, Paul states, "I know and am persuaded in the Lord Jesus that nothing is unclean in itself."[16] Thus, in a similar vein to Acts 10:15 and Mark 7:19, Paul believes that all of God's creatures are clean and edible.[17] Paul corroborates himself in Colossians 2:20, saying, "Let no one pass judgment on you in questions of food and drink," as well as 1 Timothy 4:4 with "Nothing is to be rejected if it is received with thanksgiving." Thus, food was a means of identification. But Paul was not the only Church Father struggling with Judaizers in separating Christian food practices from the "other."

For example, Justin Martyr (c. 100–165) discusses the same issue in his *Debate with Tryphon.*[18] Toward the end of the dialogue, Tryphon, a rabbi, asks, if he were to become a Christian, would he be required to give up kosher practices and other parts of the Jewish law? Justin replies by saying that Christians are not agreed on this, which causes confusion for Tryphon. According to Justin, some Christians would say that one must give them up, while others would allow a convert to observe the laws of Moses, provided that one did not try to compel other converts to do similarly. Justin Martyr finishes this discussion by saying that it is only Christ who saves one, which helps justify the church's disorganized stance.[19] Thus, yet again, the early church struggled in differentiating its identity from Judaism, as seen in the light of food practices.

As the early church developed, so, too, did its practice of sharing a weekly meal. The *Didache*, which is also referred to as "The Teachings of the Twelve Apostles," is the oldest surviving written catechism in Christianity, dating to the mid to late first century AD.[20] In the *Didache*, the anonymous author discusses at length the proper procedures for sharing a weekly meal in the Eucharist.[21] The ritual greatly resembles that of the Last Supper, which is followed by a meal. This meal was typically done in secret, since Christianity was not a *religio licita* (Latin for "permitted religion").[22] Thus, Christians worshiped and ate this meal secretly to avoid persecution. As a result, Christianity became known for these secret and mysterious meals. Similarly, from the opposite perspective, pagan sources on Christian food practices also corroborate this and provide insights into Christianity's emerging identity.

Pliny's famous letter to Trajan and Trajan's response shed great light on how the Romans viewed these secret Christian meals.[23] In Pliny's letter, he informs Emperor Trajan that certain Christians are holding secret meetings "on a fixed day before dawn and sing responsively a hymn to Christ."[24] When this meeting was over, "it was their custom to depart and to assemble again to partake of food—but ordinary and innocent food." Pliny decreed that such secret meetings should end. Yet Pliny was still suspicious of these food cults, so he captured two Christian deacons and tortured them in order to discover more information about their practices; however, this was to no avail. Here, again, we see food practices as an integral part of the early Christian identity.

ANTHONY AND THE DESERT FATHERS (c. AD THIRD TO SEVENTH CENTURIES)

In the third century, a new food cult evolved in early Christianity among the Desert Fathers and ascetics that would further Christian practices from the "other."[25] These men and women set off into the desert in search of a stricter life in which to imitate God.[26] Thus, in following the famous words of Matthew 19:21[27] that urges one to sell all of one's possessions and follow Jesus, several figures such as Anthony the Great would do so. Athanasius, the bishop of Alexandria and author of *The Life of Anthony*, recalls Anthony's austere food practices, which several other Christians followed.[28] Moreover, beyond those immediately with Anthony in the desert, Athanasius's *Life of Anthony* was influential in exposing the Western non-Greek world regarding such desert tendencies; this, in turn, resulted in the spread of asceticism in the West as well, such as with Jerome.[29]

In terms of Anthony's food practices, Athanasius describes it as being rather meager. Anthony typically ate only one meal a day after sunset, although at times he would go several days without eating.[30] He only consumed bread and salt, and he exclusively drank water.[31] Anthony would expand his diet slightly as he got older, which might also be attributed to the fact that his teeth "had become worn to the gums through the great age of the old man."[32] However, Anthony and others living in the Egyptian desert were limited concerning their resources. Thus, in order to accommodate this austere lifestyle, a network was established to bring supplies to these Desert Fathers.[33]

This network consisted of several individuals and did not have a standard operating procedure. For instance, while the young Anthony was living in abandoned tombs near a village, he had an acquaintance of his bring a loaf of bread at various intervals over several days.[34] Other systems included monasteries and hermits, with the former bringing food to the latter at set intervals; in this system, which Anthony was a part of as a hermit when he was advanced in years, he was brought bread, olives, pulse, and oil every month.[35] Yet Anthony, despite his limited food, shared what he had with visitors.[36] Moreover, as Georgia Frank successfully argues, these Desert Fathers, given their asceticism—particularly their food habits—became living pilgrimage attractions, which is seen in several early travel accounts.[37]

Palladius of Galatia (c. AD 363–420/430) discusses several of these austere practices in his *Lausiac History*. For example, Isidore and several others never ate meat.[38] To justify their diets, these figures turned to biblical passages on food, such as Hebrews 5:14, which states that solid food, such as meat, should only be consumed by the spiritually mature.[39] Thus, several Desert Fathers, such as Anthony and Dorotheus, in following these passages and trying to live a life of humility, relied heavily on bread. In fact, Dorotheus is said to have eaten only six ounces of bread a day.[40] Therefore, major monastic sites, such as at Kellia near Alexandria, which had over two thousand monks, and Nitria, which had over five thousand monks, had several bakeries but few butchers and other food producers to accommodate these bread-hungry individuals.[41] In fact, Nitria relied on seven bakeries to feed its large monastic community.[42] Yet these communities often produced more than just bread in trying to be self-sufficient.[43] Later monastic communities in the medieval West were far more open concerning their diets. These examples show the transformation of food practices within Christianity.

Females also participated in this ascetic culture, such as Amma Syncletica of Alexandria.[44] However, female monastics had a slightly different diet, and the sources about them provide far more insights into the world of fasting and feasting than males in late antiquity (c. 250–750). In terms of gendered roles, as males dominated the influential positions of the secular and spiritual worlds, females typically managed domestic matters, which included food preparation.[45] Also, as the intake of food was one of the few things females could control concerning their bodies in this period, Caroline Bynum successfully argues that fasting and feasting were far more important to medieval Christian females than males, which is reflected in the dominance of this theme in female hagiography.[46]

For example, early Christian females, such as Macrina and Eustochium, fasted so intensely that they are depicted as having physically "transformed" into male form—meaning having rid themselves of their female features.[47] This theme of starvation, or rather "lack" of food cult, is found across a vast demographic. In following this theme and as the high medieval period advanced, several females such as Catherine of Siena and Hildegard of Bingen would claim to be sustained solely on the Eucharist alone.[48] The imagery of food is also rather different when medieval authors discuss church figures and eating.

Bynum in particular demonstrates the stark differences between Francis and Clare, who both took strict vows of poverty with the same religious order—the Franciscans.[49] However, Francis of Assisi is depicted with poverty and care, while Clare's problem is food. For example, when Francis needs food, sustenance miraculously appears. Francis, and medieval males overall, usually did not lose their desire for food.[50] However, Clare is even demanded at times to eat more food, since she too severely lacks required nutrients. As seen in Clare, medieval females typically did not lose their desire for food and had to fight this demon constantly.

AUGUSTINE AND FAUSTUS

Augustine of Hippo (354–430), arguably the most influential Church Father in Western Christianity, provides great insights into what mainstream food cults and practices were in his work *Against Faustus the Manichaean*.[51] In this work, Augustine debates with a Manichaean elect named Faustus about the latter's theology and practices.[52] Here, Augustine shows us how food practices could be a major divider between Christianity and the "other." First, I shall provide a brief introduction to contextualize the Manichaeans.

The Manichaeans, to which Faustus belonged, were a dualist Christian sect, meaning that they called themselves Christians and viewed the universe as two all-powerful forces that were constantly at battle with each other—light versus dark, good versus evil.[53] They thought that everything on earth was made up of light and dark elements, including foodstuffs. For example, cucumbers were made up of light elements while wine was made from dark elements. Only those foods that were made of primarily light elements should be eaten.

The Manichaeans also believed that one would be reincarnated into something on earth until one was spiritually freed from this world and advanced into the next; this caused a tension, as human spirits could be reincarnated into various foods, such as fruits and vegetables. Thus, whenever a Manichaean ate anything, he would be torturing the spirit of that object, such as a cucumber, with his or her teeth, cutting knives, and/or digestive system. However, the only way that the spiritual component of a food item could be released from that foodstuffs was as the digested item left the body as feces out of a Manichaean's other end.[54] Therefore, the elect Manichaeans did not pick fruits from trees or kill animals, since this would injure those spirits and would cause harm to their own souls; this resulted in a two-tiered system that forced the common Manichaean to do "soul service" for the elect, meaning that they would hunt and gather food while the elect would pray for them.[55] Those who needed another reincarnation would be defecated onto the ground to start anew. Naturally, Augustine responds to these stances.

First, Augustine responds with his reading of Scripture. For starters, Augustine argues that "Christ never taught you that you should not pluck a vegetable for fear of committing homicide."[56] Here, Augustine responds to the Manichaean practice concerning the light and dark forces in all living things, even food. He also states that Jesus Christ would have chosen his words differently if the non-elect were really brought back in melons or cucumbers. According to Augustine, "Jesus should have said, not 'I was hungry and ye gave me meat'; but, 'Ye were hungry, and ye ate me,' or 'I was hungry, and I ate you.'"[57] From this passage, it is clear that Augustine is adamantly opposed to the Manichaean idea concerning food and reincarnation. In fact, Augustine is rather sarcastic with his rhetoric in terms of rejecting their food practices.

Augustine clearly opposes Manichaean dietary habits throughout *Against Faustus the Manichaean*; however, his sarcasm arguably peaks in XIII.18. Here, Augustine puts forward the idea that if the Manichaeans want their words to be pure, why not eat their books?[58] Well, Augustine even rejects this notion using their own logic, showing that they cannot do this because books are made of sheepskin, which is unclean because they are the dead hides of past souls. Moreover, books are unclean, given the darkened ink on the white pages, which has both light and dark values. At this point Augustine even wonders why Manichaeans have books, given the homicide that they must have done in their system to create such things. Here, too, we see food cults as a means of separating Catholicism from the "other." Augustine is clear and concise while closing this discussion that the Manichaeans should not be called Christians and should not eat or attend Mass with them. Although food cults provide a means of inclusiveness when done together, here, with Augustine, they provide a means of separation and exclusion.

CONCLUSIONS

Food practices were an integral part of the formation of the Christian identity. Early Christianity assimilated several food practices from early Judaism; however, these customs were debated in the era of the apostles and apologists. Here, figures such as Paul used their rhetoric on food to separate Jewish food practices from Christian ones. However, one may see the confusion in this period, as even Peter and Justin Martyr supported the dietary practices of Judaizers. As Christianity progressed throughout the centuries, new food cults developed that transformed their identity away from other religions, as seen in the Desert Fathers and Mothers. Nevertheless, some heretical sects, such as the Manichaeans, had a similar network of supporters to provide resources for their elect. Yet Augustine of Hippo responded, albeit at times sarcastically, to the obscure Manichaean rules regarding light and dark elements in food as well as how one freed an object's spiritual essence via defecation. These are only a few examples of how the rhetoric of food was used as an identity marker in Christianity and as a means to separate Christians from the "other." In the centuries after Augustine and the Desert Fathers, food cults and the rhetoric surrounding food would also cause bifurcations in the church vis-à-vis "us" versus "them."

For example, in the medieval period, Christians in the Greek East and Latin West started to debate whether the Eucharist should be made of leavened or unleavened wheat.[59] The Roman Catholic Church viewed the Last Supper as a Passover Seder meal, which would mean that Jesus and his disciples used unleavened bread for the event. However, the Greek Orthodox Church viewed the Last Supper through the lens of biblical passages such as John 18:28, which suggests that Passover was upcoming but not yet present; thus, Jesus would have used leavened bread.[60] This theological debate peaked in 1053 to 1054, when Patriarch Michael Cerularius of Constantinople closed all the Latin churches in Constantinople, which was shortly thereafter followed by his official excommunication from Catholicism via Cardinal Humbert. Moreover, Cardinal Humbert placed the excommunication on the altar in Hagia Sophia in Constantinople while the patriarch was holding Mass. This event resulted in the East-West Schism, which still separates the two churches today, and this issue of the Eucharist, concerning leavened or unleavened bread, acts as an identity marker as well.

In March 1522, Ulrich Zwingli, the grand minister of Zurich, was invited to dine at the house of Christoph Froschauer, a printer in the city, who recently helped Zwingli publish a new edition of the Epistles of Saint Paul.[61] Christoph served traditional Zurich smoked sausages, which was taboo given that Lent was a time of fasting from meats.[62] Zwingli did not eat the sausages; nevertheless, Christoph was soon arrested for his religious crimes. But Zwingli stood up for Christoph and preached his famous *Von Erkiesen und Freiheit der Speisen* (German for "Regarding the Choice and Freedom of Foods"), where Zwingli emphasized the voluntary practice of fasting from meats during Lent. As a result of this sermon, Zwingli turned away from the Catholic tradition to a closer reading of the Bible, which from the text alone does not support such a stance.[63] Thus, Zwingli allowed his flock to partake of meats during Lent, which was a departure from Catholic practices and Rome. This 1522 Sermon of the Sausages is credited in the Reformation as the turning point in Zurich. Although these are only two examples, it is clear that food practices and food cults helped shape and form the Christian identity in history and today.

NOTES

1. Ken Albala, "Historical Background to Food in Christianity," in *Food and Faith in Christian Culture*, ed. Ken Albala and Trudy Eden (New York: Columbia University Press, 2011), 8–9.

2. Nathan Mitchell, *Cult and Controversy: The Worship of the Eucharist Outside Mass* (Collegeville: Pueblo Books, 1982), 10–12; Angel Mendez Montoya, *Theology of Food: Eating and the Eucharist* (Oxford: Wiley-Blackwell, 2012), 2; Norman Wirzba, *Food and Faith: A Theology of Eating* (Cambridge: Cambridge University Press, 2011), 5.

3. Trudy Eden, "Introduction," in *Food and Faith in Christian Culture*, ed. Ken Albala and Trudy Eden (New York: Columbia University Press, 2011), 1–5.

4. Jordan Rosenblum, *Food and Identity in Early Rabbinic Judaism* (Cambridge: Cambridge University Press, 2010).

5. Peter Tomson, "Jewish Food Laws in Early Christian Community Discourse," *Semeia* 86 (1999): 193.

6. Nathan MacDonald, *Not Bread Alone: The Uses of Food in the Old Testament* (Oxford: Oxford University Press, 2008).

7. Thomas Mann, "Not by Word Alone: Food in the Hebrew Bible," *Interpretation* 67, no. 4 (2013): 354–55.

8. Albala, "Historical Background to Food in Christianity," 12.

9. Albala, "Historical Background to Food in Christianity," 11.

10. Paul, *Letter to the Galatians*. See also Tomson, "Jewish Food Laws in Early Christian Community Discourse," 202.

11. Walter Bauer, *Orthodoxy and Heresy in Earliest Christianity* (Philadelphia: Fortress Press, 1971), 1–5; Bart Ehrman, *Lost Christianities: The Battles for Scripture and the Faiths We Never Knew* (New York: Oxford University Press, 2003), 1–4; Karen King, *What Is Gnosticism?* (Cambridge, MA: Harvard University Press, 2005), 55–56.

12. Michele Murray, *Playing a Jewish Game: Gentile Christian Judaizing in the First and Second Centuries CE* (Waterloo: Wilfried Laurier University Press, 2004), 29–31.

13. Tomson, "Jewish Food Laws in Early Christian Community Discourse," 195.

14. Albala, "Historical Background to Food in Christianity," 10.

15. John Brunt, "Rejected, Ignored, or Misunderstood? The Fate of Paul's Approach to the Problem of Food Offered to Idols in Early Christianity," *New Testament Studies* 31 (1985): 113–24.

16. Aaron Eby, *Biblically Kosher: A Messianic Jewish Perspective on Kashrut* (New York: Fruits of Zion, 2012).

17. Tomson, "Jewish Food Laws in Early Christian Community Discourse," 198.

18. Murray, *Playing a Jewish Game*, 73–74; Thomas B. Falls, trans., *Writings of Saint Justin Martyr* (Washington, DC: Catholic University of America Press, 2008), 139–40.

19. Justin Martyr, *Debate with Tryphon the Jew*, 46–47.

20. Willy Rordorf and André Tuilier, *La Doctrine des Douze Apôtres: Didachè* (Paris: Editions Du Cerf, 1978), 9–11.

21. Huub Van de Sandt, "'Do Not Give What Is Holy to the Dogs' (Did 9:5D and Matt 7:6A): The Eucharistic Food of the Didache in Its Jewish Purity Setting," *Vigiliae Christianae* 56 (2002): 223.

22. Justo Gonzalez, *The Story of Christianity: The Early Church to the Dawn of the Reformation* (New York: Harper One, 2010), 83.

23. Pliny, *Letter to Trajan* (*Epistula* 10.96–97).

24. Gonzalez, *The Story of Christianity*, 49–50.

25. Gonzalez, *The Story of Christianity*, 161–64.

26. Warren Treadgold, *A History of the Byzantine State and Society* (Palo Alto: Stanford University Press, 1997), 30–31.

27. Matthew 19:21 (NIV): "Jesus answered, 'If you want to be perfect, go, sell your possessions and give to the poor, and you will have treasure in heaven. Then come, follow me.'" Michael David Coogan, trans., *The New Oxford Annotated Bible* (Oxford: Oxford University Press, 2007).

28. Athanasius, *Life of Anthony*. See also David Brakke, *Athanasius and Asceticism* (Baltimore: Johns Hopkins Press, 1998); David Brakke, *Athanasius and the Politics of Asceticism* (Oxford: Oxford University Press, 1995).

29. Philip Rousseau, *Ascetics, Authority, and the Church in the Age of Jerome and Cassian* (Notre Dame: University of Notre Dame Press, 2010).

30. Athanasius, *Life of Anthony*, 7.

31. Athanasius, *Life of Anthony*, 7.

32. Athanasius, *Life of Anthony*, 93.

33. Brakke, *Athanasius and Asceticism*, 22.
34. Athanasius, *Life of Anthony*, 8.
35. Athanasius, *Life of Anthony*, 50–51.
36. Athanasius, *Life of Anthony*, 50.
37. Georgia Frank, *The Memory of the Eyes: Pilgrims to Living Saints in Late Antiquity* (Berkeley: University of California Press, 2000), 171–73.
38. Palladius of Galatia, *Lausiac History* 1 and 21.
39. Paul, Hebrews 5:14 (NIV): "But solid food is for the mature, who by constant use have trained themselves to distinguish good from evil." Michael David Coogan, trans., *The New Oxford Annotated Bible* (Oxford: Oxford University Press, 2007).
40. Palladius of Galatia, *Lausiac History* 2.
41. Palladius of Galatia, *Lausicac History* 7; Roger Bagnall and Dominic Rathbone, eds., *Egypt from Alexander to the Early Christians: An Archaeological and Historical Guide* (Los Angeles: J. Paul Getty Museum Press, 2004), 108–12.
42. Palladius of Galatia, *Lausiac History* 2, 7, and 33.
43. This theme of work and labor—*ora et labora*—would be the cornerstone of later monastic rules, such as the *Benedictine Rule*. These monasteries similarly had an emphasis on working and praying to maintain their lifestyle.
44. *Sayings of the Desert Fathers 3.* See also Palladius of Galatia, *Lausiac History* 6, 41, 46, 47, 63, and 69.
45. Caroline Walker Bynum, *Holy Feast and Holy Fast: The Religious Significance of Food to Medieval Women* (Berkeley: University of California Press, 1987), 23–30.
46. Bynum, *Holy Feast and Holy Fast*, 11–12.
47. Jerome, *Epistula* 22; Gregory of Nyssa, *Life of Macrina.*
48. Bynum, *Holy Feast and Holy Fast*, 102.
49. Bynum, *Holy Feast and Holy Fast*, 102; Regis Armstrong, *Francis and Clare: The Complete Works* (New York: Paulist Press, 1982).
50. Bynum, *Holy Feast and Holy Fast*, 104.
51. Gonzalez, *The Story of Christianity*, 241–51; Peter Brown, *Augustine of Hippo: A Biography* (Berkeley: University of California Press, 2000), 1–5.
52. Jacobus van Amersfoort, "Some Remarks on the Gospel Tradition in the Anti-Manicean Writings of Augustine of Hippo," *Studia Patristica* (2001): 324–30.
53. Iain Gardner and Samuel Lieu, trans., *Manichaean Texts from the Roman Empire* (Cambridge: Cambridge University Press, 2004), 11.
54. Gardner and Lieu, *Manichaean Texts from the Roman Empire*, 22–23.
55. Augustine, *Against Faustus the Manichaean* II.5; Gardner and Lieu, *Manichaean Texts from the Roman Empire*, 24.
56. Augustine, *Against Faustus the Manichaean* V.6.
57. Augustine, *Against Faustus the Manichaean* V.10.
58. Augustine, *Against Faustus the Manichaean* XIII.18.
59. Thomas Herman, *The History of the Christian Church until the Great Schism in 1054* (New York: Author House, 2004), 480–82; Gonzalez, *The Story of Christianity*, 393–411.
60. Christopher David Schabel, "The Quarrel over Unleavened Bread in the Western Theology, 1234–1439," in *Greeks, Latins, and Intellectual History 1204–1500*, ed. Martin Hinterberger, Christopher David Schabel, and Panepistemio Kyprou (Leuven: Peeters, 2011), 85–87.
61. G. R. Potter, *Zwingli* (Cambridge: Cambridge University Press, 1976), 75.
62. Potter, *Zwingli*, 76.
63. Gonzalez, *The Story of Christianity*, 60–62.

BIBLIOGRAPHY

Albala, Ken. "Historical Background to Food in Christianity." In *Food and Faith in Christian Culture*, edited by Ken Albala and Trudy Eden, 7–20. New York: Columbia University Press, 2011.

Amersfoort, Jacobus van. "Some Remarks on the Gospel Tradition in the Anti-Manicean Writings of Augustine of Hippo." *Studia Patristica* (2001): 324–30.

Armstrong, Regis, trans. *Francis and Clare: The Complete Works*. New York: Paulist Press, 1982.

Athanasius of Alexandria. *Life of Anthony.*

Augustine of Hippo. *Against Faustus the Manichaean.*

Bagnall, Roger, and Dominic Rathbone, eds. *Egypt from Alexander to the Early Christians: An Archaeological and Historical Guide*. Los Angeles: J. Paul Getty Museum Press, 2004.

Bauer, Walter. *Orthodoxy and Heresy in Earliest Christianity.* Philadelphia: Fortress Press, 1971.

Brakke, David. *Athanasius and Asceticism.* Baltimore: Johns Hopkins Press, 1998.

Brakke, David. *Athanasius and the Politics of Asceticism.* Oxford: Oxford University Press, 1995.

Brown, Peter. *Augustine of Hippo: A Biography.* Berkeley: University of California Press, 2000.

Brunt, John. "Rejected, Ignored, or Misunderstood? The Fate of Paul's Approach to the Problem of Food Offered to Idols in Early Christianity." *New Testament Studies* 31 (1985): 113–24.

Bynum, Caroline Walker. *Holy Feast and Holy Fast: The Religious Significance of Food to Medieval Women.* Berkeley: University of California Press, 1987.

Coogan, Michael David, trans. *The New Oxford Annotated Bible.* Oxford: Oxford University Press, 2007.

Eby, Aaron. *Biblically Kosher: A Messianic Jewish Perspective on Kashrut*. New York: Fruits of Zion, 2012.

Eden, Trudy. "Introduction." In *Food and Faith in Christian Culture*, edited by Ken Albala and Trudy Eden, 1–5. New York: Columbia University Press, 2011.

Ehrman, Bart. *Lost Christianities: The Battles for Scripture and the Faiths We Never Knew.* New York: Oxford University Press, 2003.

Falls, Thomas B., trans. *Writings of Saint Justin Martyr.* Washington, DC: Catholic University of America Press, 2008.

Frank, Georgia. *The Memory of the Eyes: Pilgrims to the Living Saints in Late Antiquity.* Berkeley: University of California Press, 2000.

Gardner, Iain, and Samuel Lieu, trans. *Manichaean Texts from the Roman Empire.* Cambridge: Cambridge University Press, 2004.

Gonzalez, Justo. *The Story of Christianity: The Early Church to the Dawn of the Reformation.* New York: Harper One, 2010.

Gregory of Nyssa. *Life of Macrina.*

Herman, Thomas. *The History of the Christian Church until the Great Schism in 1054.* New York: Author House, 2004.

Jerome. *Letter 22.*

Justin Martyr. *Debate with Tryphon the Jew.*

King, Karen. *What Is Gnosticism?* Cambridge, MA: Harvard University Press, 2005.

MacDonald, Nathan. *Not Bread Alone: The Use of Food in the Old Testament.* Oxford: Oxford University Press, 2008.

Mann, Thomas. "Not by Word Alone: Food in the Hebrew Bible." *Interpretation* 67, no. 4 (2013): 351–63.

Mendez Montoya, Angel. *Theology of Food: Eating and the Eucharist.* Oxford: Wiley-Blackwell, 2012.

Mitchell, Nathan. *Cult and Controversy: The Worship of the Eucharist Outside Mass.* Collegeville: Pueblo Books, 1982.

Murray, Michele. *Playing a Jewish Game: Gentile Christian Judaizing in the First and Second Centuries CE.* Waterloo: Wilfried Laurier University Press, 2004.

Palladius of Galatia. *Lausiac History.*

Paul. *Letter to the Galatians.*

Pliny. *Letter to Trajan.*

Potter, G. R. *Zwingli.* Cambridge: Cambridge University Press, 1976.

Rordorf, Willy, and André Tuilier. *La Doctrine des Douze Apôtres: Didachè*. Paris: Editions Du Cerf, 1978.

Rosenblum, Jordan. *Food and Identity in Early Rabbinic Judaism.* Cambridge: Cambridge University Press, 2010.

Rousseau, Philip. *Ascetics, Authority, and the Church in the Age of Jerome and Cassian*. Notre Dame: University of Notre Dame Press, 2010.

Sayings of the Desert Fathers.

Schabel, Christopher David. "The Quarrel over Unleavened Bread in the Western Theology, 1234–1439." In *Greeks, Latins, and Intellectual History 1204–1500*, edited by Martin Hinterberger, Christopher David Schabel, and Panepistemio Kyprou, 85–127. Leuven: Peeters, 2011.

Tomson, Peter. "Jewish Food Laws in Early Christian Community Discourse." *Semeia* 86 (1999): 193–211.

Treadgold, Warren. *A History of the Byzantine State and Society.* Palo Alto: Stanford University Press, 1997.

Van de Sandt, Huub. "'Do Not Give What Is Holy to the Dogs' (Did 9:5D and Matt 7:6A): The Eucharistic Food of the Didache in Its Jewish Purity Setting." *Vigiliae Christianae* 56 (2002): 223–46.

Wirzba, Norman. *Food and Faith: A Theology of Eating*. Cambridge: Cambridge University Press, 2011.

Chapter Four

Longevity Diets in Historical Perspective

Ken Albala

Since the nineteenth century, advances in modern medicine, improved nutrition and hygiene, and a better understanding of the aging process have all tended to confirm our persistent belief that the average life expectancy has been rising and will continue to rise in coming years. It is not uncommon to hear predictions that in the next century humans can expect to live well into their nineties or even to a hundred years old. Even our official government-sponsored guidelines make explicit claims that through careful dieting and exercise we might avoid heart disease, cancer, and other ailments that would otherwise cut our lives short. But such desires are in fact nothing new. The dream of extending life by means of diet or drugs is perennial, oftentimes leading aspirants to frame complex regimens promising extreme longevity. Followers throughout history have adopted radical lifestyle habits that sometimes constitute a formal cult, meaning a type of special devotional practice geared toward transformative goals. Like all food ideologies, the cult of longevity often includes a kind of epiphany and conversion experience—an abandonment of former habits and social ties, if necessary, to achieve their goals. Devotees also form a type of community of believers, sharing their experiences and ideally congratulating each other for their accomplishments, if not collective salvation, which come in the form of ripe old age. History also records success stories, hearty ancient souls who serve as inspiration for those still on the path, much as saints and prophets have in the context of religion.

However, the idea of extending life indefinitely has had many conceptual roadblocks in the Western tradition. Surprisingly, the possibility of achieving extreme longevity runs counter to the prevailing notion in both the Judeo-Christian and the Greco-Roman traditions that humans nowadays live significantly fewer years than their ancient ancestors. It was believed that humans in their pristine state understood more about the physical universe in its concrete earthly workings as well as its hidden mystical secrets, which meant that they could also harness its forces more effectively to prolong their lives by means of the *prisca scientia* or original knowledge. On top of that, the "natural" diet and simple habits of the ancients automatically promoted long life. Whether one is speaking of Eden, the Golden Age, or a modern notion of what our Paleolithic predecessors ate, the idea that we now live a corrupted existence and fewer years has been a consistent thread in Western thought.

Our fall from the natural state and longevity was not merely a change of habits, though, it was also a loss of knowledge. Adam, whose wisdom was derived directly from God, conceived Seth at 130 years old and continued to beget children for another 800 years until his death at 930. He was outdone by Methuselah, who lived to 969. According to the Greeks, particularly Hesiod in the *Theogony*, humans in the Golden Age living closely in tune with nature never grew old, and after several hundred years they passed away gently as though they were overcome with sleep.[1] Ancient sages and magi such as Orpheus and Hermes Trismegistus and even more semihistorical figures such as Pythagoras lived for several hundred years precisely because they understood the mystical forces of the universe, how to eat well, and how to use therapeutic herbs so as to live in harmony with the cosmos. In ancient China a parallel tradition surrounds the Taoist sages, and in most cultures there is a similar notion of the wise ancestors whose longevity sprang from their understanding of natural and supernatural forces. Brahmins also had a reputation for longevity due to their abstemious diet and lifestyle habits. These, of course, were formal types of worship rather than cults in the figurative sense.

In the Western tradition humankind was to fall from its exalted position, and the punishment both for Adam and his progeny and for humans in the corrupt Iron Age would be labor, suffering and death, and (most important for our discussion) a loss of the pristine knowledge that enabled humans to prolong life by hundreds of years. Thus, opposite to our own intuitions, both the Hebrew and Greek traditions posit that the further we get from our origins, the more base, ignorant, and unhealthy is the human condition and, consequently, the shorter our life span.

Nonetheless, the possibility of reacquiring ancient wisdom and unlocking nature's secrets remained a tantalizing possibility for Western thinkers, and through their alchemical and magical inquiries they sought to rediscover the elixir of life, the fountain of youth, and the key to longevity that had been lost so many generations before. It should be pointed out, though, that life cannot be extended indefinitely. Immortality is by definition reserved for the gods or God and to acquire immortality is to become a god. Adam and Eve, after eating from the tree of knowledge of good and evil, were specifically banished from Eden to prevent them from eating from the tree of life. God says, "What if he now reaches out his hand and takes from the tree of life and also eats it and lives forever?" Similarly, the Greeks' conception of divine immortality was derived from the unique diet of the gods, who lived off ambrosia and nectar and the smoke of sacrificial victims. According to Pindar, a god who tasted of human food would be demoted and mortals who shared a divine repast would become by definition gods. This is precisely why Odysseus, though he shares the goddess Calypso's bed (mortals and gods can mate, after all), does not eat with her, because then he would become a god and never return to Ithaca.

Apart from food of the gods, mortals can make better use of earthly foods and medicines to prolong their lives and can seek out natural, mystical truths that would enable them to extend their stay on earth. Built into the basic tenets of Western medicine stemming from Hippocrates and Galen is the idea that health and life span are directly related to what we might call lifestyle choices and diet. Following the most popular metaphor, human life is like a burning oil lamp provided at birth of an ample supply of oil (or radical moisture in physiological terms). The heat of the flame slowly consumes the fuel throughout one's life. This fuel can be replenished via foods that are digested and ultimately converted into our own flesh and spirits, but because our capacity to digest and convert food slowly diminishes as we age, it becomes increasingly difficult to fully replenish the burning lamp; eventually we are totally unable, and then we die. Nonetheless, life can be prolonged, according to the Greek physicians, by carefully moderating dietary intake to prevent premature wasting of vital heat and radical moisture. In practical terms this means that while in youth the body can digest large amounts of relatively course foods, as we grow older both the quantity of intake must be reduced as well as the consistency of foods, which must be more subtle and easily digested. Moreover, physical exercise and sexual activity must be gradually reduced so as not to overburden the system and artificially extinguish the flame of life. Much like any fire, the amount of fuel must be proportionate to the flame's intensity—too little and the flame burns up quickly, too much and it is snuffed out.

Therefore, most medical prescriptions for longevity involved eating less, eating lighter foods, and strangely enough getting less exercise. It also involved eating foods that are qualitatively warmer to offset the naturally colder complexion of the aged. According to the Regimen Sanitatis Salernitanum, old people should drink wine, which is both easily digested and, as an analog of blood, easily transforms into it. *Vinum lac senum* (Wine is the milk for old folks).[2]

Although there was probably some empirical basis for supporting such claims originally, it should be stressed that it was a theoretical system and principles deduced from that system led physicians to specific dietary recommendations. For example, when a physician recommended eggs, milk, and broth for his elderly patients, it was based on the theoretical assumption that these provide the lightest and most easily assimilated form of nutrition. And just as mother's milk is the most appropriate food for toothless infants, it once again provides ideal nutrition for the equally weak and often toothless elderly patients. According to Platina, the best prescription was to drink human milk from a cheerful, young, and beautiful woman, warm and directly from the source.[3] One can easily understand the popularity of this therapy. It also bears saying that for Western physicians the process of aging was a natural process of becoming colder and drier, and therefore it was inevitable. Galen claimed that aging should not be considered a disease because it is not contrary to nature. Still, the process may be slowed somewhat through careful attention to regimen, though never wholly averted.

When this Greek medical tradition fused with the Judeo-Christian tradition, not surprisingly a number of nearly insoluble problems arose. First, it is clear from the passages in Genesis and Job in particular that God has ordained the number of days allotted to each individual: "His days are determined and the number of his months is with thee and thou has the appointed his bound that he cannot pass."[4] Psalms gives us threescore and ten, or at most fourscore.[5] Even the conscious attempt to extend life implicitly contradicts God's will. Furthermore, in the New Testament, with its focus on salvation and the afterlife, the desire to prolong the soul's entrapment in physical form becomes positively suspect. If this world involves suffering and sin, and if the body and what happens to it are of little importance compared to everlasting life, then why would one want to spend a few more miserable years on earth? For Paul, there was a serious dilemma between choosing the obviously preferable afterlife with Christ and staying on earth to fulfill His divine mission. In Philippians 1: "What I should like to do is to depart and be with Christ; that is better by far; but for your sake there is greater need for me to stay on in the body."[6]

Thus, even in the Christian context there could be a legitimate excuse to try to prolong life even if not for its own sake or to enjoy a few more years but to do God's work. This was precisely the same logic John Calvin used when confronted with the question of why our life on earth matters if our salvation is out of our hands and entirely predestined. In any case, it was up to God and His Providence when the final hours should come, and such matters are ultimately out of our control. But could one be blamed for trying to extend life? When motivated by pride and love of earthly objects, yes, but as part of God's plan, why not?

There also runs through Judeo-Christian thought another theme directly related to this idea: that in the full cyclical development of God's plan humans will once again enjoy life after the coming of the Messiah, after which an earthly paradise will be founded in a New Jerusalem. According to John, the author of the book of Revelation, after the second coming of Christ there will be ushered in the Millennium, a thousand years of peace, freedom from sickness, and life spans comparable to those of the first humans. This notion, however, suggests that extending life and the current world of sin is ultimately futile. That is, except for those who held the idea that there might be some earthly spot where people presently enjoy an existence comparable to paradise, where people still live in the state of nature and have not yet fallen in with corrupt civilization.

For the Greeks, this "heaven on earth" was the land of the Hyperboreans, which means "beyond Boreas" (the north wind). This is a basic theme in most folk tales around the world: the Isles of the Blessed, Atlantis, Shangri-La, Tir na Nog (the land of youth) for the Celts, St. Brendan's Island, or Avalon. In all of these, pristine humans in their original natural state still enjoy extraordinarily long lives, and sometimes this is explained by their simple diet of fruits and vegetables that are spontaneously produced by the earth. Most Adamic diets are also vegetarian. But frequently there's also some miraculous substance, some quasi-ambrosial food or a fountain of youth that prevents the inhabitants from aging. Ponce de Leon was searching for precisely this legendary fountain of youth in 1513 when he accidentally bumped into Florida. His efforts prompted serious debate back in Rome on whether God could have provided man with such a miraculous substance, and most agreed that it was possible. Nobody contested the benefit of therapeutic waters. It made perfect sense that there could be certain waters with the power to restore youth or even confer immortality. This was also the power attributed by many medieval romances to wine drunk directly from the Holy Grail.

There were also other miraculous substances that were said to prolong life. According to the Neoplatonic philosopher Marsilio Ficino, any incorruptible substance such as precious gems or especially gold when consumed or drunk in the form of *aurum potabile* has the power to render the human body significantly impervious to corruption.[7] Equally, the flesh of many animals thought to enjoy long life (such as stag) was believed to confer longevity. According to European folk traditions, following the logic of direct transference of material properties whereby lion's flesh increases courage and rabbits cause timidity, long-lived animals should extend human life when consumed.

There was also a related theme that aging can be temporarily suspended when the subject undergoes intense hibernation-like sleep. Sleeping Beauty was suspended for one hundred years in the original non-Disney version of the tale, and Rip Van Winkle slept for thirty. Needless to say, cryogenics is just a modern incarnation of the fascination with staving off death and awaking in the future when the ability to cure all diseases has been discovered, and perhaps there is even a means of reviving the dead. The Woody Allen movie *Sleeper* is just another version of the story, but many people have willingly had themselves frozen.

Medieval alchemists undertook the most sustained and systematic effort in the West to prolong life. This ancestor to modern chemistry was not primarily designed to transmute base metals into gold; instead, alchemists sought to understand and control natural forces both seen and unseen—what were referred to as the *occult*. This word did not have the sinister connotations it does today. It simply meant forces that cannot be perceived or explained through human senses or reason. Magnetism, for example, was considered an occult force. Using these forces to aid humans in extending life was one among many goals of the alchemists.

Roger Bacon was explicit in stating that Western medicine and diet could only aid humans to a certain degree but that "experimental art supplies the defect of medicine in this particular."[8] In other words, there is much more that we can do with science. In this case, experimental procedures involved concentrating and rarefying natural substances to increase their potency. Among these was distillation, which can extract and purify the essence of wine, yielding alcohol or aqua vitae, the water of life. Akvavit and usque beatha (whiskey) are also derived from the same word. This was one of the most potent pro-longevity drugs of the era. This is because if hot and moist wine fortifies the vital heat and radical moisture of our bodies, then it does so even more forcefully when reduced to its essence or elixir without demanding energy in digestion.

The procedures for refining such substances, although in ways anticipating straightforward laboratory methods, also involved what we might call mysticism and deliberately obscure language. As revived ancient wisdom, it should be anything but immediately comprehensible. That is probably why alchemy has often become synonymous with charlatanism and quackery, but seemingly unfairly. These procedures were seen as a way to tap into the divine forces of the universe long forgotten by mortals, and, of course, it would be strange and perplexing as a consequence. Furthermore, the alchemists sought out as authoritative sources the oldest possible writings on the topic because these were considered more true and closer to the origin of all knowledge. These texts were often written in the first and second century AD in Hellenistic Egypt by figures such as Zosimus, but they were attributed to much older authors such as Hermes, Isis, and even Moses.

In fact, Western alchemy has its roots in late Greek science in Egypt (which of course had a long fascination with immortality). It was later adopted and expanded by Arabic authors, especially in ninth- and tenth-century Baghdad among figures such as Jabir and al-Razi. But it is really only in the Latin West that it became preoccupied with longevity per se. This began in the twelfth century as classical Greek medical texts, science, and philosophy all began to be translated from Arabic sources into Latin. Alchemy came along with it, as did the word *alembic*, which was used to distill these substances, and many other Arabic scientific words such as *alkali* and *algebra*.

The most important alchemists in Europe at the time were Roger Bacon, Arnold of Villanova, and Raymond Lull. The latter were Catalonian and most interested in extracting the life-promoting quintessence, or fifth element. Bacon, who hailed from Oxford, was the first to argue explicitly that the current shortness of life is only accidental rather than essential or fixed.

He pointed specifically to the biblical patriarchs after the Fall, who lived hundreds of years. He figured there must be something we are doing wrong today. Later alchemists, most notably Paracelsus, argued that the critical event that changed the human life span was the flood. Presumably plants and vegetables in the antediluvian state were far more concentrated and nutritious and provided humans with everything they needed to live hundreds of years, but after being soaked with the floodwaters they became practically useless, which is why we now have to eat meat. It is also why plant-based medicines no longer suffice. A meat-based diet causes its own problems as well. Being much more difficult to digest than the Edenic vegetables, meat taxes the system more rigorously and ages us prematurely. But if the ancient super vegetables are no longer available, there might be a way to artificially manufacture superfoods and drugs that extend life. These ideas resonate in so many fascinating ways with our own obsession to identify superfoods, functional foods, and neutraceuticals.

Another argument that Bacon made is that we ourselves have become corrupt and immoral compared to the ancients and far less conscious of hygiene. In this case it really is just sin that debilitates the body as well as luxury and excess and poor habits. These are all the curses of civilization. Moreover, weakened parents naturally conceive impaired children, so the tendency to live shorter and shorter lives is passed on through each succeeding generation. It is therefore only those people who reject all luxury such as ascetics or perhaps Brahmins who can live past one hundred years.

Given all these impediments, the secret arts might still be employed to restore longevity, and Bacon was fond of stories of peasants accidentally discovering golden phials of miraculous concoctions. There is one about an English woodsman who found a strange ointment and, after using it, lived for three hundred years. Another recounts the story of Artephius, who discovered the secret of long life and lived for 1,025 years. Bacon, diverging from standard Galenic medicine, proposed that life can be comfortably extended not just a few years but, with the right miraculous substances, up to 100 or 150 years for his own generation, and probably much longer down the road. Unlike physicians, he went far beyond standard diet and hygiene by focusing on pharmaceuticals and even natural substances that confer longevity such as pearls, coral, rosemary, serpent's flesh, ambergris, gold, and a bone from a stag's heart. All of these contain an ample supply of vital spirit. Vital spirit is normally brought in through the lungs and mixes with our blood and in a sense nourishes or brings life to various parts of our body. It's not quite oxygen, because that had not been discovered yet, but something vaguely analogous that we get from the air. The advantage of superdrugs is that these supply vital spirit in a much more potent and concentrated form and thus rekindle our own innate force.

Another far less expensive source is the breath of a young virgin. This is an odd example but one that illustrates this logic nicely. Because youth have an ample supply of the vital principal not yet wasted by sexual activity, directly inhaling their breath provides a concentrated shot to promote longevity. Again, you have to wonder about these peoples' motives, and Roger Bacon expresses this idea in very cautious and veiled language so as not to be taken the wrong way, but it is indeed mouth to mouth. Apart from these, the most typical longevity drug is gold, specifically because it is incorruptible and can't be destroyed or created by any element—fire, air, water, or earth. It is therefore analogous to or sympathetically linked to the sun, the paramount provider of life, and thus the conservator of life when taken internally.

The alchemists were also fascinated with the Philosopher's Stone, which not only can transmute base metals into gold but also refines and fortifies the vital spirits in the human body. The great Elizabethan alchemist John Dee had such a Philosopher's Stone, which was on display in the British Museum. Bacon says, "This is the secret of secrets the most noble matter which transforms any metallic body into very pure gold which conserve the body in their essence, fortifies them in their virtue, which makes an old man young and drives out all sickness of the body." The difficult thing was, of course, making it properly. It involved a long, torturous set of procedures: distillations, dissolving, precipitations, burning (usually of mercury) to approximate the very substance that will preserve us after the resurrection, keeping in mind that our bodies are restored after the final judgment. This was called the quintessence, or the elixir of life, unlike substances made up of the four elements, which are subject to decay. If one could properly prepare the most refined form of the Philosopher's Stone in assimilate form (usually potable), then you would have the key to longevity.

It was never really clear, though, which kind of chemicals one should start with—gold, mercury, ammonia, wine—and the result of all these experiments was a variety of pharmaceutical products such as sel ammoniac, aqua vitae, aurum potabile, and various mercurial salts that were increasingly seen not as the panacea but as drugs for specific ailments. This, of course, was the beginning of pharmaceutical chemistry, which emerged in the course of the sixteenth century with one of the most fascinating figures in the history of medicine—Paracelsus. On the one hand, he was the last of the great medieval alchemists and, on the other, strangely enough, the father of modern pharmacy. As a branch of medicine, pharmacy obviously departed from the dietary regimen almost completely.

Did these alchemical practices constitute a kind of cult? It seems apparent that this is a special kind of devotion—secretive, mystical—and indeed it does promise transformation and ideally promotes longevity. Like any other food cult in the past, it is difficult to gauge exactly how widespread it was and how seriously its followers believed in it. But insofar as the popular writings suggest an ardent interest, we can consider this a dietary cult.

Alchemy was not the only dietary cult, though. As we have seen, standard Galenic medicine discussed longevity even if it did not promise it explicitly. New iatrochemical and iatromechanical theories appeared in the seventeenth century, which opened up new possibilities, and new longevity diets appeared in the early modern period, often quite separate from professional medical circles. The most influential of these was one by Alvise Cornaro, a self-avowed octogenarian who, after becoming gravely ill in midlife, decided to abandon his profligate lifestyle and thereafter enjoyed robust good health. As he reported in his widely published account, the key was a temperate diet and trusting his own experience in avoiding foods that caused him to suffer: strong wines, melons and other fruits, lettuce, fish, pork, sausages, legumes, cake—all he imagined to be cold foods that upset his humorally cold constitution. More important, he also reduced the quantity of his intake, and, completely contrary to the standard medical theory of his day, he ate only twelve ounces of solid food and fourteen ounces of liquid. When in his seventies friends convinced him to increase his diet by two ounces, which made him sick again until he reverted to his former diet. He then lived on to 98, or, according to some sources, 102. In all likelihood Cornaro suffered from diabetes, and there is even a passage where he mentions his intense thirst.[9]

The move toward quantification of nutrition took another century with the work of Santorio Santorio and his *Dietetica Statica*, in which for thirty years the author weighed himself, his food, and his excreta to determine which foods offered the most nutrition and which were ideal for maintaining weight and promoting health.[10] This was the first study that implied that nutrition and, indirectly, the length of life could be measured.

In the meantime, Cornaro served as the prime example of a person who could extend life simply through temperance and sobriety and calorie reduction. Many people were said to have read and been inspired by his writings, including Benjamin Franklin. And naturally, various health food movements in the following centuries pointed to Cornaro's autobiographical account. But the idea of a calorie restriction diet for longevity received focused attention once again only in the twentieth century. Mary Crowell and Clive McKay at Cornell University in the 1930s experimented with severely restricting the quantity of food fed to laboratory rats and found that it extended their life span as long as certain nutrients weren't lacking.[11] Roy Walford and Richard Weindruch followed up these experiments with mice in the 1980s and in their book *The Retardation of Aging and Disease by Dietary Restriction.* While never becoming a widespread diet phenomenon, there have been many people who trust in its application to humans, and results of the first clinical trials published only a decade ago have suggested great promise.[12] We may, in time, see a popular diet specifically promoting longevity through eating less. One such title by Brian M. Delaney and Lisa Walford released recently promotes calorie restriction (CR).[13]

Far more common than calorie restriction is the notion that particular foods will promote longevity because they either help prevent disease or are themselves conducive to long life. Yogurt gained an avid following, which it still enjoys, after the work of Elie Metchnikoff early in the twentieth century. Metchnikoff claimed to have identified "good bacteria" in the gut prevalent in the yogurt enjoyed by Bulgarian herdsmen, who were often centenarians.[14] His book *The Prolongation of Life* popularized the idea, and products soon appeared on grocery shelves laden with *Lactobacillus bulgaricus*. As late as the 1970s one could see commercials on TV advertising yogurt as a promoter of longevity. Although scientific research has not upheld the claim for longevity, the recent mapping of the human gut biome does suggest that bacteria play a much greater role in human health and physiology than ever suspected.

Related to those diets explicitly geared toward longevity are several, popular since the time of Sylvester Graham in the United States, that promoted health food, vitality, and, coincidentally, long life. These might be classified as basic health food diets, but at times they did become rigorous in the extreme. Take, for example, the work of Bernarr Macfadden in the early twentieth century, who promoted physical perfection, rigorous fasting, and other questionable dieting practices. He, too, claimed that they would help him live to 150.

Generic longevity diets have come and gone in the past century, but many have gained some legitimacy in professional circles. Studies of Okinawans, farmers in the Caucasus, vegetarian Seventh-Day Adventists, and the entire Mediterranean diet phenomenon inspired by Ancel Keys not only greatly influenced popular ideas of nutrition but also kept alive the idea that life could be extended through diet. And of course superfoods are marketed with explicit health claims; note the resurgence in nuts, kale, and blueberries that promise to prevent disease and extend life. A recent title by Dan Buettner, *The Blue Zones Solution*, examines various peoples around the globe who often live past one hundred and simply sees what they do right, which basically boils down to a simple plant-based diet, moderate alcohol, exercise, and little stress.

We must again consider whether devotion to these ideas constitutes a cult. Listening to devotees, watching them shop, eat, and of course commend each other for their wise choices, one would think so. A conversion experience is not unusual. Nor are the movement's leaders, who provide inspiration extending from yoga instructors to modern health gurus. The firm belief that we have the power to extend life by means of diet and medicine seems as strong today as it was among the medieval alchemists.

NOTES

1. Gerald J. Gruman, *A History of Ideas about the Prolongation of Life*, transactions of the American Philosophical Society, vol. 56, part 9 (1966) (Reprint, New York: Springer, 2003), 12.
2. Regimen Sanitatis Salernitanum, "Vinum lac senum, iuvenis venenum." https://archive.org/stream/schoolofsalernum00hariiala/schoolofsalernum00hariiala_djvu.txt.
3. Platina (Bartolomeo Sacchi), *De honesta voluptate* (Rome, 1470).
4. Job 14:5, as quoted in Gruman, *A History of Ideas*, 7–18.
5. Psalms 90:5–6.
6. Phillippians 1:23.
7. Marsilio Ficino, *Three Books on Life*, trans. Carole V. Kaske and John R. Clark (Binghamton, NY: Medieval and Renaissance Texts and Studies, 1989).
8. Roger Bacon, *Opus Majus*, https://archive.org/stream/opusmajusofroger002065mbp/opusmajusofroger002065mbp_djvu.txt.
9. D. Schäfer, "Aging, Longevity, and Diet: Historical Remarks on Calorie Intake Reduction," *Gerontology* 51 (2005): 126–30.
10. Santorio Santorio, *Medicina Statica* (Venice: N. Polo, 1614).
11. Roger B. McDonald and John J. Ramsey, "Honoring Clive McKay and 75 Years of Calorie Restriction Research," *Journal of Nutrition* 140, no. 7 (July 2010): 1205–10.
12. S. K. Das, C. H. Gilhooly, J. K. Golden, A. G. Pittas, P. J. Fuss, R. A. Cheatham, S. Tyler, M. Tsay, M. A. McCrory, et al., "Long-Term Effects of 2 Energy-Restricted Diets Differing in Glycemic Load on Dietary Adherence, Body Composition, and Metabolism in CALERIE: A 1-y Randomized Controlled Trial," *American Journal of Clinical Nutrition* 85 (2007): 1023–30.

13. Brian M. Delaney and Lisa Walford, *The Longevity Diet: The Only Proven Way to Slow the Aging Process and Maintain Peak Vitality through Caloric Restriction*, 3rd ed. (New York: Da Capo Lifelong Books, 2010).

14. Harvey Levenstein, *Fear of Food* (Chicago: University of Chicago Press, 2012), 27–35.

BIBLIOGRAPHY

Bacon, Roger. *Opus Majus*. https://archive.org/stream/opusmajusofroger002065mbp/opusmajusofroger002065mbp_djvu.txt.

Das, S. K., C. H. Gilhooly, J. K. Golden, A. G. Pittas, P. J. Fuss, R. A. Cheatham, S. Tyler, M. Tsay, M. A. McCrory, et al. "Long-Term Effects of 2 Energy-Restricted Diets Differing in Glycemic Load on Dietary Adherence, Body Composition, and Metabolism in CALERIE: A 1-y Randomized Controlled Trial." *American Journal of Clinical Nutrition* 85 (2007): 1023–30.

Delaney, Brian M., and Lisa Walford. *The Longevity Diet: The Only Proven Way to Slow the Aging Process and Maintain Peak Vitality through Caloric Restriction*. 3rd ed. New York: Da Capo Lifelong Books, 2010.

Ficino, Marsilio. *Three Books on Life*. Translated by Carole V. Kaske and John R. Clark. Binghamton, NY: Medieval and Renaissance Texts and Studies, 1989.

Gruman, Gerald J. *A History of Ideas about the Prolongation of Life*. Transactions of the American Philosophical Society, vol. 56, part 9 (1966). Reprint, New York: Springer, 2003.

Levenstein, Harvey. *Fear of Food.* Chicago: University of Chicago Press, 2012.

McDonald, Roger B., and John J. Ramsey. "Honoring Clive McKay and 75 Years of Calorie Restriction Research." *Journal of Nutrition* 140, no. 7 (July 2010): 1205–10.

Platina (Bartolomeo Sacchi). *De honesta voluptate*. Rome, 1470.

Regimen Sanitatis Salernitanum. English translation by John Harrington. New York: Hoeber, 1920. https://archive.org/stream/schoolofsalernum00hariiala/schoolofsalernum00hariiala_djvu.txt.

Santorio Santorio. *Medicina Statica.* Venice: N. Polo, 1614.

Schäfer, D. "Aging, Longevity, and Diet: Historical Remarks on Calorie Intake Reduction." *Gerontology* 51 (2005): 126–30.

Chapter Five

Juicing

Language, Ritual, and Placebo Sociality in a Community of Extreme Eaters

Samuel Veissière and Liona Gibbs-Bravo

WHAT DO CULTURES, CULTS, FOOD BELIEFS, AND PLACEBOS HAVE IN COMMON?

In this chapter, we present ethnographic, cognitive, and social neuroscientific insights on the culture of *juicing*, a practice that consists of extracting juice from fruits and vegetables to produce liquid with no pulp or solid matter. As an emerging cultural practice, juicing is grounded in beliefs concerning pollution and purity and is enacted through a set of highly prescriptive and extreme rituals to "flush" out undesirable substances and achieve "cleansing." Theorizing how juicers come to desire and work toward historically, culturally, and ideologically specific body types, we focus on the role of ritual, language, and sociality in mediating the ways of "feeling clean" that characterize juicer experiences. Juicers' success in being thin or feeling clean, we argue, has little to do with intrinsic properties of any specific foods or ways of preparing and consuming them. We propose, rather, that these positive responses are rooted in the pro-social rewards of constructing a juicer identity and are primarily enabled by ritual, the performative nature of language, and the embodied character of collectively held beliefs. Indeed, as we will argue, the "juice" dimension in juicing culture can be understood as a semantic filler for a set of identity-constructing rituals, but as a chemical substance in and of itself it is causally irrelevant.

As anthropologists and cognitive scientists, studying juicing provides us with a fascinating case study into fundamental questions on the very nature and emergence of culture and subjectivity.

In our analysis, we introduce the notion of *placebo sociality* to describe the physiological effects of language, belief, and expectations mediated through collective ritual practice that eventually give rise to specific ways of experiencing one's body.

As we will show, placebo sociality properly understood is a pleonasm: culture by definition produces placebo effects. Culture *is* placebo. What we believe and expect, as the well-known story goes, affects how we feel. In this chapter, we offer a precise account of how these processes come into being socially, cognitively, and phenomenally.

We begin with a simple working definition of culture borrowed from the biological sciences. When members of the same species develop *group-specific ways of feeling and doing things*, we can speak of culture.[1] We then proceed to unravel something of an old anthropological mystery: How and why do people who mostly don't interact with one another in the flesh develop standardized, scripted ways of being that feel so real and personal to them? How and why do cultural differences take hold with such strange phenomenal ("what it feels like") stability? Why is this process largely unconscious for humans?

The cultlike dimension of juicing culture, as we will argue, provides further clues into these mechanisms. Indeed, we insist that the collective mediation and embodiment of food beliefs within the context of emergent cultlike social iterations offer something of a recipe for unpacking highly efficient forms of placebo sociality—and embodied cultural mechanisms in general.

At its core, we understand the difference between a *cult* and a *culture* as one of degrees but not of kind. Like "cultures," cults are characterized by a preexisting imagined order ready to be integrated by human hosts; an imagined order that, as the old sociological adage goes, prescribes manners of thinking, desiring, feeling, and moving in the world. Unlike the cultures we inherit through the accident of birth, however, cults offer a stronger illusion of choice and rationality. They offer the illusion of a fresh, new, formal worldview that seems more rational, appealing, and rewarding to social subjects. By accepting cult beliefs and engaging in new—often extreme—practices, one is afforded the "choice" to abandon certain aspects of cultural life one feels most disgruntled with. Theorizing why certain people and not others partially abandon their old ways in search of new ones is beyond the scope of this chapter. This seems, in any case, to have characterized the human experience ever since our species entered a symbolic niche and began fashioning cumulative cultural worlds.[2] While individual psychological dispositions may play a part in this process, we must also note, as social scientists, that cult formations invariably take place as a response to historical, economic, social, and cultural forces that mostly lie beyond the conscious reach of the people who maintain those institutional worlds through collective convention and action.[3] But cults, we insist, offer a stronger illusion of choice and purpose than those aspects of our life (such as nationality, social status at birth, dominant values, the economic order, etc.) that are *obviously* not chosen by social subjects.

Cults also afford something uniquely appealing to humans; a crucial ingredient of successful sociality that has long been understood by demagogues, marketing specialists, extremists, and gurus of all kinds: they offer *hardship.* This insight seems counterintuitive and will require a whole chapter to unpack. Humans, as we hope to demonstrate, do not simply desire safety, freedom from want, and the satisfaction of basic physiological and social needs: they also thrive on a sense of *purpose* and *sacrifice.*[4] They like to work hard for rare, hard-to-reach, highly arousing, often esoteric experiences—experiences that will give a select few the full satisfaction of having entered higher realms of truth, entitlement, prestige, and solidarity. Many of our "primitive" ancestors understood this and incorporated extremes rites of passages for a select few members of their society who would be endowed with prestige and prepared for leadership roles. These often involved extreme sensory deprivation, flesh cutting, and survival scenarios requiring cooperation in harsh environments.[5] Military training the world over—particularly of "elite corps"—is still based on this simple recipe. When successfully orchestrated, these scenarios will produce subjects ready to die for their peers and the imagined social order but who have achieved a maximal sense of *having chosen and earned* this "privilege"!

A fully embodied placebo response, as we will see, entails the onset of measurable physiological responses triggered by symbolic cues.[6] As we will argue, however, an undertheorized aspect of such responses is that they require total surrender to an *epistemic authority*—that is, to something or someone representing a body of knowledge one can entirely trust. This is why human children, who are socialized to trust adults and defer to their authority, are particularly receptive to placebo effects. A headache that goes away with a sugar pill or a feeling of elation arising from drinking a specifically prepared juice are both physiological responses to symbolic cues that have acquired authority in a ritual context. The most successful of such responses, we claim, are produced when humans operate under the illusion that they have undergone hard intellectual, moral, emotional, and physical work to *choose* and *earn* the otherwise opaque symbolic order that will condition their embodied response.

This brief ethnography of juicing culture will tell the story of this strange but universally human mechanism. Telling this full story will also require detours through the cognitive science and anthropology of religion and ritual,[7] the philosophy and anthropology of language,[8] and the emerging social neuroscience of placebo.[9] But first, we begin with an ethnographic window into juicing culture, written in the voice of the ethnographer.[10]

A HAPPIER, CLEANER PERSON: AUTOETHNOGRAPHY OF A JUICE CLEANSE (LIONA GIBBS-BRAVO)

Juicing, which has become increasingly popular—even over the short period of time I have been studying it (January 2015–January 2016)—is the practice of extracting juice from fruits and vegetables to produce liquid with no pulp or solid matter, oftentimes consumed in a period known as *cleansing*.

Like other "food cults" that have gained increased popularity in recent years (e.g., the cults of paleo diets [Bell, this volume] and gluten-free eating [Martin, this volume]), the culture of juicing presented me with clear examples of extreme food beliefs and practices.

Over the span of three months, I spent much of my time in juice bars of Montreal and Toronto, which all offered a similar atmosphere and array of products.

The first of these juice havens I visited was attached to one of the most popular juice brands in Montreal. Although it operates mainly online, the brand at the time of my research had begun distributing their juices in cafés and food shows throughout the city. The tagline "Nothing Else" had first greeted me on the company's website, wrapped in a mostly empty and white minimal aesthetic.

The company's owner, in a series of ethnographic conversations echoing the vision outlined on the website, explained that the practice was grounded in "transparency and simplicity, and taking control of what we consume."

The local store's atmosphere paralleled that of the website in an array of minimalist details I soon began to recognize as the hallmarks of juice bars and juicing culture at large. Located at the bottom of a business tower, the small shop had a constant flow of people wearing suits and spandex, hurriedly taking a break from their work to buy juice products and paraphernalia.

The owner was busy with the flow of customers, but in between explaining the health benefits of juice and greeting devoted regulars, he invited me into the juicing world.

I was told about the importance of the process used to make juice, the differences between juicing and blending, his personal philosophy toward health and juice, and the controversial topic of cleansing.

Cold-pressed juices, which are preferred over pasteurized or blended juices, are made without heat generated from the friction of blades, allegedly preserving the maximum amount of nutrients and vitamins in the juice. Incorporating juice into a diet, as the businessman explained, capitalizes on ingesting fruits and vegetables in their "purest" form, thereby intaking the "maximal amount of nutrients possible." The introductory cleanse offered by the business, in turn, was judiciously named the "Purity Cleanse."

The notion of detoxifying and cleansing one's body of unwanted elements, as I came to learn, is visible and central in every aspect of juicing culture. This is a theme I consistently encountered in every juice bar I visited in Montreal and Toronto. The importance placed on cold pressing and cleansing bodies to reach optimal purity, as I discovered, go hand in hand. By ingesting food in its "purest form," so the story goes, one can similarly achieve an optimally pure form of bodily health. Along with the emphasis on cold pressing, many other aspects of the juice experience are outlined in order to maintain the highest level of purity.

This offering of *order*, *clarity*, and *control* in juice cleanses provides an opportunity to create order in the otherwise ambiguous world of health. The "unhealthy" individual, in the model offered by juicing culture, is segregated for an initial period of days to follow a strict juice diet and subsequently emerges as a healthy individual through this highly controlled and methodical process.

From what type of juice is best suited for what hour of ingestion to the amount of time between pressing and ingesting, there is an exhaustive list of cleansing prescriptions, as well as pre- and postcleanse rules outlining what to cut out and what to increase to ensure maximal benefits—whatever those may be: higher energy, better skin, clearer thoughts, detoxification, and weight loss.

It took me some time, many store visits, and countless hours of reading juicing web forums before deciding to try the products. By then, it may be more accurate to say that I wanted in on juicing power.

As I left the store with my $10 juice in hand, I was congratulated for taking care of my body and encouraged to let my new fellow juicers know how I felt in the subsequent days. Yet, as critical as I was inclined to be, I couldn't shake off the increasingly pervasive thoughts that *I* was feeling a little more energetic. It seemed, I couldn't help noticing, that my skin already looked a bit brighter. As I felt invited into this clean, white world, I began to give serious thought to undergoing a cleanse.

My ethnographic self was beginning to merge with my wanting-to-cleanse self. I wanted to better understand the cleansing concept, but a part of me wanted in on the enthusiastic list of benefits. I decided to go for it. I was no longer sure why.

I decided on a three-day cleanse and weighed the options of either buying juice from a program or making it myself. The cheapest program I could find began at $60 a day, in a package that included a variety of juice blends to be ingested in a specific order. I opted for the homemade option.

I soon found out that time and mental and physical investments were far outweighed by financial investments. Preparing for the cleanse required three hours of reading on proper juicing techniques and grocery items. The online world of juicing is extensive, and the more I researched, the more I felt I needed to learn more about all aspects, from the best temperature to store juice to the benefits of prolonging one's cleanse. I then spent five hours grocery shopping in different parts of the city and another five hours making all my juices for the next three days. I was consumed by the endless list of rules outlining how to properly execute not only the cleanse itself but also all the pre- and postrequirements for maximal effects. This left little time to think about much other than cleansing. Whether I was pondering the effects on my body and trying to notice changes or thinking about my next juice because I was hungry, I was consumed by thoughts of my food intake and purification. I became very focused on all the details regarding how many hours apart I was drinking my juice and which type (more fruit heavy, green, detoxifying) I was drinking at what time of day. As these ritualistic behaviors consumed me, I felt the desire to share them with other people who understood the difficulty of what I was undertaking. I craved a like-minded community to reinforce what I was feeling, to motivate me, and a place to share my success. I turned to Instagram, where juice cleansers are abundant. Gaining followers and the approval of the Instagram community strangely absorbed me and added to the amount of mental time invested in cleansing. I discovered which hashtags would gain me more followers (#kale was rather popular that week), as well as which one would lead me to the most interesting content posted by others (#livecleanordie, #deathbyginger, #karmicjuice). A lot of people in my friend group were quite skeptical of the process, and while I was initially equally skeptical, I became aware of my blossoming belief in juicing principles and the social symbol juice had offered me. I was engaged with the juicing community through Instagram and felt the cosmology reinforced and supported, which drew me to focus more on my Instagram interactions than on interactions with my friends. On the second night of my cleanse, I found myself sitting at a barbecue sipping my Mean Green juice while my friends ate their burgers, scrolling through Instagram to see what other juicers were up to. I felt a quiet satisfaction in knowing that by giving up that burger I was becoming a healthier, *better person*. This intense feeling of self-satisfaction and moral superiority in my deprivation in fact remained as a strong undercurrent throughout my cleanse process. When I was staring at the clock with my stomach growling waiting desperately for the time I could start my next juice, or having trouble falling asleep because I was so hungry, I felt I would be rewarded for this work by emerging as a cleaner, happier person.

DISCUSSION: SYMBOLS, LANGUAGE, AND RITUAL IN PLACEBO SOCIALITY

Gibbs-Bravo's account of transitioning from ethnographer to juicer with precise embodied efficacy (her sense of elation, cleanliness, and reward in particular) neatly illustrates the "placebo" mechanisms we introduced in the opening section. These mechanisms, we insist, are made salient in cultlike forms of sociality but are ultimately intrinsic to all forms of socioculturally patterned human practice.

In this section, we expand on Gibbs-Bravo's autoethnography to flesh out some of the cognitive, symbolic, political, and ritualistic aspects of these mechanisms.

To understand how a seemingly arbitrary symbolic convention (like the meaning and alleged effects attributed to ways of talking about certain foods) can take hold with such precision, we should begin with a discussion of what Veissière has termed the "hypnotic" quality of sociality.

In a series of recent articles,[11] Veissière and colleagues have theorized the embodied effects of large-scale, linguistically, and symbolically mediated joint attention through the lens of hypnosis. Drawing on recent theoretical and empirical work on hypnosis, they have highlighted the relation between epidemics of shared expectations and representations[12] and regimes of attention.[13] They have based their argument on recent work in cultural neuroscience that departs from reductionist models in which dissociation, trance, and hypnosis are understood as distinct (or "altered") states of consciousness.[14] In these new minimal models, hypnosis is understood as any intense, or "atypical," form of attention that mobilizes pre-reflective, nonconscious cognitive resources and triggers strong modes of affect or readiness-to-action in response to contextual cues and prompts. "Hypnosis," thus, refers to forms of largely automatized selective attention that recruit meta-expectative mechanisms and trigger specific modes of affect and readiness-to-action implicitly learned in patterned sociocultural practice. "Culture," in this view, is understood as a shared repertoire of *expectations* (expectations about how the world is and how the world should be), themselves implicitly nested in expectations about others' expectations—that is, expectations about how others expect us to behave, think, and feel from moment to moment and context to context.[15] Cultural ontogeny and hypnotic induction, in this view, both entail the outsourcing of relevant action-generating information to an *epistemic authority*—that is, to a person, cue, prompt, or symbol that has acquired high attentional relevance. A successful "hypnotic" social enactment, in other words, is not unlike the experience of surrendering to the symbolically constituted epistemic authority of a therapist, or an experimenter in a placebo study. In the ongoing enactment and reenactment of cultural ontogeny, however, the "epistemic authorities" to which we outsource attentional relevance need not entail the presence of actual human agents—the process, as Veissière and colleagues have argued, entails largely implicit expectations about (relevant and "authoritative") others' expectations.[16] In this view, humans are understood as behaving *according to the way they expect others to expect them to behave* in any given situation. Appreciating this basic joint-intentional formula for sociality requires a little more detail. Humans, to be precise, mostly operate pre-reflectively within the field of possibilities for *variations in action* modeled on their expectations of what others expect of them in specific contexts—in other words, on what these meta-expectations *afford.*

All forms of sociality, thus, run off the background of a basic cognitive formula requiring three orders of automatic intentionality—that is to say, an implicit, non-narrative, hypothesis-generating, error-reduction scenario of the "I think they think I think" variety that can be translated as "what would relevant others expect me to think/feel/do in this situation?" The notion of *variation* in action within a convention is very important. Humans do not simply obey prescribed expectations but also transgress them, improvise, and iterate in various ways. A red traffic light, for example, is a form of conventional meaning that has acquired stability as a cultural cue that affords "stopping" or "not going through." A red light late at night on a deserted street, however, may also afford "going through" given a certain set of cues. In this case, it is the physical absence of other agents, but inferences about the content of other imagined minds nonetheless, that prescribes this shift in conventional meaning.

Specific fields of semantic affordances, thus, invariably entail different licenses for transgressing expected behavior. The background formula for action is not simply "what would others expect me to do or feel here?" but also *"how much licensing can I get away with here given what the set of local cues tells me about others' likelihood to be able to judge me against and enforce the set of expectations that should otherwise govern my behavior in this specific situation?"*

Juicers in their process of enculturation, as we will explain, similarly model their affective and bodily response to dieting rituals—down to precise feelings of elation and moral arousal—against the background of implied expectations about other juicers' experiences in a similar context.

Our work on food ritual, as we hope will become apparent, aims to contribute to these emerging insights on the hypnotic nature of sociality, the physiological malleability of these processes, and the implicit joint intentional mechanisms that make them possible.

It may very well be that, as the famous quote often attributed to the renegade psychiatrist R. D. Laing goes, "We all live in a state of hypnotic trance induced in early infancy."[17] Rather than being determined in the synchronically and diachronically limited sphere of early home socialization, however, this hypnotic process should be understood as ontogenetically continuous, and intrinsic to the field and landscape of cultural affordances more generally.[18]

All social experiences in this model are always "hypnotically induced" in the sense that they entail preconscious surrender to epistemic authorities governing a set of expectations. Hypnotic sociality, thus, is another oxymoron, as the vast majority of our behaviors is socially learned, and involves selective joint-attentional mechanisms that eventually govern intuition and patterns of readiness-to-action. By this account, humans operate in joint-intentional, joint-attentional contexts, and invariably "hypnotize" one another in culture-general and context-specific ways. In a particular place and time, one may learn to encode the landscape of a poorly lit street at night as affording danger, and the presence of a particular kind of symbolically encoded agent (based on such arbitrary conventions as phenotype, styles of dress, and manners of walking) as affording fear and prescribing a flight response.

Cultlike social iterations like juicing culture, we argue, present a clear framework for studying the socialization of new embodied responses to symbolic conventions. As we will see, they also clearly point to the role of ritual in this mediation.

We now turn to anthropological analyses of the cognitive and sociopolitical foundations of ritual as a key ingredient in the mediation of sociality.[19]

Cognitive anthropologist Harvey Whitehouse,[20] building on his studies of rites of passage in Papua New Guinea, has identified what he terms *doctrinal* and *imagistic* modes of religiosity and theorized their role in the mediation of social solidarity and the large-scale spread of representations and symbolic conventions. Here, we draw on Veissière's reading of Whitehouse and his suggestion to think of imagisticity and doctrinality more generally as modes of *ritual performativity* and correlative modes of *social learning*.

In the original "religious" formulation of the idea, Whitehouse hypothesized that the rise of centralized and organized forms of religiosity in the Neolithic period played an important role in the spread of relatively homogenous mental representations that enabled large and increasingly anonymous groups of people to internalize similar cosmological views and organize themselves in what we would now recognize as "societies" or imagined communities. Here, we needn't be concerned with the difficult-to-define set of practices and beliefs of "religiosity," but rather ask how beliefs, representations, and behaviors of any kind can remain stable over time and space. How do people become and remain "literate" in all these conventions? Whitehouse directs our attention to the ritual shaping of memory.

First, we should distinguish between two basic types of memories or memory systems. Leaving aside broader questions of working and implicit memory, we can describe *explicit* memory as all that is consciously retrievable, or that we can recall. *Episodic memory* can be recalled with minimal efforts and pertains to specific sequences of events, states of affairs, peoples, and other autobiographical details.[21] By definition, episodic recalls afford remembrance of what was learned when, from whom, and with whom. *Semantic memory*, by contrast, houses all the "encyclopedic" knowledge with which we furnish our mental worlds—all the kinds, kinds of kinds, and their properties. I can recall, episodically, that I met Natasha in a green taxi on Sunday, and I can recall the scent of her perfume and how I felt that day. But I also semantically recall what taxis, perfumes, the color green, and Sundays "are," even if I cannot recall when I learned that a car was a car, a Sunday was Sunday, and green was green. I also cannot recall how I may have internalized culturally specific ways of gendering scent and olfactorizing gender and emotions, and so on.

Whitehouse, then, has identified doctrinal and imagistic modes of religiosity and ritual action and theorized their role in consolidating episodic and semantic memory. Doctrinal modes entail actions performed at high, routine frequency under relatively centralized, "expert," dependent, hierarchical divisions of epistemic labor and power. Going to church every Sunday, being formally instructed by religious experts, and performing daily religious rituals alone and with others is an example of doctrinal religiosity. High frequency and repetition, Whitehouse explained, favor low emotional arousal, which does not facilitate episodic recall but tends to build semantic memory through reiteration and reinforcement.

Imagistic modes, however, entail rituals performed very rarely, or other rites that involve extreme hardship, danger, and deprivation. Rites of passages like a communion, a bar mitzvah, a wedding, or a funeral are examples of imagistic modes. Whitehouse identified a strong correlation between low frequency in ritual performance and high emotional arousal, which in turn greatly facilitate episodic recall. Any break in routine, in this view, will trigger high arousal, negative or positive. Any rarely performed or hard-to-get experience, further, will tend to be marked with high desirability, afford high arousal, and be easy to recall once attained. Extreme rituals such as those found in military training, or rites of boyhood or girlhood involving humiliation, deprivation, or mutilation, will trigger even higher forms of arousal, which will tend to leave indelible marks on episodic memory and foster very strong bonds between people who share the experience.

Key to Whitehouse's theory is an appreciation of the basic formula of (1) high-frequency, low-arousal, semantic memory-building, and (2) low-frequency, high-arousal, episodic memory-building.

It would take me great cognitive effort, for example, to summon a detailed list of all the foodstuffs that I ingested in the past week alone. However, I can easily recall what I ate on my birthday or my friend's graduation dinner, including who was at the dinner table and how the general events of both evenings unfolded.

Doctrinal and imagistic modes of ritual of social learning, as we will see, most often coexist in any given society or social iteration. The presence of doctrinal modes, indeed, is a requirement for the rapid and efficient spread of homogenous representations in large and anonymous groups. Imagistic modes vary greatly from context to context and initially produce a highly individualized, or pseudo-individualized, interpretive response, which in turn are not epidemiologically efficient for the large-scaled spread of representations. In other words, the relative lack of prescriptions (as compared to the social norm departed from), the intensity, and the high levels of arousal experienced in this mode enable high individual variations in the meaning (or interpretation) ascribed to imagistic events. Doctrinal routines, however, demand and produce conformity in meaning and interpretation. Where imagisticity produces and encourages critical thinking, doctrinality suppresses it.

In the case of cults, we need to understand how imagisticity, or pseudo-imagisticity, necessarily recedes into doctrinality in order to (1) afford the illusion of personal "critical" exegetic choice and (2) effectively suppress critical thinking and promote conformity.

The recruitment and microsocialization of agents in cultlike social iterations like juicing thus entails the coexistence of both modes of ritual performativity and social learning. This microsocialization process, we claim, presents a condensed microcosm of the process of social ontogeny itself.

On the one hand, as Gibbs-Bravo's ethnography has shown, most of the language, cues, and practices used to recruit members (notions of purity and pollution; known foodstuffs; color schemes; taste and cultural capital conventions; Internet forums; hashtags; high-tech, industry-heavy culture disguised as minimalism, etc.) draw almost exclusively on what is already publicly available semantically to potential members. The iteration begins with a *slight shift in value and status-function assignment* in existing cultural ingredients, that are then made more salient and desirable through a set of obscure, difficult, and often physically taxing imagistic practices. In the case of juicing, certain "rare" ingredients (e.g., kale) are semantically reencoded with higher-purity status and desirability through the alleged existence of a hard-to-reach "essence" (in this particular case, a "liquid" essence). The resemanticization process, in other words, is made desirable through imagistic rituals involving food deprivation, high and financially hard-to-reach technological sophistication, and esoteric recipes. As Gibbs-Bravo's compelling autoethnographic account demonstrated, these processes typically activate high-arousal modalities, which rapidly acquire strong meaning and rewarding value as a function of the small-scale solidarity-building effects of imagistic ritual. The novice juicer, in this model, experiences high arousal as a simple function of break in routine and minimal sensory deprivation. The sense of reward that ensues feels deeply personal, but it can in fact only acquire meaning in a social context in which the meaning is already constructed. In the case of such a pseudoimagistically constituted cult, the sense of "privilege," prestige, and "select-fewness" affords long-lasting high arousal, with strong effects on episodic memories. One is likely never to forget, thus, how one became a juicer.

In order for the symbolic and performative scheme to endure, however (in order for juicing culture, or any cult, to be epidemiologically successful), members must also be enculturated through highly prescriptive, high-frequency, low-arousing practices. This is when doctrinality enters the scene. In juicing culture, the mix of modalities between imagisticity and doctrinality is judiciously engineered. Detailed prescriptions, as Gibbs-Bravo described, are woven into juicing practice from the very beginning. As the novelty and high arousal wears off, the new routine is successfully ingrained, and elation gradually recedes into a "new," imagistically enriched affective baseline. At this point, the recruitment process is successful.

Before concluding with general comments on the placebolike effects of cult formations and all forms of sociality, we should briefly review how doctrinality operates in any social setting in a little more detail. For this, we need to appreciate how the *compulsive*, repetitive, and literal aspects of collectively enacted ritual action are rooted in cognitive-affective biases that are universal to the human species.

In an influential essay in cognitive anthropology, Pascal Boyer and Pierre Liénard[22] expanded on a model first outlined by Roy Rappaport[23] on what they termed the "obvious" aspects of ritual. In doing so, they sought to take the anthropological analysis of ritual beyond the context of formal religiosity or other extreme (but equally formal) rites of passage and examined the psychological foundations of everyday modes of action. By their account, most of what humans do is ritualistic in nature. Most of what we do and feel, in this model, is socially scripted, on the one hand, and psychologically reinforced, on the other. They identified key dimensions in this process. Any ritual (or, with very few exceptions, any action) usually entails the following components:

1. *No obvious goals, meaning, or empirically demonstrable efficacy*: Individuals may rationalize their participation in a ritual in myriad ways, but it remains that most humans raised in similar contexts perform exactly the same rituals every day in almost exactly the same way (e.g., brushing teeth twice a day, three meals a day, bedtime protocols, turn-taking protocols, etc.). The action in this model is understood as encoded in the social script itself, though not in individual rational decisions.
2. *Compulsion*: Everyday rituals provide a sense of meaning and comfort, and they cause great discomfort when not performed or performed wrongly. One will typically feel a compulsive urge to perform a habitual ritual when circumstances prevent us from doing so (e.g., not being able to brush one's teeth when sleeping away from home).
3. *Literalism and rigidity*: Rituals have to be performed *the right way* (as per the terms of arbitrary convention X). Cross-cultural situations typically demonstrate this key dimension of ritual, when extreme modes of negative arousal and arguments arise around "the right way" or "the right time" for the performance of habitual domestic rituals (e.g., children's bedtime and meal frequency, meal content, cooking and cleaning protocols, etc.).
4. *Repetition, reiteration, redundancy*: Rituals have to be performed *the right way*, over and over again, and so on.
5. *Order and boundaries*: There are always highly specific themes, times, places, contexts, and protocols for the *right* performance of a ritual, which in turn triggers highly specific modes of affect and readiness-to-action for a network of social actors (e.g., once a certain mark of industrial time is reached in a given cultural context, a child's bedroom [assuming a culture with ritual spaces marked as BEDROOM and CHILD'S BEDROOM] will lose its PLAY function and

> acquire a GOING-TO-BED function; this will trigger a highly standardized set of action and modes of affect, with gender-specific story reading and affection-demonstration roles from parents and a series of enacted responses from the child—in such a case, we may note a series of latent, but equally prescribed, actions such as a child's fussiness and reluctance to sleep, her response to the room now marked as SCARY, and subsequent rituals of parental threat, negotiations, and exasperations).

Gibbs-Bravo's socialization into juicing culture, as her story eloquently demonstrated, equally entailed a set of goal-demoted, compulsive, repetitive, redundant, specifically themed and ordered actions. Had she continued to find meaning and reward in her juicer identity, she would soon have found herself in an everyday ordeal of seeking and avoiding the *right* and *wrong* foods, and the right way and sequence of acquiring, preparing, ingesting, and digesting them.

This specific ordeal, however, is only extreme and exotic because it *appears to differ* from what most of us ascribe meaning and value to. What we have argued in this chapter, however, is that being a happily compulsive juicer is not behaviorally different from what it is like to be a social being in any context. The basic sociocognitive recipe we have outlined in this chapter (one of hypnotic, ritualistic, doctrinal, compulsive, collectively scripted affect and action), we insist, is intrinsic to all forms of sociality regardless of semantic content.

We now conclude with general comments on the relationship between these processes and the placebo effect.

CONCLUSION: PLACEBO IS NOT A BAD NAME FOR CULTURE

The role of placebo in diet efficacy, and in physiological responses to foodstuffs in general, has recently come under investigation in social neuroscience. Biochemist Cory Harris, a leading scholar in the field, began to examine placebo effects more closely while studying plant-based traditional medicines in laboratory and naturalistic settings in collaboration with indigenous healers in Canada. The therapeutic efficacy of traditional healing, as he began to see it, extended far beyond the properties of bioactive molecules. Similar mechanisms were at stake, he rationalized, in the otherwise chemical, immunological, and metabolic processes recruited in many food allergies and intolerances. His recent work has documented how personal beliefs and expectations (at conscious and unconscious levels) operate as strong factors in the mediation of food allergies, intolerance, and healing.[24] But the "personal" at the level of beliefs, as the old anthropological story goes, is cultural through and through. Culturally bound food taboos, to be sure, have been documented as producing strong physiological responses. For Harris, these processes most often have "no basis in biology" and should be understood as "richly embedded within personal and cultural beliefs."[25]

How foods are inscribed, anticipated, and experienced as "comfort" foods, or as sacred, magical, curative, repulsive (and, in some cases, allergenic), is largely a matter of cultural variation. Foods, in other words, regardless of specific cultural value, should also be understood as symbols.

As cognitive anthropologists, we are concerned with the *culture-general process* (that is, a process intrinsic to the form of life we call "culture") of assigning largely implicit symbolic function to foodstuffs, and with the powerful physiological effects of this process.

If there is a biological dimension to the kinds of placebo responses to foods documented by Harris and colleagues, it should be understood as a biological effect *produced by culture*, or, in less dualistic terms, as a part of the inextricable puzzle of nature-nurture that makes human biology so culturally enriched.[26]

An exhaustive discussion of the placebo effect and its hypothesized neurocognitive mechanisms is beyond the scope of this chapter.[27] In this chapter, we are concerned with the *sociocognitive* and embodied dimensions of such responses, or, in other words, with the strange mind-over-matter power of words, symbols, and symbolically encoded contexts and protocols. "Appreciating the potential of expectations, suggestions, context, symbolic thinking, framing, cultural biases, and related psychosocial factors," indeed, is currently a key question in the social neuroscience of placebo.[28]

Our approach to the ritual semanticization and embodiment of symbolic convention, we hope, will help shed light on these sociocognitive, socioaffective, biocultural processes.

To simplify the problem, we return to our comments on the hypnotic nature of socialization processes and propose to think of this dynamic as placebolike. A successful "hypnotic" social enactment, recall, is not unlike the experience of surrendering to the symbolically constituted epistemic authority of an experimenter in a placebo study. We have argued, moreover, that such embodied postexpectation mechanisms need not entail actual agents and are most often grounded in implicit expectations about others' expectations and validated in the implicit reassurance that those to whom we outsource our beliefs have the authority to justify the validity of those beliefs.

Recent literature on the placebo effect, in turn, has similarly emphasized responses that do not entail surrendering to the epistemic authority of *actual* agents and are instead enacted from broader imagined expectations in and *about* collectively held beliefs.[29] Psychologist Irving Kirsch, for example, famously debunked the chemical efficacy of SSRI antidepressant medications (and by extension, the serotonin hypothesis for depression at large) by pointing out that while enough evidence was available to show that SSRI medications did not outperform placebos in clinical trials, the medications appeared to have become more "effective" over time due to the increased power of (1) collective belief in the existence of depression as a brain disease and (2) belief in the fact that many people who suffer from depression and take SSRIs have gotten better.[30]

In an influential review of seventy-five published trials of various antidepressants (tricyclics and SSRIs) compared with placebo, a group of psychiatrists from Columbia University recorded that the effectiveness of drug treatment for depression had trended up from about 40 percent to about 55 percent between 1981 and 2000; the proportion of patients responding to placebos, in the meantime, had increased from about 20 percent to about 35 percent. At the time, the researchers concluded that "[s]ome factor or factors associated with the level of placebo response must therefore have changed significantly during this period. Unfortunately, we were not able to identify these factors."[31] For the medical anthropologist Daniel Moerman, there is no mystery surround this "missing" factor. The collective response, in his view, is clearly grounded in collective belief, and a notable "shift in consciousness among doctors, patients, friends, and, generally, everyone, to the effect that depression can be treated with drugs."[32] This shift toward biomedicalized understandings of mental illness, and a related shift toward the existence of mental illness as a natural kind, in turn, has been well documented. A longitudinal study conducted in Australia on changes in awareness and attitudes toward depression from 1995 to 2004, for example, reported a steady increase in the percentage of people who said that they or their family or friends had depression-related problems. The study, which analyzed data from national surveys of mental health literacy, found a greater increase in the brain-disease model of "mental health literacy" in states that had received high exposure to the Australian beyondblue mental health literacy campaign.[33]

This analysis of cultural shifts in ways of understanding and embodying idioms of distress, as we hope becomes evident, will assist us in our theorizing of the relationship between sociality and placebo responses in general, and ritualistically enacted food beliefs specifically. Dramatic shifts in "ways of being mad" over time, as it turns out, have also been well documented. The medical philosopher Ian Hacking has dedicated a long career to the analysis of what he terms the "looping effect" between categories of belief and language, and humans who are recruited into those categories, an ontological position he has termed *dynamic nominalism*. Hacking has minutiously documented ways of being mad that have appeared and disappeared over time, such as neurasthenia, hysterical paralysis, fugue states, and multiple personality disorders, to name but a few. Of late, he has turned his attention to such new kinds of people as those said to suffer from autism, attention deficit disorders, obesity, and child abuse.[34] Hacking's analysis goes beyond an otherwise important appreciation of the role of the myriad technologies; industries; educational, medical and paramedical professions; and structures and practices designed to "treat" (or, more to the point, "produce") these ways of being abnormal. On his "dynamic" view, these categories constructed in language, and the ways of talking about, believing in, and expecting meaning and results from these categories as though they were natural kinds, have a tendency to become reified in embodied practice. Rocks, quarks, and nebulae, in Hacking's model, are clearly natural kinds; they are *indifferent* or immune to the language that describes them. Humans, however, are not simply natural or "indifferent kinds"; they are an *interactive kind.* Ours, recall, is a culturally enriched biology; we are a kind of kind, in other words, that is strangely responsive to categories and labels of our own imaginings that may otherwise only exist in language and belief. This is an old insight on the performative power of language. In J. L. Austin's and John Searle's famous formulation of speech-act theory, language not only describes states of affairs (e.g., the cat is in the sink) but also *produces states of affairs* (e.g., "I pronounce you man and wife" or "I guess we are dating now").[35] In Judith Butler's famous retelling of that formula, a doctor's seemingly neutral utterance of the phrase "it's a girl" upon facilitating a birth is not simply descriptive: it also brings forth a historically and culturally specific *performance* of particular ways of being gendered.[36] Hacking's basic recipe for interactive kinds, in systems' theoretic terms, can be understood as feedback loops between name and thing-named, or as map-territory feedback loops.

Hacking, however, has notoriously refrained from speaking of innate human universals, or from discussing the cognitive mechanisms that may facilitate the *learning* of such behavioral responses to public language. The compelling stories of "made up people" and "new ways of being persons" he has documented, then, still beg for an explanation.

For Pascal Boyer,[37] the looping mechanisms between name and thing-named described by Hacking are best understood as "feed-forward mechanisms" of epidemiological cultural transmission. In Boyer's view from cognitive anthropology, we need to explain how certain representations that become widespread in a particular group acquire predictable effects in their subsequent transmission.[38] A simple mechanistic explanation, for Boyer, is to be found in our relevance-seeking, admittedly "lazy" cognitive architecture and in what has been termed "frequency bias"[39] (that is, in our tendency to favor, adopt, and transmit representations *that are already widespread*). Names, linguistic kinds, and behaviors that "fit a pre-existing schema," in this view, can be said to enjoy clear epidemiological advantage in terms of comprehension, acceptability, and memorability. Anything that departs too much from what is already epidemiologically successful in any given context, thus, will require greater cognitive effort to consider; it will tend to be interpreted as "deviant" and be dismissed as "noise."[40] The looping effect of widely shared (but ultimately arbitrary) concepts and norms, Boyer reminds us, has been documented in such domains as "race" concepts,[41] religious and supernatural beliefs,[42] and many others.[43]

How some (by most accounts, infinitely few) novel representations, but not others, become adopted, embodied, widespread, and passed on may be a matter of chance, existing power structures, or both. We have pointed to the role of language, resemanticization, and imagistic-doctrinal ritual modalities in the facilitation of new iterations from existing shared cultural repertoires. We have seen how such iterations build a sense of solidarity and group identity in new members united by highly arousing extreme practices and are then solidified doctrinally by feeding on the human need for compulsion, reiteration, and redundancy.

We discussed cult formations, extreme food beliefs, and emerging juicing culture as a case in point for the study of these mechanisms. In doing so, we proposed that theorizing the efficacy of food cults, and by extension the efficacy of any symbolic scheme governing collective belief and readiness-to-action, should entail a fine-grained account of implicit mechanisms of expectation and joint attention best described as "hypnotic." We concluded, finally, that all successful regimes of sociality that eventually govern intuitively enacted modes of affect with physiological precision can be described as placebo-like. If we have been successful in our argument, then the reader might conclude that *placebo* is not a bad word for *culture*.

NOTES

1. Michael Tomasello, *Why We Cooperate* (Cambridge, MA: MIT Press, 2009); Samuel Veissière, "Varieties of Tulpa Experiences: The Hypnotic Nature of Human Sociality, Personhood, and Interphenomenality," in *Hypnosis and Meditation: Towards an Integrative Science of Conscious Planes*, edited by Amir Raz and Michael Lifshitz (Oxford: Oxford University Press, 2016).

2. Kim Sterelny, *The Evolved Apprentice: How Evolution Made Humans Unique* (Cambridge, MA: MIT Press, 2012); Michael Tomasello, *Origins of Human Communication* (Cambridge, MA: MIT Press, 2008).

3. John R. Searle, *The Construction of Social Reality* (New York: Free Press, 2001).

4. Scott Atran, *In Gods We Trust: The Evolutionary Landscape of Religion* (Oxford: Oxford University Press, 2002); Scott Atran, *Talking to the Enemy: Faith, Brotherhood, and the (Un)Making of Terrorists* (New York: Ecco Press, 2010).

5. Harvey Whitehouse, *Arguments and Icons: Divergent Modes of Religiosity* (Oxford: Oxford University Press, 2000); Harvey Whitehouse, *Modes of Religiosity: A Cognitive Theory of Religious Transmission* (Walnut Creek, CA: AltaMira Press, 2004); Harvey Whitehouse and Robert N. McCauley, *Mind and Religion: Psychological and Cognitive Foundations of Religiosity* (Walnut Creek, CA: AltaMira Press, 2005).

6. Amir Raz and Cory S. Harris, eds., *Placebo Talks: Modern Perspectives on Placebos in Society* (Oxford: Oxford University Press, 2016).

7. Atran, *In Gods We Trust*; Pascal Boyer, *Religion Explained: The Evolutionary Origins of Religious Thought* (New York: Basic Books, 2001); Pascal Boyer and Pierre Liénard, "Ritual Behavior in Obsessive and Normal Individuals: Moderating Anxiety and Reorganizing the Flow of Action," *Current Directions in Psychological Science* 17, no. 4 (2008): 291–94; Veissière, "Varieties of Tulpa Experiences"; Whitehouse, *Arguments and Icons*; Whitehouse, *Modes of Religiosity*; Whitehouse and McCauley, *Mind and Religion*.

8. John L. Austin, James O. Urmson, and Marina Sbisà, *How to Do Things with Words* (Cambridge, MA: Harvard University Press, 1975); Don Kulick and Bambi B. Schieffelin, "Language Socialization," *Blackwell Publishing Ltd.* (2007): 347–68.

9. Raz and Harris, *Placebo Talks*; Daniel Moerman, "Looking at Placebos through a Cultural Lens and Finding Meaning," in Raz and Harris, *Placebo Talks*; Laurence J. Kirmayer and Maxwell J. D. Ramstead, "Embodiment and Enactment in Cultural Psychiatry," in *Embodiment, Enaction, and Culture: Investigating the Constitution of the Shared World*, edited by Christoph Durt, Thomas Fuchs, and Christian Tewes (Cambridge, MA: MIT Press, 2016); Marie Prevost and Amir Raz, "Trust and the Placebo Effect," in Raz and Harris, *Placebo Talks*; Stewart Justman, "Pills in a Pretty Box: Social Sources of the Placebo Effect," in Raz and Harris, *Placebo Talks*.

10. "We" in this chapter refers to the authors, Veissière and Gibbs-Bravo. "I" in the following section refers to Gibbs-Bravo.

11. Maxwell J. D. Ramstead, Samuel Veissière, and Laurence J. Kirmayer, "Cultural Affordances: Scaffolding Local Worlds through Shared Intentionality and Regimes of Attention," *Frontiers in Psychology* 7 (2016).

12. Dan Sperber, *Explaining Culture: A Naturalistic Approach* (Oxford: Blackwell, 1996).

13. Veissière, "Varieties of Tulpa Experiences."

14. Etzel Cardeña and Michael Winkelman, *Altering Consciousness: Multidisciplinary Perspectives* (Santa Barbara, CA: Praeger, 2011); Rebecca Seligman and Laurence J. Kirmayer, "Dissociative Experience and Cultural Neuroscience: Narrative, Metaphor and Mechanism," *Culture, Medicine and Psychiatry: An International Journal of Cross-Cultural Health Research* 32, no. 1 (2008): 31–64; Veissière, "Varieties of Tulpa Experiences."

15. Kirmayer and Ramstead, "Embodiment and Enactment in Cultural Psychiatry"; Ramstead, Veissière, and Kirmayer, "Cultural Affordances."

16. Kirmayer and Ramstead, "Embodiment and Enactment in Cultural Psychiatry"; Ramstead, Veissière, and Kirmayer, "Cultural Affordances."

17. Swami Ajaya, *Psychotherapy, East and West: A Unifying Paradigm* (Honesdale, PA: Himalayan International Institute of Yoga, Science, and Philosophy of the U.S.A., 1983), 168.

18. Ramstead, Veissière, and Kirmayer, "Cultural Affordances."

19. Whitehouse, *Modes of Religiosity*.

20. Whitehouse, *Arguments and Icons*; Whitehouse, *Modes of Religiosity*; Whitehouse and McCauley, *Mind and Religion*.

21. Pascal Boyer and James V. Wertsch, *Memory in Mind and Culture* (New York: Cambridge University Press, 2009).

22. Boyer and Liénard, "Ritual Behavior in Obsessive and Normal Individuals."

23. Roy A. Rappaport, *Ecology, Meaning, and Religion* (Richmond, CA: North Atlantic Books, 1979).

24. Cory Harris and Timothy Jones, "Placebolicious: The Many Flavours of Placebo in Diet and Food Culture," in Raz and Harris, *Placebo Talks*.

25. Harris and Jones, "Placebolicious," 174.

26. Augustín Fuentes, *Race, Monogamy, and Other Lies They Told You: Busting Myths about Human Nature* (Berkeley: University of California Press, 2012).

27. For a more comprehensive review, see Raz and Harris, *Placebo Talks*.

28. Natasha Campbell and Amir Raz, "Placebo Science in Medical Education," in Raz and Harris, *Placebo Talks*, 93.

29. Justman, "Pills in a Pretty Box"; Laurence J. Kirmayer, "Unpacking the Placebo Response: Lessons from Ethnographic Studies of Healing," in Raz and Harris, *Placebo Talks*; Moerman, "Looking at Placebos through a Cultural Lens and Finding Meaning"; Raz and Harris, *Placebo Talks*.

30. Irving Kirsch, *The Emperor's New Drugs: Exploding the Antidepressant Myth* (New York: Basic Books, 2010); Irving Kirsch, "Antidepressants and the Placebo Effect," in Raz and Harris, *Placebo Talks*.

31. Timothy Walsh et al., "Placebo Response in Studies of Major Depression: Variable, Substantial, and Growing," *JAMA* 287, no. 14 (2002): 1844; cited in Moerman, "Looking at Placebos through a Cultural Lens and Finding Meaning," 110.

32. Moerman, "Looking at Placebos through a Cultural Lens and Finding Meaning," 110.

33. Anthony F. Jorm, Helen Christensen, and Kathleen M. Griffiths, "Changes in Depression Awareness and Attitudes in Australia: The Impact of Beyondblue: The National Depres-

sion Initiative," *Australian and New Zealand Journal of Psychiatry* 40, no. 1 (January 1, 2006): 42–46.

34. Ian Hacking, *Rewriting the Soul: Multiple Personality and the Sciences of Memory* (Princeton, NJ: Princeton University Press, 1995); Ian Hacking, "Kinds of People: Moving Targets," *Proceedings of the British Academy* 151 (January 1, 2007): 285–318.

35. J. L. Austin, *How to Do Things with Words* (Cambridge, MA: Harvard University Press, 1962); John R. Searle, *The Construction of Social Reality* (New York: Free Press, 2007).

36. Don Kulick and Bambi B. Schieffelin, "Language Socialization," in *A Companion to Linguistic Anthropology*, edited by Alessandro Duranti (Malden, MA: Blackwell, 2007), 349–68; Judith Butler, *Gender Trouble: Feminism and the Subversion of Identity* (New York: Routledge, 1999).

37. Pascal Boyer, "Intuitive Expectations and the Detection of Mental Disorder: A Cognitive Background to Folk-Psychiatries," *Philosophical Psychology* 24, no. 1 (2011): 95–118.

38. Boyer, "Intuitive Expectations and the Detection of Mental Disorder."

39. Robert Boyd and Peter J. Richerson, *Culture and the Evolutionary Process* (Chicago: University of Chicago Press, 1985).

40. Boyer, "Intuitive Expectations and the Detection of Mental Disorder."

41. Lawrence A. Hirschfeld and Susan A. Gelman, *Mapping the Mind: Domain Specificity in Cognition and Culture* (Cambridge: Cambridge University Press, 1994).

42. Boyer, *Religion Explained.*

43. Hirschfeld and Gelman, *Mapping the Mind.*

BIBLIOGRAPHY

Ajaya, Swami. *Psychotherapy, East and West: A Unifying Paradigm*. Honesdale, PA: Himalayan International Institute of Yoga, Science, and Philosophy of the U.S.A., 1983.

Atran, Scott. *In Gods We Trust: The Evolutionary Landscape of Religion*. Oxford: Oxford University Press, 2002.

Atran, Scott. *Talking to the Enemy: Faith, Brotherhood, and the (Un)Making of Terrorists*. New York: Ecco Press, 2010.

Austin, John L., James O. Urmson, and Marina Sbisà. *How to Do Things with Words*. Cambridge, MA: Harvard University Press, 1975.

Boyd, Robert, and Peter J. Richerson. *Culture and the Evolutionary Process*. Chicago: University of Chicago Press, 1985.

Boyer, Pascal. "Intuitive Expectations and the Detection of Mental Disorder: A Cognitive Background to Folk-Psychiatries." *Philosophical Psychology* 24, no. 1 (2011): 95–118.

Boyer, Pascal. *Religion Explained: The Evolutionary Origins of Religious Thought*. New York: Basic Books, 2001.

Boyer, Pascal, and Pierre Liénard. "Ritual Behavior in Obsessive and Normal Individuals: Moderating Anxiety and Reorganizing the Flow of Action." *Current Directions in Psychological Science* 17, no. 4 (2008): 291–94.

Boyer, Pascal, and James V. Wertsch. *Memory in Mind and Culture*. New York: Cambridge University Press, 2009.

Butler, Judith. *Gender Trouble: Feminism and the Subversion of Identity*. New York: Routledge, 1999.

Campbell, Natasha, and Amir Raz. "Placebo Science in Medical Education." In *Placebo Talks: Modern Perspectives on Placebos in Society*, edited by Amir Raz and Cory S. Harris. Oxford: Oxford University Press, 2016.

Cardeña, Etzel, and Michael Winkelman. *Altering Consciousness: Multidisciplinary Perspectives*. Santa Barbara, CA: Praeger, 2011.

Fuentes, Augustín. *Race, Monogamy, and Other Lies They Told You: Busting Myths about Human Nature*. Berkeley: University of California Press, 2012.

Hacking, Ian. *Historical Ontology*. Cambridge, MA: Harvard University Press, 2002.

Hacking, Ian. "Humans, Aliens & Autism." *Daedalus* 138, no. 3 (October 12, 2009): 44–59.

Hacking, Ian. "Kinds of People: Moving Targets." *Proceedings of the British Academy* 151 (January 1, 2007): 285–318.

Hacking, Ian. *Rewriting the Soul: Multiple Personality and the Sciences of Memory*. Princeton, NJ: Princeton University Press, 1995.

Harris, Cory, and Timothy Jones. "Placebolicious: The Many Flavours of Placebo in Diet and Food Culture." In *Placebo Talks: Modern Perspectives on Placebos in Society*, edited by Amir Raz and Cory S. Harris. Oxford: Oxford University Press, 2016.

Hirschfeld, A. Lawrence, and Susan A. Gelman. *Mapping the Mind: Domain Specificity in Cognition and Culture*. Cambridge: Cambridge University Press, 1994.

Jorm, Anthony F., Helen Christensen, and Kathleen M. Griffiths. "Changes in Depression Awareness and Attitudes in Australia: The Impact of Beyondblue: The National Depression Initiative." *Australian and New Zealand Journal of Psychiatry* 40, no. 1 (January 1, 2006): 42–46.

Justman, Stewart. "Pills in a Pretty Box: Social Sources of the Placebo Effect." In *Placebo Talks: Modern Perspectives on Placebos in Society*, edited by Amir Raz and Cory S. Harris. Oxford: Oxford University Press, 2016.

Kirsch, Irving. *The Emperor's New Drugs: Exploding the Antidepressant Myth*. New York: Basic Books, 2010.

Kirsch, Irving. "Antidepressants and the Placebo Effect." In *Placebo Talks: Modern Perspectives on Placebos in Society*, edited by Amir Raz and Cory S. Harris. Oxford: Oxford University Press, 2016.

Kirmayer, J. Laurence. "Unpacking the Placebo Response: Lessons from Ethnographic Studies of Healing." In *Placebo Talks: Modern Perspectives on Placebos in Society*, edited by Amir Raz and Cory S. Harris. Oxford: Oxford University Press, 2016.

Kirmayer, J. Laurence, and Maxwell J. D. Ramstead. "Embodiment and Enactment in Cultural Psychiatry." In *Embodiment, Enaction, and Culture: Investigating the Constitution of the Shared World*, edited by Christoph Durt, Thomas Fuchs, and Christian Tewes. Cambridge, MA: MIT Press, 2016.

Kulick, Don, and Bambi B. Schieffelin. "Language Socialization." In *A Companion to Linguistic Anthropology*, edited by Alessandro Duranti, 349–68. Malden, MA: Blackwell, 2007.

Liénard, Pierre, and Pascal Boyer. "Whence Collective Rituals? A Cultural Selection Model of Ritualized Behavior." *American Anthropologist* 108, no. 4 (January 1, 2006): 814–27.

Moerman, Daniel. "Looking at Placebos through a Cultural Lens and Finding Meaning." In *Placebo Talks: Modern Perspectives on Placebos in Society*, edited by Amir Raz and Cory S. Harris. Oxford: Oxford University Press, 2016.

Prevost, Marie, and Amir Raz. "Trust and the Placebo Effect." In *Placebo Talks: Modern Perspectives on Placebos in Society*, edited by Amir Raz and Cory S. Harris. Oxford: Oxford University Press, 2016.

Ramstead, Maxwell J. D., Samuel Veissière, and Laurence J. Kirmayer. "Cultural Affordances: Scaffolding Local Worlds through Shared Intentionality and Regimes of Attention," *Frontiers in Psychology* 7 (2016).

Rappaport, Roy A. *Ecology, Meaning, and Religion*. Richmond, CA: North Atlantic Books, 1979.

Raz, Amir, and Cory S. Harris, eds. *Placebo Talks: Modern Perspectives on Placebos in Society*. Oxford: Oxford University Press, 2016.

Raz, Amir, and Michael Lifshitz, eds. *Hypnosis and Meditation: Towards an Integrative Science of Conscious Planes*. Oxford: Oxford University Press, 2016.

Searle, John R. *The Construction of Social Reality*. New York: Free Press, 2001.

Seligman, Rebecca, and Laurence J. Kirmayer. "Dissociative Experience and Cultural Neuroscience: Narrative, Metaphor and Mechanism." *Culture, Medicine and Psychiatry: An International Journal of Cross-Cultural Health Research* 32, no. 1 (March 1, 2008): 31–64.

Sperber, Dan. *Explaining Culture: A Naturalistic Approach*. Oxford: Blackwell, 1996.

Sterelny, Kim. *The Evolved Apprentice: How Evolution Made Humans Unique*. Cambridge, MA: MIT Press, 2012.

Tomasello, Michael. *Origins of Human Communication*. Cambridge, MA: MIT Press, 2008.

Tomasello, Michael. *Why We Cooperate*. Cambridge, MA: MIT Press, 2009.

Veissière, Samuel. "Varieties of Tulpa Experiences: The Hypnotic Nature of Human Sociality, Personhood, and Interphenomenality." In *Hypnosis and Meditation: Towards an Integrative Science of Conscious Planes*, edited by Amir Raz and Michael Lifshitz. Oxford: Oxford University Press, 2016.

Walsh, Timothy B., Stuart N. Seidman, Robyn Sysko, and Madelyn Gould. "Placebo Response in Studies of Major Depression: Variable, Substantial, and Growing." *JAMA* 287, no. 14 (2002): 1840–47.

Whitehouse, Harvey. *Arguments and Icons: Divergent Modes of Religiosity*. Oxford: Oxford University Press, 2000.

Whitehouse, Harvey. *Modes of Religiosity: A Cognitive Theory of Religious Transmission*. Walnut Creek, CA: AltaMira Press, 2004.

Whitehouse, Harvey, and Robert N. McCauley. *Mind and Religion: Psychological and Cognitive Foundations of Religiosity*. Walnut Creek, CA: AltaMira Press, 2005.

Chapter Six

Contemporary Superfood Cults

Nutritionism, Neoliberalism, and Gender

Tina Sikka

In this chapter, I argue that the contemporary superfood movement, which is currently embraced by a strata of the financially well off in North America and Western Europe, is not socially, politically, or economically progressive. I also argue this movement fails in its stated objective to change the quality of our food, transform the consolidated food production system, and improve the state of public health. Rather, I contend that superfood companies like Navitas Naturals, Naturya, and Raw Revolution, through a variety of discursive strategies, work to visually and linguistically construct their products as progressive in order to mask an underlying reliance on neoliberal business practices, nutritionism, and gendered stereotypes.[1] It also relies on the harnessing of discursive strategies in order to build a kind of tribe or cultlike social identity around the sustained consumption of superfoods. In supporting this position, I begin this chapter with a description of what superfoods are, how they differ from functional foods, and provide a brief background into the companies taken up in this piece. I then discuss critical discourse analysis (CDA), which I then use to unpack the ways in which neoliberalism, nutritionism, and gender bias function in superfood discourse, with specific attention paid to how these food products are advertised.

There is a large degree of descriptive confusion among consumers and scholars with respect to the difference between so-called functional foods and superfoods. For the purposes of this chapter, superfoods are treated as a subset of the larger category of functional foods. According to current statistics, the functional food industry is expected to reach approximately $130 billion per year and, according to IndustryARC, will likely exceed $305.4 billion by 2020.[2] As a foodstuff category, functional foods can be defined as foods that are fortified with "special constituents that possess advantageous physiological effects."[3] Health claims related to these products range from disease treatment and illness prevention to weight loss and anti-aging.[4] There are efforts in a number of countries to establish and/or strengthen laws regulating the health claims on packaged functional foods, with the EU leading the charge.[5]

As a business category, functional foods refer to sports drinks, energy drinks, nutritional shakes, healthy snacks, and breakfast products that have been popularized by the likes of PepsiCo's Gatorade, Coca-Cola's Powerade, and Abbot Nutrition's EAS. In relation to food products, functional foods include items from such companies as Nestle S.A., Kraft Foods, Kellogg Company, and General Mills. These items, often based on cereal and grain, are typically fortified with vitamins and minerals as well as, more recently, probiotics and prebiotics.

Superfoods, on the other hand, do not have a precise legal or scientific definition but can be loosely defined as foods that are thought to be particularly nutritious and energy dense. According to Lunn,

> By far the most well known definition of a superfood relates to the fruit and vegetable section of most supermarkets. Here, superfood describes a food that is especially rich in phytochemicals. The idea is that by highlighting a number of foods that are very good sources of antioxidant micronutrients or other classes of plant bioactives, their levels in the diet can be boosted.[6]

Foods that fall into this category include chia seeds, acai berries, blueberries, pomegranates, beetroot, soy, green tea, goji berries, coconut oil, salmon, dark chocolate, cacao, and kale.

Overwhelmingly, highly concentrated corporate actors dominate the ownership structure of functional foods while smaller private companies control the manufacture of the superfoods. My criteria for choosing which superfood brands to focus on came down to the core factor of media presence—where media refers to predominantly American and British health and beauty magazines, in both print and digital versions, as well as noted beauty blogs. Comprehensive business information on each of the chosen companies was difficult to gather since they are largely privately held and therefore unlisted. As such, precise details on revenues and number of employees were difficult to verify. The following is a brief snapshot of each company based on what could be collected from public sources and their websites.

Naturya is a UK company founded in 2009 with revenues under $500,000 and approximately ten employees. It produces ten superfood products grown just outside Bath in Wales. These include acai powder, chia seeds, wheatgrass powder, and chlorella powder, to name a few.[7] Navitas Naturals, the second company discussed in this chapter, is a California-based group created in 2003 that sells a large variety of superfoods to customers in the United States and Canada, including organic acai powders, raw cacao, raw cashew nuts, camu powders, raw chia seeds and powders, chocolate kits, coconut oil, sprouted flax seed powders, raw goji berries, and raw goldenberries. Estimated annual revenue for Navitas Naturals ranges from $25 to $50 million, while the cited number of its employees varies from 100 to 250 depending on the source.[8] Finally, Raw Revolution is a U.S. company that incorporates superfoods such as spirulina, nuts, raspberries, and dark chocolate into nutritional bar form. Its products are produced at a factory just outside of New York City. Financial information for this company is unavailable.[9]

Over the past few years there has been a sharp rise in coverage of superfoods in beauty, health, and nutrition magazines as well as blogs. What is unique about these particular products is the way in which companies have chosen to market them. In opposition to traditional branded food products, corporations such as Navitas Naturals and Naturya do not take out conventional print ads in magazines or pay for advertisements on television. Rather, these products are integrated into the very stories and recipes that form the content of magazines such as *Shape*, *Health*, and *Women's Fitness*. Marketing one's product in this way entails pitching products and associated stories to magazines and food/health writers. Similarly, reviews posted on popular health and beauty blogs often involve the companies themselves sending products to the owners of the blogs with the hope that their product will appear within the context of a post—most often as a review.

In order to investigate the principles, assumptions, and norms that constitute the visual and discursive representation of these products, I subject each of these company's websites and product advertorials to multiple readings through CDA.[10] What makes CDA uniquely suited to the analysis of how superfoods are discursively framed and marketed is that it not only describes the constructed values, conventions, and understandings that are reinforced by self-descriptions and advertorials but also connects said visual and textual representations to larger "social processes and structures which give rise to the production of a text, and of the social structures and processes within which individuals or groups as social historical subjects create meanings in their interaction with texts."[11] As such, CDA works to reveal taken-for-granted political, economic, and sociocultural assumptions while also considering the power relationships that constitute and divide interested parties. Because of the focus on food and health, I draw on Ferree and Merrill's inverted pyramid model of critical discourse analysis specifically. At the top of this structure is discourse, understood as a collection of conflicting and inconsistent but interconnected ideas, followed by ideologies, "conceptualized as coherent systems of related ideas that combine explanation with normative prescriptions,"[12] and frames. Frames are a kind of snapshot of the principal ideas, norms, and structures that "shape interpretation and understanding of specific issues."[13] They are actively constituted through the process of framing—a social and strategic practice by which groups actively struggle to produce dominant frames.

In drawing on this method, and by specifically focusing textual, discursive, *and* contextual significations of superfoods established by Navitas Naturals, Raw Revolution, and Naturya,[14] I have come to the conclusion that the discursive frames of neoliberalism, gender, and nutritionism constitute the most significant ideational structures that comprise superfood discourse. I discuss each of these in kind.

NEOLIBERALISM

Neoliberalism, at its core, can be defined as a coherent ideology that aims to promote consumerism and consumption in place of participatory democratic engagement.[15] The ascendancy of neoliberal discourse in politics and social life have, according to Henri Giroux, replaced civic discourse with "the language of commercialism, privatization, and deregulation" wherein "individual and social agency are defined largely through market-driven notions of individualism, competition, and consumption."[16]

The neoliberal dispotif works through superfood companies in a highly contradictory way. On the one hand, these corporations aptly present themselves as working against the traditional neoliberal, mass-produced, globalized, energy-intensive, environmentally and personally harmful production and consumption practices that characterize contemporary food and nutrition industries. However, at the same time, their positioning within this paradigm works to perpetuate traditional capitalist economic structures.

That is, the media messages shaped by companies like Naturya, Raw Revolution, and Navitas Naturals, and the discursive corporate framing of the companies themselves, reproduces the neoliberal subject through a variety of tropes and strategies embedded in how their brand is presented and products advertised. Specifically, neoliberalism is repackaged by these companies and sold as a progressive social movement that embraces social enlightenment, localism, and good works. For example, their websites make high hat of their founders' origin stories as they relate to the early development of their respective companies. (I return to this idea below.) Overall, what is troubling about these firms is that despite constructing themselves as progressive, they in fact fundamentally and uncritically work to replicate neoliberal ideas like consumer choice, value chains, and individual striving. They also promote the idea that resolving the problems inherent in the food system lies within the domain of individual responsibility while simultaneously "underemphasiz[ing] structural fixes" to ill health, nutritional deserts, and the lack of affordable access to healthy food.[17]

As stated, the most palpable example of this kind of framing begins with the narratives that describe how these companies were founded and the ideals that constitute their present and future development. The brand that most exemplifies this neoliberal version of individual striving is that of Raw Revolution. Raw Revolution, according to its website, was created in the kitchen of founder Alice Benedetto. The "Our Story" narrative goes on to describe how

> Alice started slowly, feeding her delicious, natural snacks to friends and family, and then started selling small batches through local stores near her suburban home. When the first bars sold out within days, Alice knew that she was on to something.

Further on, the website details how Alice and her husband purchased used cooking equipment and are now producing millions of bars that are sold globally but all made at their family-owned factory outside New York City. The narrative closes by observing that "a lot has changed in the last decade, but some things are the same as they have always been. The ingredients are fresh. The taste is revolutionary. And the story is just beginning."[18]

This narrative fulfills one of the primary tenets of neoliberalism, which reduces individuals to rational economic actors whose "capacity for 'self-care'—their ability to provide for their own needs and service their own ambitions, whether as welfare recipients, medical patients, consumers of pharmaceuticals, university students, or workers in ephemeral occupations" becomes the primary measure of their moral autonomy as well.[19]

In addition to the "pull oneself up by one's bootstraps" entrepreneurial ethos illustrated by the Raw Revolution narrative, a problematic neocolonial form of capitalist neoliberalism also persists in the marketing of many superfoods. Navitas Naturals, for example, which also prides itself on being family owned, roots its history in its founder Zach Adelman's experience of encountering and then beginning to import maca, a root vegetable used by the indigenous peoples of Peru, into the United States while on a trip to Peru in 2003. As the website proudly asserts, "Our organic superfoods come from ancient cultures around the world where they are traditionally used for both nutritional and medicinal purposes."[20] This form of cultural appropriation has the effect of commodifying, and profiting off of, indigenous knowledge in a manner that preserves Eurocentric views of the world. It also imposes Western legal concepts like ownership onto traditional knowledge in ways that are "inherently predatory and harmful to the interests, worldviews, and self-determination of the Third World."[21] In fact, there are a number of patent applications that have been filed aimed at gaining intellectual property rights over the herbal-derived extracts of superfoods like goji berries. Finally, this appropriation can also be read as a type of corporatized multiculturalism that allows for a form of experiencing the other safely, as a commodified product, "without ever coming into contact with actual, potentially fear-invoking racialized bodies."[22]

Navitas Naturals describes itself as committed to socially responsible business practices including fair trade, food safety, and direct purchasing. Currently the company imports acai from Brazil, mulberries from Turkey, goldenberries from Colombia, and chia seeds from Mexico and Chile. The company reassures the reader on its website that traditional farming practices and local customs have been preserved through the use of photographic images of pristine Andean Mountains, productive yet rural farm land, and working indigenous farmers.[23]

The problem with this description and these images is that it depoliticizes the farmers from these countries, who are discursively and visually constructed as docile workers, and further on, requiring help from benevolent external actors. Zach goes on in the interview to state that, in Peru,

> our partner Carlos was in need of financial support to complete the new state-of-the-art facility his company is building in Concepcion, so we stepped in to help them finish the job by the end of the year. The expansion project will help

> us keep up with growing demand and allow us to maintain even better quality control, and it will create room for future growth. Our growing sales, new financial investment and noticeable economic impact that Carlos's business has had in the local community are an even bigger deal than I had first realized.[24]

There is often also the effect, as in the case of quinoa, that demand for superfoods in the West pushes up prices so that items that are considered staples in places like Peru and Bolivia become unaffordable for local populations.[25]

Finally, the success with which superfood companies have co-opted the "alternative food networks" (AFN) movement—which is a food production paradigm that advocates for more traditional modes of farming based on trust, transparent provenance, and includes "farmers' markets, allotments, urban permaculture, community supported agriculture and organic box schemes"—is disquieting.[26] The primary result of this neoliberal co-optation is that these movements have, in opposition to their rhetoric, become part of the dominant food system. As such, the majority of these food products, like many organic foods, will, in the future, likely also be "sourced through global commodity chains dominated by the same agrifood TNCs as the conventional system."[27] There is already an established trend of large companies like Monsanto and Proctor and Gamble (P&G) beginning to buy up health and superfood companies. P&G, for instance, recently acquired New Chapter, a superfood supplement company that has also branched out to personal and homecare products.

GENDER

With respect to gender, superfood advertorials are overwhelmingly targeted to women. Gender, in this context, is understood as a social construct where hegemonic understandings of masculinity and femininity are shaped by a given society's dominant norms and values. Much of the discourse surrounding superfoods serves to reinforce expectations around perceived masculine and feminine interests, behaviors, and concerns with respect to health and food. CDA is particularly useful in this context, as it not only recognizes how gender norms work to organize experience and knowledge but also reveals the interests and "investedness" that constitute these standards.[28]

A large majority of branded superfood tie-ins and general media coverage can be found in women's magazines and blogs/websites with a large female viewership. A focus on Western beauty norms, weight loss, and celebrity association is particularly evident in relation to how superfoods are framed. Raw Revolution's press coverage in particular is highly gendered and featured exclusively in women's magazines, blogs, and websites. The specific blogs that feature their products include *The Hip Hostess*, *Peace, Love and Nutrition*, *The Healthy Helper*, and *Blondies, Bakes and Bites*, which all present themselves as blogs oriented to female self-improvement and empowerment through nutrition, diets, cooking, crafting, exercise, and fashion in a manner that has a "strong tendency to privilege norms of physical attractiveness and the presentation of one's body for appreciation."[29] These blogs also contain strong elements of nurturing maternalism in that they thematize women's roles as primary caregivers, nurturers, cookers, and bakers.

As a result, superfood marketing has come to frame its products as not only a means through which to attain the ideal body type (even if it is promoted using the language of health, fitness, and well-being) but also a source of the nutrition and energy needed for women to take on the busy, multitasking, caretaker roles they have traditionally been associated with. In the blog *Chic & Sweaty*, formerly known as *Peace, Love and Nutrition*, Raw Revolution's superfood bars are positively reviewed by blogger Jocelyn Steiber as "VERY convenient and easy to fit into my busy lifestyle," and, "because they are raw," they are able "to give your body more nutrients and enzymes." Finally, in a nod to body maintenance, she notes that although these bars are "the perfect blend of carbs, fat and protein," one should be careful since, as Steiber warns, "because of the nut content they are high in calories/fat."[30]

Assumptions around gender-normative taste preferences are also present in the marketing of superfoods. What is most interesting about this form of gendering is that it is highly paradoxical and persists concurrently on opposite ends of the health and taste spectrum. Traditionally, the foods associated with women and the food choices they make center on lighter fare ("for example salad . . . [which is known] as a feminized and feminizing dish,"[31] as well as items categorized as "light," "low calorie," and "diet foods"[32]) *or the complete opposite*. Within the first category, superfoods of the seed and nut variety are often suggested as good additions to salads, as in the Dragonfruit Salad recipes from Navitas Naturals. In fact, the recipe section for Navitas Naturals is filled with an entirely vegan menu that fits the normative expectations of women's food choices. Recipes for butternut squash soup, goldenberry pilaf, pineapple tofu kabobs, and spinachadillas are described as *elegant*, *vibrant*, *green*, *meatless*, and *in style* by the website.[33]

At the same time, superfood manufacturers target a further, entirely different, taste profile—namely, sweets. Historically, the consumption of sweet foodstuffs like desserts, baked goods, and chocolate by women has been identified as sources of pleasure, sex, desire, and lust. Kathleen Banks Nutter points out that chocolate in particular has had a strong association with women and sex since the sixteenth century, stating that "even before women's lust for chocolate was recognized, the connection between chocolate and lust was made."[34] Susan Bordo states that "mythological, artistic, polemical, and scientific discourses from many cultures and eras certainly suggest the symbolic potency of female hunger as a cultural metaphor for unleashed female power and desire."[35] In addition, many junk food ads targeted to women play on the perception that women have a highly tormented relationship with food and where "giving in" is oftentimes framed as a form of empowerment or way to attain comfort.

Also of note is the historical development of cultural expectations and norms that aim to police feminine sexuality and associated eating practices. These expectations were formed ostensibly to protect women from engaging in hedonistic, overindulgent, vulgar, and sinful activities.[36] This is a significant sociological phenomenon that plays out in superfood advertising as well. These companies, whose products are constituted by this peculiar admixture of "light" and "sweet" items, are able to safely sell their sweeter superfoods by discursively framing them as "light" and "healthy." Navitas Naturals products, for instance, include cacao butter and cacao sweet nubs as recommended additions to listed recipes like Coconut Cupcake Bites and Judy's Cacao Truffles.[37] Naturya also performs this form of double-taste gendering in its recipe section with decadent-sounding recipes and flavors like Very Berry Sunshine, Nana Ice Cream, Avocado Lime Cheesecake, Sweet Potato Brownies, and Superfood Chocolate Porridge that exist in tandem with its lighter fare. Similarly, Raw Revolution's bar flavors include Chocolate Crave, Heavenly Hazelnut Chocolate, and Chocolate Coconut Bliss.[38] Even the names connote desire and indulgence in the forbidden—yet the byline assures the reader these bars are "high protein, high fiber, low sugar, all vegan," and, therefore, acceptable.[39] Superfood marketing, in this sense, appears to have found a solution to the highly confusing message women are given with respect to the need to maintain a thin body at the same time as giving in to junk food.

It is also significant to note that superfoods are increasingly being promoted in men's health magazines as well, but in a rather distinctive way with respect to visuals, number of product tie-ins, and health claims. To begin with, the promotion of superfood to men is often done without reference to a specific branded product—with the exception of health food drinks and nutritional sports bars. Although these bars also tend to be on the sweet side, they are often marketed as "hearty," "filling," and "performance enhancing." Interestingly, however, in a recent article the *Wall Street Journal* discusses how male athletes who favor savory bars will now be able to buy ones that taste like pizza or even French fries.[40] This further genders these products.

Furthermore, the foods given the label *superfood* in men's magazines are also distinct from those in women's magazines in that they are focused on whole foodstuffs rather than on branded products. As such, the types of foods that fall under the superfoods label targeted at men include milk, eggs, almonds, chicken, beef, as well as unbranded quinoa, green tea, and chia seeds. Men's magazines also draw on and market superfoods in the context of health, energy, and athletic performance, with some even including references to medical journals, rather than beauty, body maintenance, and indulgence. Yet it is also important to note that the ways in which superfoods are marketed to men, even if it is without reference to specific brands, also works to reinforce dominant gender norms and expectations—this time in relation to masculinity. As such, meat in particular figures prominently in all of the lists of superfoods recommended in men's health magazines. The focus on meat plays into normative assumptions about masculinity.[41] According to Twigg,

> Men in particular are thought in some sense to need meat, especially red meat, and a series of masculine qualities are encapsulated in the idea of red bloodedness. It is part of the traditional image of John Bull, the beer-quaffing, beef-eating, fine figure of a man, and negative perceptions of vegetarianism within the dominant culture echo these ideas.[42]

For example, in an article for *Men's Health* titled "40 Age-Erasing Superfoods: Look, Feel and Stay Young," beef is highlighted as a superfood crucial to building muscle. Grass-fed beef in particular, the article explains, contains omega-3 fatty acids that limit inflammation as well as "conjugated linoleic acid (CLA), which studies have shown help reduce belly fat and build lean muscle."[43] This gendered framing demonstrates how men, as well as women, are being incorporated into the youth-oriented food and beauty industry.

NUTRITIONISM

Nutritionism is the third and final discursive frame used in the promotion of superfood products across media platforms. This paradigm articulates a view of food that emphasizes the "*nutri-biochemical level of engagement with food and the body*, and on identifying relationships between nutrients on the one hand, and particular health conditions, biological markers (i.e., biomarkers), and biochemical processes of the body on the other."[44] This reductionist perspective first articulated by nutritonists, according to Scirinis, has been co-opted by food companies to market products in terms of their perceived nutritional benefits and ability to obviate disease. Critiques of this approach toward food and health include the problematic assumption that nutritional content is vital to understand the value of food and that, since nutrition profiling is a scientific process, the public needs "experts to explain the hidden reality of food to us."[45] What is most pernicious about this approach is that it decontextualizes food from the context of its production, and eventual consumption, as well as erasing the difference between whole and processed foods, which, for superfood manufacturers, has the benefit of presenting their highly processed nutritional bars and drinks as functionally and nutritionally equivalent, or superior, to unprocessed whole foods. According to Anne Barhill, this kind of nutritionism "is the quasi-scientific ideology that underlies the commercial approach to nutrition."[46]

All three superfood companies taken up in this chapter draw on the discourse of scientific nutritionism to sell their products. Navitas Naturals, in describing its products, is conspicuous in highlighting the nutritional benefit of superfoods—primarily through the use of keywords popularly associated with health. For instance, its Acai Powder is described as containing all the "vital nutrients and flavour of the fresh fruit" while providing "vibrant antioxidants, omega fats, and fiber."[47] Similarly, the Blueberry Hemp Power Snacks are described as being a rich source of omega-3 and omega-6 fatty acids, iron, magnesium, zinc, and potassium, all balanced in an "ideal ratio to support human health."[48] The use of scientific keywords like these are representative of how language and discourse can be used ideologically through "reconfiguring and conditioning society and culture, creating and perpetuating power relationships" and normative understandings of food and health.[49]

A similar use of framing terms can be found in the way Raw Revolution, on its website, has included a detailed list of ingredients and a precise nutritional breakdown below each of the products. Additionally, the FAQ page is filled with questions related to nutritional content, including how raw its products are, whether they are gluten-free, what isomaltooligosaccharides (IMO) are, and whether agave syrup is "bad" for you.[50]

Additionally, nutritionism, as it relates to superfoods in particular but also on a larger level, has the effect of constructing a highly rigid hierarchy of moral consumption. The formation of norms around consumption has a rich history in seeking to regulate both the qualities of food and the quantities eaten. These norms can be thought of as technologies of the self that encourage self-regulation through the wedding of medicalized science with social concerns that "encourage communities to do the 'right' thing and behave in a 'proper' way."[51]

Ruth Wodak calls this strategy *referentialism*, in which in- and out-groups are constructed through the use of language that sees the meaning of words as fixed.[52] This approach, which leads to the labeling of some consumers—for example, those who eat superfoods—as virtuous and those who do not as possessing negative traits by virtue of their food choices, has the effect of constructing the consumption of superfoods as an inherently moral act. Other kinds of food choices are thus seen as inferior, less than, and (in some cases) even sinful. Much like the stratagems observed in traditional religious cults, this moralizing enables the dissemination of a "dogma of virtue" that solidifies a feeling of emotional solidarity and dedication among superfood adherents.[53]

This discourse also often feeds into and is supported by governmental public health advice that reinforces a cultural shift "from eating food to eating nutrients" in a way that, again, "has turned eating into a science rather than part of a pleasant social event."[54] A focus on dietary guidelines, sodium levels, fat content, and the much-maligned food pyramid, rather than on the quality and source of foods, is widespread. As it relates to superfoods, there are instances in which governments have incorporated nutritionism into their own recommendations about health. The British National Institutes of Health (NIH), for instance, in a section of its website on food and balance, states the following: "Super Foods are a component of the Balanced Choices program and will highlight foods that promote health benefits above and beyond the basic nutrients,"[55] followed by a list of such items as cranberries, kiwi, fish, tea, yogurt, and dark chocolate. While the recommended superfoods on the list are all unprocessed and whole, the definitional slippage involved in relying on the word *superfood* by the NIH serves to extend the putative benefits of these foods to other commercial products like those sold by Raw Revolution, Naturya, and Navitas Naturals. Recently, however, government health bodies have begun to crack down on the health claims made by companies selling superfood products. Most notably, the European Union has banned the use of *superfood* in product claims unless it is accompanied by an approved statement that explains precisely how the product is good for one's health (since 2007).

Finally, the distorted and misleading media coverage of the nutritional claims of superfoods also serves to perpetuate the ideology of nutritionism and furthers the relegation of a sociocultural relationship with food to science. Health information about what we should eat is presented in magazines, on television, and online in ways that are often contradictory, confusing, decontextualized, and even false. Yet it is important to acknowledge that presenting information about the miraculous benefits of superfoods in a dramatic fashion is effective in attracting and retaining viewers/readers and advertisers. Edgley and Brissett point out:

> Few scientific studies accompany their cassandras with a sense of perspective—a gentle reminder that there is a difference between statistical and personal risk. . . . Perhaps we do this because the language of crisis and imminent doom seem in a mass society to be the only way to get anyone's attention.[56]

In a news story that figures prominently on its Facebook and home page, Naturya products are mentioned in the *Daily Mail*, a British tabloid with upward of two million daily readers, as used by two prominent celebrity chefs who, in the piece, outline their "no rule rules" for eating well and like a celebrity. The chefs recommend a Naturya product as an ingredient in their Go-To Green Smoothie. They suggest "1 teaspoon of super green powder (chlorella, spirulina, etc.)—we like Naturya." The context in which the recipe is given supports the celebrity nutritionists' goal advocating for the consumption of "organic, homemade food without grain, gluten, high starch or refined sugar" as the best way to achieve optimal health.[57] The identical recipe, with the same ingredient recommendation, also appears in a blog post for *Vogue*'s Arts and Lifestyle section, written by the chefs personally.[58]

A similar approach is taken by a story on Raw Revolution's superfood bars written for *Organic Spa* magazine, which is an upscale American lifestyle magazine that focuses on advice related to living an "organic way of life." In 2012, the magazine featured an article on "Buying the Best Bar," in which Raw Revolution bars were given the stamp of approval for being "packed with raw all-natural ingredients like hemp protein and sprouted flax seeds."[59]

While it could be argued that the underlying philosophy of superfood and other food trend movements might "be commended, as the belief that food is necessary for health is reaffirmed," in addition to the fact that it has motivated governments, scientists, and nutritionists to "disseminate nutritional findings beyond the walls of the laboratory,"[60] as I have illustrated in this chapter there are considerable problems with the discursive construction of the superfood category as it relates specifically to the frames of corporate neoliberalism, gender, and nutritionism. Together, these frames produce a superfood discourse that masks its neoliberal foundations beneath a veneer of progressive politics, perpetuates a highly gendered image of women as fixated on diet and beauty, as well as drawing on a functional form of scientific nutritionism to equate the consumption of these foodstuffs with disease mitigation and attaining optimal health rather than on enjoyment, community building, and general well-being.

Moreover, on a purely consumer protection and regulatory level, the validity of superfood health claims made by companies that produce these products need to be verified. Interestingly, there has been a considerable rise in the number of articles from these same magazines—*Shape*, *Women's Fitness*, and *Health*—that focus on debunking nutrition myths with such titles as "The 10 Biggest Nutrition Myths," "Healthy Diet Myths Debunked," and "Nutrition Myths—Food Trends You Should Ignore." Perhaps a move toward transparent nutritional communication, coupled with an embrace of connected and nonexploitative food production practices, will form the next new trend? Here's hoping.

NOTES

1. Navitas Naturals, http://navitasnaturals.com, accessed November 15, 2015; Naturya, https://naturya.com, accessed November 15, 2015; Raw Revolution, http://www.rawrev.com, accessed November 15, 2015.

2. IndustryARC, "Functional Food and Nutraceuticals Market—by Type (Foods, Beverages, Supplements); Benefits (Health and Wellness, Disease Prevention, Fitness, Beauty); Origin & Ingredient—Forecast (2015–2020)," 2014, http://industryarc.com/Report/99/Functional-Food-and-Nutraceuticals-Market-Size.html.

3. Istvan Siro, Emese Kapolna, Beata Kapolna, and Andrea Lugasi, "Functional Food: Product Development, Marketing and Consumer Acceptance—a Review," *Appetite* 51 no. 3 (2008): 457.

4. Lilsa Kotilainen, Riikka Rajalahti, Catherine Ragasa, and Elija Pehu, "Health Enhancing Foods: Opportunities for Strengthening the Sector in Developing Countries," *World Bank Agriculture and Rural Development Discussion Paper 30* (2006); C. Stanton, R. P. Ross, G. F. Fitzgerald, and D. Van Sinderen, "Fermented Functional Foods Based on Probiotics and Their Biogenic Metabolites," *Current Opinion in Biotechnology* 16 (2005); C. Side, "Overview on Marketing Functional Foods in Europe," *Functional Food Network General Meeting* (2006).

5. Patrick Coppens, Miguel Fernandes Da Silva, and Simon Pettman, "European Regulations on Nutraceuticals, Dietary Supplements and Functional Foods: A Framework Based on Safety," *Toxicology* 221 (2006); Bebasis Bagchi, "Nutraceuticals and Functional Foods Regulations in the United States and Around the World," *Toxicology* 221 (2006).

6. J. Lunn, "Superfoods," *Nutrition Bulletin* 31 (2006): 171.

7. Naturya, https://naturya.com, accessed November 15, 2015.

8. Navitas Naturals, http://navitasnaturals.com, accessed November 15, 2015.

9. Raw Revolution, http://www.rawrev.com, accessed November 15, 2015.

10. Advertorials are newspaper and magazine content that give the reader information about a particular product or service in a manner that replicates the "objective" style of traditional journalism.

11. Ruth Wodak, "Critical Discourse Analysis," in *Qualitative Research Practice*, ed. Clive Seale, Giampietro Gobo, Jaber F. Gubrium, and David Silverman (Thousand Oaks, CA: Sage, 2004): 3.

12. Myra Ferree and David A. Merrill, "Hot Movements, Cold Cognition: Thinking about Social Movements in Gendered Frames," *Contemporary Sociology* 29, no. 3 (2000): 455–56.

13. Jossee Johnston and Shyon Baumann, *Foodies: Democracy and Distinction in the Gourmet Foodscape* (New York: Routledge, 2010), 40; Pamela E. Oliver and Hank Johnston, "What a Good Idea! Ideology and Frames in Social Movement Research," *Mobilization* 5, no. 1 (1999).

14. Norman Fairclough and Ruth Wodak, "Critical Discourse Analysis," in *Discourse as Social Interaction (Discourse Studies: A Multidisciplinary Introduction, Volume 2)*, ed. T. A. Van Dijk (London: Sage, 1997); Norman Fairclough, *Analysing Discourse: Textual Analysis for Social Research* (Abingdon: Routledge, 2003).

15. Robert W. McChesney, "Introduction," in *Profit over People: Neoliberalism and Global Order*, ed. Noam Chomsky (New York: Seven Stories Press, 1999); Arthur MacEwan, *Neoliberalism or Democracy? Economic Strategy, Markets, and Alternatives for the 21st Century* (New York: Zed Books, 1999); Noam Chomsky, *Profit over People: Neoliberalism and Global Order* (New York: Seven Stories Press, 1999).

16. Henry Giroux, "Neoliberalism, Corporate Culture, and the Promise of Higher Education: The University as a Democratic Public Sphere," *Harvard Educational Review* 72, no. 4 (2002): 426.

17. Gerardo Otero, Gabriela Pechlaner, and Efe Can Gürcan, "The Neoliberal Diet: Fattening Profits and People," in *Routledge Handbook of Poverty and the United States*, ed. Stephen Haymes, Maria Vidal de Haymes, and Reuben Miller (New York: Routledge, 2015), 4, http://www.sfu.ca/~otero/docs/NeoliberalDietInUSRoutledge-Final.pdf.

18. Raw Revolution, "Our Story: The Raw Revolution Story," http://www.rawrev.com/#!our-story/cvk8, accessed November 15, 2015.

19. Wendy Brown, "American Nightmare Neoliberalism, Neoconservatism, and De-democratization," *Political Theory* 34, no. 6 (2006): 694.

20. Navitas Naturals, "About Us," http://navitasnaturals.com/about.html, accessed November 18, 2015.

21. Ikechi Mgbeoji, *Global Biopiracy: Patents, Plants, and Indigenous Knowledge* (Vancouver: University of British Columbia, 2006), 8.

22. Laura Lindenfeld, "Visiting the Mexican American Family: Tortilla Soup as Culinary Tourism," *Communication and Critical/Cultural Studies* 4 (2007): 303.

23. Navitas Naturals, "Superfood News," http://navitasnaturals.com/newsletters/Jul12.html, accessed November 18, 2015.

24. Navitas Naturals, "Superfood News."

25. Joanne Blythman, "Can Vegans Stomach the Unpalatable Truth about Quinoa?" *The Guardian*, January 16, 2013, http://www.theguardian.com/commentisfree/2013/jan/16/vegans-stomach-unpalatable-truth-quinoa; Marygold Walsh-Dilley, "Negotiating Hybridity in Highland Bolivia: Indigenous Moral Economy and the Expanding Market for Quinoa," *Journal of Peasant Studies* 40, no. 4 (2013).

26. Carol Richards, Geoffrey Lawrence, and David Burch, "Supermarkets and Agro-Industrial Foods," *Food, Culture & Society* 14, no. 1 (2011): 31.

27. Douglas H. Constance, Mary Hendrickson, and Philip H. Howard, "Agribusiness Concentration: Globalization, Market Power and Resistance," in *The Global Food System: Issues and Solutions*, ed. William D. Schanbacher (Santa Barbara, CA: Praegar, 2014), 51.

28. Deborah Cameron, *On Language and Sexual Politics* (London: Routledge, 2006); Gabriele Griffin, "The Uses of Discourse Analysis in the Study of Gender and Migration," unpublished paper, University of New York, 2007.

29. Kyra Hunting, "Fashioning Feminine Fandome: Fashion Blogging and the Expression of Mediated Identity," in *Cupcakes, Pinterest, and Ladyporn: Feminized Popular Culture in the Early Twenty-First Century*, ed. Elana Levine (Champaign: University of Illinois, 2015), 120.

30. Jocelyn Steiber, "Product Review—Raw Revolution Bars," *Chic & Sweaty* (blog), April 14, 2010, https://peacelovenutrition.wordpress.com/2010/04/14/product-review-raw-revolution-bars/. It is important to acknowledge the literature and studies that suggest there are tangible benefits to blogging with respect to their ability to provide an outlet for creative expressiveness and identity formation. As Hunting argues, while fashion is "seen as frivolous and anti-intellectual" by many scholars, it can in fact be an "important space for self-expression." The same can be said about lifestyle, food, health, and beauty blogs. Hunting, "Fashioning Feminine Fandome," 122.

31. Deborah McPhail, Brenda Beagan, and Gwen E. Chapman, "'I Don't Want to Be Sexist But . . . ,'" *Food, Culture & Society* 15, no. 3 (2012): 478.

32. McPhail, Beagan, and Chapman, "'I Don't Want to Be Sexist But . . . ,'" 475; Brendan Gough, "'Real Men Don't Diet': An Analysis of Contemporary Newspaper Representations of Men, Food and Health," *Social Science & Medicine* 64, no. 2 (2007).

33. Navitas Naturals, "Recipes," http://navitasnaturals.com/recipes.html, accessed November 18, 2015.

34. Kathleen Banks Nutter, "From Romance to PMS," in *Edible Ideologies: Representing Food and Meaning*, ed. Kathleen LeBesco and Peter Naccarato (Albany: State University of New York, 2008), 199.

35. Susan Bordo, *Unbearable Weight: Feminism, Western Culture and the Body* (Berkeley: University of California Press, 1993), 116.

36. Bordo, *Unbearable Weight*, 116; Elspeth Probyn, *Carnal Appetites: FoodSexIdentities* (London: Routledge, 2000); Paul Messaris, *Visual Persuasion: The Role of Images in Advertising* (Thousand Oaks, CA: Sage, 1997).

37. Navitas Naturals, "Recipes," http://navitasnaturals.com/recipes.html, accessed November 18, 2015.

38. Raw Revolution, "Products," http://www.rawrev.com/#!products/c1bl9, accessed November 22, 2015.

39. Naturya, "Recipes," https://naturya.com/recipes/recipe-list/category/joysbreakfastlunch-dinner, accessed November 25, 2015.

40. Frederick Dreier, "For Athletes Who Don't Savor Sweets, How about a Squeeze of Pizza?" *Wall Street Journal*, January 22, 2015, http://www.wsj.com/articles/from-sweet-to-savory-energy-bars-taste-more-like-meat-and-potatoes-1421968613.

41. Jemal Nath, "Gendered Fare? A Qualitative Investigation of Alternative Food and Masculinities," *Journal of Sociology* 47, no. 3 (2010).

42. Julia Twigg, "Vegetarianism and the Meanings of Meat," in *The Sociology of Food and Eating: Essays on the Sociological Significant of Food*, ed. A. Murcott (Aldershot: Gower, 1983), 24.

43. "40 Age-Erasing Superfoods," *Men's Health*, April 21, 2015, http://www.menshealth.com/nutrition/age-erasing-superfoods.

44. Gyory Scrinis, "On the Ideology of Nutritionism," *Gastronomica: The Journal of Food and Culture* 8, no. 1 (2008): 40; Allison Hayes-Conroy and Jessica Hayes-Conroy, *Doing Nutrition Differently: Critical Approaches to Diet and Dietary Intervention* (Farnham: Ashgate, 2013); Gyorgy Scrinis, *Nutritionism: The Science and Politics of Dietary Advice* (New York: Columbia University Press, 2013).

45. Michael Pollan, "Unhappy Meals," *New York Times* [serial on the Internet], January 28, 2007, http://michaelpollan.com/articles-archive/unhappy-meals/.

46. Anne Barnhill, "Nutritionism, Commercialization and Food Comment on 'Buying Health: The Costs of Commercialism and an Alternative Philosophy,'" *International Journal of Health Policy Management* 1, no. 3 (2013): 225.

47. Navitas Naturals, "Acai Powder," http://navitasnaturals.com/product/432/Acai-Powder.html, accessed November 22, 2015.

48. Navitas Naturals, "Blueberry Hemp Power Snacks," http://navitasnaturals.com/product/497/Snack-Blueberry-Hemp.html, accessed November 22, 2015.

49. Ruth Breeze, "Critical Discourse Analysis and Its Critics," *Pragmatics* 21, no. 4 (2011): 489.

50. Raw Revolution, "FAQ," http://www.rawrev.com/#!faq/ccjp, accessed November 22, 2015.

51. J. Coveney, "The Government and Ethics of Health Promotion: The Importance of Michel Foucault," *Health and Education Research, Theory & Practice* 13, no. 3 (1998): 466; Michel Foucault, "Technologies of the Self," in *Technologies of the Self: A Seminar with Michel Foucault*, ed. L. Martin, H. Gutman, and P. Hutton (Amherst: University of Massachusetts, 1988).

52. Wodak, "Critical Discourse Analysis."

53. Jeff Goodwin, James M. Jasper, and Francesca Polletta, *Passionate Politics: Emotions and Social Movements* (London: University of Chicago Press, 2001).

54. Anne Marie Rieffestahl, "Super-Healthy Families," *Food, Culture & Society* 17, no. 4 (2014): 616.

55. National Institutes of Health, "Food," Office of Research Services, http://www.ors.od.nih.gov/pes/dats/food/balance/Pages/superfoods.aspx, accessed July 17, 2015.

56. Charles Edgley and Dennis Brissett, "Health Nazis and the Cult of the Perfect Body: Some Polemic Observations," *Symbolic Interaction* 13, no. 2 (1990): 268.

57. Toni Jones, "Slow Down, Chew, Make Friends with Fat and Start Spiralizing: How to Eat Now by this Year's Hottest Celebrity Chefs, Stunning Sisters Hemsley + Hemsley," *Daily Mail*, February 6, 2015, http://www.dailymail.co.uk/femail/food/article-2940670/How-eat-year-s-hottest-celebrity-chefs-stunning-sisters-Hemsley-Hemsley.html.

58. Melissa Hemsley and Jasmine Hemsley, "Go-To Green Smoothie," *Vogue: Food and Lifestyle*, August 9, 2013, http://www.vogue.co.uk/arts-and-lifestyle/2013/08/hemsley-and-hemsley-go-to-green-smoothie-recipe, accessed July 16, 2015.

59. "Buying the Best Bar," *Organic Spa*, May 3, 2012, https://www.organicspamagazine.com/buying-the-best-blog/.

60. Lois D. McBean and Elwood W. Speckmann, "Food Faddism: A Challenge to Nutritionists and Dietitians," *American Journal of Clinical Nutrition* 27 (1974): 1077.

BIBLIOGRAPHY

Bagchi, Debasis. "Nutraceuticals and Functional Foods Regulations in the United States and Around the World." *Toxicology* 221 (2006): 1–3.

Barnhill, Anne. "Nutritionism, Commercialization and Food Comment on 'Buying Health: The Costs of Commercialism and an Alternative Philosophy.'" *International Journal of Health Policy Management* 1, no. 3 (2013): 223–25.

Blythman, Joanne. "Can Vegans Stomach the Unpalatable Truth about Quinoa?" *The Guardian*, January 16, 2013. http://www.theguardian.com/commentisfree/2013/jan/16/vegans-stomach-unpalatable-truth-quinoa. Accessed January 2016.

Bordo, Susan. *Unbearable Weight: Feminism, Western Culture and the Body*. Berkeley: University of California Press, 1993.

Breeze, Ruth. "Critical Discourse Analysis and Its Critics." *Pragmatics* 21, no. 4 (2011): 493–525.

Brown, Wendy. "American Nightmare Neoliberalism, Neoconservatism, and De-democratization." *Political Theory* 34, no. 6 (2006): 690–714.

Cameron, Deborah. *On Language and Sexual Politics*. London: Routledge, 2006.

Chomsky, Noam. *Profit over People: Neoliberalism and Global Order*. New York: Seven Stories Press, 1999.

Constance, Douglas H., Mary Hendrickson, and Philip H. Howard. "Agribusiness Concentration: Globalization, Market Power and Resistance." In *The Global Food System: Issues and Solutions*, edited by William D. Schanbacher, 31–49. Santa Barbara, CA: Praegar, 2014.

Coppens, Patrick, Miguel Fernandes Da Silva, and Simon Pettman. "European Regulations on Nutraceuticals, Dietary Supplements and Functional Foods: A Framework Based on Safety." *Toxicology* 221 (2006): 59–74.

Coveney, J. "The Government and Ethics of Health Promotion: The Importance of Michel Foucault." *Health and Education Research, Theory & Practice* 13, no. 3 (1998): 459–68.

Dreier, Frederick. "For Athletes Who Don't Savor Sweets, How about a Squeeze of Pizza?" *Wall Street Journal*, January 22, 2015. http://www.wsj.com/articles/from-sweet-to-savory-energy-bars-taste-more-like-meat-and-potatoes-1421968613. Accessed July 25, 2015.

Edgley, Charles, and Dennis Brissett. "Health Nazis and the Cult of the Perfect Body: Some Polemic Observations." *Symbolic Interaction* 13, no. 2 (1990): 257–79.

Editors of Men's Health. "40 Age-Erasing Superfoods." *Men's Health*, April 21, 2015. http://www.menshealth.com/nutrition/age-erasing-superfoods. Accessed July 14, 2015.

Fairclough, Norman. *Analysing Discourse: Textual Analysis for Social Research*. Abingdon: Routledge, 2003.

Fairclough, Norman, and Ruth Wodak. "Critical Discourse Analysis." In *Discourse as Social Interaction (Discourse Studies: A Multidisciplinary Introduction, Volume 2)*, edited by T. A. Van Dijk. London: Sage, 1997.

Ferree, Myra, and David A. Merrill. "Hot Movements, Cold Cognition: Thinking about Social Movements in Gendered Frames." *Contemporary Sociology* 29, no. 3 (2000): 454–62.

Foucault, Michel. "Technologies of the Self." In *Technologies of the Self: A Seminar with Michel Foucault*, edited by L. Martin, H. Gutman, and P. Hutton, 16–49. Amherst: University of Massachusetts, 1988.

Giroux, Henry. "Neoliberalism, Corporate Culture, and the Promise of Higher Education: The University as a Democratic Public Sphere." *Harvard Educational Review* 72, no. 4 (2002): 425–64.

Goodwin, Jeff, James M. Jasper, and Francesca Polletta. *Passionate Politics: Emotions and Social Movements*. London: University of Chicago Press, 2001.

Gough, Brendan. "'Real Men Don't Diet': An Analysis of Contemporary Newspaper Representations of Men, Food and Health." *Social Science & Medicine* 64, no. 2 (2007): 326–37.

Griffin, Gabriele. "The Uses of Discourse Analysis in the Study of Gender and Migration." Unpublished paper, University of New York, 2007.

Hayes-Conroy, Allison, and Jessica Hayes-Conroy. *Doing Nutrition Differently: Critical Approaches to Diet and Dietary Intervention*. Farnham: Ashgate, 2013.

Hemsley, Melissa, and Jasmine Hemsley. "Go-To Green Smoothie." *Vogue: Food and Lifestyle*. August 9, 2013. http://www.vogue.co.uk/arts-and-lifestyle/2013/08/hemsley-and-hemsley-go-to-green-smoothie-recipe. Accessed July 16, 2015.

Hunting, Kyra. "Fashioning Feminine Fandome: Fashion Blogging and the Expression of Mediated Identity." In *Cupcakes, Pinterest, and Ladyporn: Feminized Popular Culture in the Early Twenty-First Century*, edited by Elana Levine, 116–37. Champaign: University of Illinois, 2015.

IndustryARC. "Functional Food and Nutraceuticals Market—by Type (Foods, Beverages, Supplements); Benefits (Health and Wellness, Disease Prevention, Fitness, Beauty); Origin & Ingredient—Forecast (2015–2020)." 2014. http://industryarc.com/Report/99/Functional-Food-and-Nutraceuticals-Market-Size.html. Accessed June 12, 2015.

Johnston, Jossee, and Shyon Baumann. *Foodies: Democracy and Distinction in the Gourmet Foodscape*. New York: Routledge, 2010.

Jones, Toni. "Slow Down, Chew, Make Friends with Fat and Start Spiralizing: How to Eat Now by this Year's Hottest Celebrity Chefs, Stunning Sisters Hemsley + Hemsley." *Daily Mail*, February 6, 2015. http://www.dailymail.co.uk/femail/food/article-2940670/How-eat-year-s-hottest-celebrity-chefs-stunning-sisters-Hemsley-Hemsley.html. Accessed September 1, 2015.

Kotilainen, Lilsa, Riikka Rajalahti, Catherine Ragasa, and Elija Pehu. "Health Enhancing Foods: Opportunities for Strengthening the Sector in Developing Countries." *World Bank Agriculture and Rural Development Discussion Paper 30*, 2006.

Lindenfeld, Laura. "Visiting the Mexican American Family: Tortilla Soup as Culinary Tourism." *Communication and Critical/Cultural Studies* 4 (2007): 303–20.

Lunn, J. "Superfoods." *Nutrition Bulletin* 31 (2006): 171–72.

MacEwan, Arthur. *Neo-liberalism or Democracy? Economic Strategy, Markets, and Alternatives for the 21st Century*. New York: Zed Books, 1999.

McBean, Lois D., and Elwood W. Speckmann. "Food Faddism: A Challenge to Nutritionists and Dietitians." *American Journal of Clinical Nutrition* 27 (1974): 1071–78.

McPhail, Deborah, Brenda Beagan, and Gwen E. Chapman. "'I Don't Want to Be Sexist But . . .'" *Food, Culture & Society* 15, no. 3 (2012): 473–89.

McChesney, Robert W. "Introduction." In *Profit over People: Neoliberalism and Global Order*, edited by Noam Chomsky. New York: Seven Stories Press, 1999.

Messaris, Paul. *Visual Persuasion: The Role of Images in Advertising*. Thousand Oaks, CA: Sage, 1997.

Mgbeoji, Ikechi. *Global Biopiracy: Patents, Plants, and Indigenous Knowledge*. Vancouver: University of British Columbia, 2006.

Nath, Jemal. "Gendered Fare? A Qualitative Investigation of Alternative Food and Masculinities." *Journal of Sociology* 47, no. 3 (2010): 261–78.

National Institutes of Health. "Food." Office of Research Services. http://www.ors.od.nih.gov/pes/dats/food/balance/Pages/superfoods.aspx. Accessed July 17, 2015.

Nutter, Kathleen Banks. "From Romance to PMS." In *Edible Ideologies: Representing Food and Meaning*, edited by Kathleen LeBesco and Peter Naccarato, 199–221. Albany: State University of New York, 2008.

Oliver, Pamela E., and Hank Johnston. "What a Good Idea! Ideology and Frames in Social Movement Research." *Mobilization* 5, no. 1 (1999): 37–54.

Organic Spa. "Buying the Best Bar." *Organic Spa*, May 3, 2012. http://www.organicspamagazine.com/buying-the-best-blog/. Accessed July 30, 2015.

Otero, Gerardo, Gabriela Pechlaner, and Efe Can Gürcan. "The Neoliberal Diet: Fattening Profits and People." In *Routledge Handbook of Poverty and the United States*, edited by Stephen Haymes, Maria Vidal de Haymes, and Reuben Miller. New York: Routledge, forthcoming. http://www.sfu.ca/~otero/docs/NeoliberalDietInUSRoutledge-Final.pdf. Accessed July 20, 2015.

Pollan, Michael. "Unhappy Meals." *New York Times* [serial on the Internet], January 28, 2007. http://michaelpollan.com/articles-archive/unhappy-meals/. Accessed September 10, 2015.

Probyn, Elspeth. *Carnal Appetites: FoodSexIdentities*. London: Routledge, 2000.

Richards, Carol, Geoffrey Lawrence, and David Burch. "Supermarkets and Agro-Industrial Foods." *Food, Culture & Society* 14, no. 1 (2011): 29–47.

Rieffestahl, Anne Marie. "Super-Healthy Families." *Food, Culture & Society* 17, no. 4 (2014): 616–27.

Scrinis, Gyorgy. *Nutritionism: The Science and Politics of Dietary Advice*. New York: Columbia University Press, 2013.

Scrinis, Gyorgy. "On the Ideology of Nutritionism." *Gastronomica: The Journal of Food and Culture* 8, no. 1 (2008): 39–48.

Side, C. "Overview on Marketing Functional Foods in Europe." *Functional Food Network General Meeting*, 2006.

Siro, Istvan, Emese Kapolna, Beata Kapolna, and Andrea Lugasi. "Functional Food. Product Development, Marketing and Consumer Acceptance—a Review." *Appetite* 51, no. 3 (2008): 456–67.

Stanton, C., R. P. Ross, G. F. Fitzgerald, and D. Van Sinderen. "Fermented Functional Foods Based on Probiotics and Their Biogenic Metabolites." *Current Opinion in Biotechnology* 16 (2005): 198–203.

Steiber, Jocelyn. "Product Review—Raw Revolution Bars." *Chic & Sweaty* (blog). April 14, 2010. https://peacelovenutrition.wordpress.com/2010/04/14/product-review-raw-revolution-bars/.

Twigg, Julia. "Vegetarianism and the Meanings of Meat." In *The Sociology of Food and Eating: Essays on the Sociological Significant of Food*, edited by A. Murcott, 18–30. Aldershot: Gower, 1983.

Walsh-Dilley, Marygold. "Negotiating Hybridity in Highland Bolivia: Indigenous Moral Economy and the Expanding Market for Quinoa." *Journal of Peasant Studies* 40, no. 4 (2013): 659–82.

Wodak, Ruth. "Critical Discourse Analysis." In *Qualitative Research Practice*, edited by Clive Seale, Giampietro Gobo, Jaber F. Gubrium, and David Silverman, 197–213. Thousand Oaks, CA: Sage, 2004.

Chapter Seven

Gluttons Galore

A Rising Faction in Food Discourses and Dining Experiences

Carlnita P. Greene

There is a rising faction found within our food discourses and dining experiences that many of us neither notice nor stop to consider. Ranging from innumerable blogs presenting colossal meals to television shows featuring a gamut of eating competitions, every day we are bombarded with excessiveness and overindulgence. Within "today's 'eat more' environment," "the food industry spends billions of dollars a year to encourage people to buy its products," urges us to dine out more often than in the past, and offers us considerable portions of "low nutrient density and high-calorie junk foods."[1] Likewise, countless restaurants across the country tout their "all-you-can-eat" menus, brimming with an assorted plethora of food, seemingly prepared to assuage their customers' appetites. Yet, when considered together, all of these various facets point to the fact that there also is a rapidly growing "cult" of gluttony in American society.

Although some people may believe that it is far-fetched to define this current emphasis on gluttony as a "cult," I propose that there are several reasons why we can label it as such. Certainly, today's focus on gluttony is not based on religion, nor do most people consider "gluttons" to be "fanatics." However, whereas in the past some people regarded gluttony as a "sin" or as taboo, now it is a pervasive ideology within contemporary culture, which acts as a key form of influence in our lives.

Rather than existing on the fringes of society or within its margins, today gluttony is firmly situated within the mainstream with a cadre of loyal followers. As a group, "gluttons" comprise many members, both young and old, with diverse genders, races, ethnicities, ages, abilities, and sexual orientations. It even includes people with disparate incomes, ranging from the extremely wealthy to the working classes, because, whether on a grand or a small scale, they often engage in gluttony according to their relative means.

Despite the fact that we are aware of the food industry's marketing ploys that implore us to purchase more goods and know about the detrimental health effects of overeating, many of us, nevertheless, still continue to engage in this kind of overindulgence. Similarly, while many people also are acutely aware of the environmental impact of overconsumption and waste, we still frequently dine at "all-you-can-eat" restaurants or regularly purchase "supersized" portions. For all of these varied reasons, not only is this group of "gluttons" growing exponentially, but also, increasingly, we *all* are encouraged to become ardent members of "the club." Moreover, I contend that one of the primary reasons why we continue to behave in these ways largely is due to "the Glutton" and its rhetoric of excess.

"THE GLUTTON" AND THE RHETORIC OF FOOD EXCESS

In *Gourmands and Gluttons: The Rhetoric of Food Excess*, I claim that within media, popular culture, and everyday life, "the Glutton" emerges as a cultural persona found throughout food discourses.[2] Rhetorically, this persona relies on *tantalizing appeals*, which are rooted in its definition of "quantity," as linked to desire, pleasure, aesthetics, and the senses.[3] As such, "the Glutton's" appeals are steeped in meanings related to excess, such as enormous portions, fat, largess, overeating, overindulgence, and revelry to the extreme.[4] Since these appeals also tantalize us with "the promise of fulfillment" and "titillate us" with its associated pleasures, when food discourses or dining experiences feature "the Glutton," they also inadvertently encourage us to engage in gluttony or hyperconsumption.[5]

Furthermore, because "the Glutton's" rhetoric is supported by *strategies of excess*, which deflect our attention away from our consumption habits and bolster these appeals, we often overlook the fact that we actually are overeating or excessively consuming because it does not *seem* as if we are being "gluttonous" or overly indulgent.[6] When combined, these strategies, appeals, and meanings, surrounding the notion of "bigger is better," increasingly shape the ways in which we consider our relationships to food. They also regularly inform our definitions of "gluttony" and "excess," such that we are repeatedly encouraged to view gluttony as "normal" and excess as "ordinary" without critically considering how they function or their potential impact.[7] That is to say, the "Glutton's" rhetoric of excess is everywhere.

Due to its ubiquity, today gluttony has become synonymous with the larger foodscape and characterizes many of our dining experiences. As they are prime incentives for attracting and maintaining customers, food-related media, businesses, organizations, and experiences within their marketing and promotions frequently use "the Glutton's" strategies and appeals.[8] Therefore, I contend that "the Glutton's" rhetoric sways myriad followers into joining this group through its enticing appeals and strategies.

To thoroughly grasp how "the Glutton" urges us to join its ranks, I will utilize the Olive Garden as a quintessential example that demonstrates how restaurants and their food discourses tempt us into overeating when we are dining out. Specifically, I argue that by employing "the Glutton's" rhetoric in their marketing strategies, the Olive Garden, or other restaurants, may compel us to "become gluttons" because they challenge us to "up the ante" through competition and excessive portions, redefine gluttony as *value* rather than quantity, and make us feel connected to other "gluttons," who serve as a social reinforcement for engaging in this kind of behavior. Therefore, now I will provide an analysis of the restaurant chain's "Never Ending Pasta Pass" promotions.

THE APPEALS OF GLUTTONY AND THE OLIVE GARDEN'S "NEVER ENDING PASTA" PROMOTIONS

Founded in 1982, the Olive Garden is a chain of restaurants featuring cuisine "inspired by Italy" and served within casual dining settings.[9] With more than eight hundred restaurants across the country, the Olive Garden is a familiar site for most Americans and is a place where many of us eat regularly.[10] Despite its popularity, over the years the chain repeatedly has received much criticism regarding its claim that it offers customers a "genuine" Italian dining experience featuring "uniquely Italian" flavors and quality.[11] Frequently, it has been the brunt of numerous jokes and has served as the basis for media spoofs, since many people regard its food neither as Italian nor as Italian American, but rather as inauthentic, homogenized fare.[12] Regardless of the quality of its food, however, the Olive Garden still attracts diners with its large quantities.

Famous for its "never-ending" breadsticks, the Olive Garden's use of "the Glutton's" rhetoric and appeals is not entirely new. For the past twenty years, it has promoted its "all-you-can-eat" salad bars, unlimited lunches, and "endless" plates of pasta. Its long-standing, "most popular and requested promotion" is the "Never Ending Pasta Bowl," where customers can purchase bowls of pasta "which cost $9.99 and lets people eat as much pasta as they can in a single visit."[13] Due to the continual success of this promotion, which "sold over 13 million bowls" in 2013, the following year the chain launched a new, related promotion of the "Never Ending Pasta Pass."[14]

As Bruce Horowitz explains in "Olive Garden: $100 for 7 Weeks of Pasta," in 2014 the restaurant chain released "its first-ever 'Never Ending Pasta Pass,' which for $100 gives the holder the right to consume all of the pasta, bread, and Coca-Cola branded soft drinks that they can stuff down for seven weeks."[15] For this promotion, the Olive Garden only released one thousand passes for sale, which meant that "the restaurant chain sold out of all 1,000 of its Never Ending Pasta Passes *within two hours* of the promotion's 3 pm EST starting time."[16] To capitalize on its popularity with customers, in September 2015, the Olive Garden brought back the same promotion, with a slight variation, by increasing the total number of passes available to two thousand.

That is to say, aside from selling one thousand individual passes, it expanded its 2015 promotion to include an additional one thousand family passes, which "sold at $300 each and allow[ed] the cardholder to bring up to three guests."[17] Far surpassing the previous year's demand, in the 2015 promotion, the two thousand passes "sold out *in less than one second*" after they were released.[18] Yet I argue that one of the key reasons why these promotions achieved their goals is because they strategically utilized "the Glutton's" appeals of competition and "endless" portions.

The Challenge of Competition and "Endless" Portions

The "Never Ending Pasta Pass" promotions garnered publicity and spurred active participation because potential customers had to compete to "win" the passes. For example, when the passes became available in September 2015, "would-be" diners had to register online through the Olive Garden's website in the hope that they would be included among the first two thousand customers who would "win" the chance to purchase either a family or an individual pass.[19] Similarly, since there were only two thousand passes available, these limited quantities, coupled with the odds of "winning" them, may have inspired people to participate in the contest—whether merely as a game of chance or as a means of experiencing the thrill of competition.

In these ways, the promotions positioned those people who were able to buy the passes as "winners" who could share their victories with others. Simultaneously, since the passes were "won" through competition, the promotions encouraged "nonwinners" to view the passes as being more valuable, which both heightened consumer demand and created even more publicity about dining at the Olive Garden. For instance, in 2014, several people who did not "win" pasta passes retaliated against the Olive Garden by criticizing it via social media, with one person on Facebook posting that the promotion was "a scam."[20]

Responding to this accusation, an Olive Garden spokesperson stated that it was "no scam, just high demand," and suggested that the person should enter another round of competition for a pass by participating via another social media platform, Twitter.[21] Paralleling those comments from 2014, during the 2015 competition the Olive Garden's marketing team also advised people who did not "win" a pass to "follow us on social media for a chance to win one!"[22] As such, the Olive Garden's promotions fostered an ongoing cycle of consumer engagement, regardless of the outcomes.

Even when diners did not "win" passes directly from the Olive Garden, during the September 2015 promotion they still had additional opportunities to bid on passes from several "winners" who sold them on eBay. As Brad Tuttle explains in "Olive Garden's Never-Ending Pasta Passes Selling for $600+ on eBay," "In one auction for an individual pass, bids had pushed the price up to $310" while those bids on another family pass were "up over $600. Other sellers were listing passes at 'Buy It Now' prices such as $595 for an individual and $1,200 for a family of four—*for passes that originally sold for $100 and $300, respectively, remember*."[23] I propose that, when combined, these responses from both the Olive Garden and the sellers on eBay heightened levels of competition, incited consumers to invest more time in attempting to "win," and urged them to view both the passes and the ability to dine at the Olive Garden as worthy prizes. In turn, these kinds of promotions also encourage prospective and loyal customers alike to define "winning" as being directly rooted in perpetual competition or as being achieved only by continually "upping the ante" through gluttony or hyperconsumption.

When dining at the Olive Garden, customers may be enticed into overeating because they are tempted by "the Glutton's" strategy of quantity. By advertising its "all-you-can-eat" promotions, the Olive Garden may appeal to potential diners simply based on the *sheer amount* of food that it could offer to them. These large quantities of food may lure some people to visit the restaurant simply to view these enormous portions or to observe gluttony "in action" without consuming them. In contrast, other people may choose to dine there because they are attracted by the opportunity, and for the very fact that they can engage in the taboo of overeating.

The allure of copious plates or bowls full of pasta may challenge people into seeing whether they can conquer these "endless" portions by consuming as much of them as possible. Regardless of whether people order "never-ending" pasta bowls or "endless" breadsticks, or choose the "all-you-can-eat" salad bar, they concurrently are encouraged to consume more food and to "raise the stakes" when eating. As Deborah A. Cohen and Mary Story explain in "Mitigating the Health Risks of Eating Out: The Need for Standardized Portion Sizes in Restaurants," "when people are served more food than they need, they eat more than they should."[24] Therefore, the challenge of "never-ending" supplies of food urges us to "up the ante" through continual eating.

Whether intentionally or unintentionally, other diners also may inspire us to eat more food. If a person at our table has a "Never Ending Pasta Pass" or orders a "Never Ending Pasta Bowl," we also consciously or unconsciously may "compete" with that person and attempt to eat "all-you-can-eat." Extending the competition beyond the people immediately seated at our tables, there also may be an unspoken, wider competition with other restaurant goers. For instance, when we see numerous plates of pasta repeatedly being served to other customers, or view the enormous portion sizes they are consuming, we may order more food or want to have as many empty plates on our table as the one alongside us, especially if they seem to be enjoying themselves.

When these dining experiences are paired with the Olive Garden's marketing strategies, they dually situate gluttony within the context of abundance and reinforce the notion that overeating does not involve any waste. In other words, the Olive Garden stresses that it has "endless" portions, through its menu and promotions, while also *quantifying* exactly how much food it donates to charities through its marketing. In a post to its Facebook page on July 26, 2015, for example, it claims, "Last year, our restaurant donated enough meatballs to top more than 56,000 bowls of pasta."[25] This post suggests that its supply of food is so large that it can provide its customers with "endless" portions; in addition, it supposedly has such an abundance of food that it can offer this food to other people "free of charge." In turn, by revealing the specific quantities of these donations, the chain subtly implies that it sells its excessive quantities of food *without creating any waste* because it eliminates waste through the act of donating its food.

Following this logic, customers may believe that we, too, can consume as much as we want because nothing will be wasted. Therefore, when dining there, we can focus on the bounty of food piled high on our plates and presented to us instead of considering the limited global resources and human labor that went into creating them. Equally, our overeating does not seem like waste if there is an "endless" supply of food, especially because the restaurant resituates these large quantities in terms of value and connection.

Reframing Quantity as Value and Connection

While the Olive Garden's limited quantities of "Never Ending Pasta Passes" initially encouraged customers to view them as valuable because they were rare, their promotions also suggest that customers should consider the value of their meals through the lens of quantity versus price. For example, in the article "Update: Man Eating Only Olive Garden Achieves His Goal, Eats $1,840 Worth of Food," Joanna Rothkopf features Alan Martin, who ate 115 meals during the 2014 promotion, which were worth $1,840 total.[26] To many people, it may seem as if Martin consumed a considerable amount of food as compared to his expenses, because he ate sixteen meals total in seven weeks, which cost him around $16 per meal. Outwardly, these large quantities of food sold by the Olive Garden, as compared to their prices, also may lead people to assume that they are getting a bargain when dining there through inferring the idea that "a lot of something . . . means it must be good."[27]

Perhaps the most alluring appeal, which encourages us to view our dining experiences as "valuable," is the impression that by participating in its promotions or by dining there we will be able to make connections with other people. If we extend our examination of the Olive Garden's "Never Ending Pasta Pass" promotions beyond their popular appeals of competition and excessive servings, we also can see how these kinds of promotions encouraged both loyal and potential customers to feel connected to other Olive Garden patrons when they participated in the 2014 and 2015 competitions via social media. Regardless of whether they "won" passes, ultimately, "winners" and "losers" *all* could dine "together" at the Olive Garden.

Furthermore, the Olive Garden's marketing strategies strongly encouraged its patrons to view themselves as "fans" who were connected both to the other customers and to the chain itself. Reframing its promotions, not as an endorsement of gluttony, but rather as a perk for being loyal fans, in a 2014 interview the chain's executive vice president of marketing suggested that these promotions were not "about gorging, but about fun. 'We're trying to make our fans feel like VIPs . . . That's one reason that up to seven guests who eat with the passholder will receive freebee Coca-Cola branded drinks.'"[28] In this sense, diners could regard themselves as "VIPs," and, whether dining in person or participating online, they also could imagine themselves as belonging to a much larger group of "fans" with whom they could share eating adventures.

For example, when Alan Martin was interviewed in 2014 and asked whether his participation in this promotion was valuable, he explained:

> It was worth it for the first bite of spaghetti and meatball! But it was worth it in more ways than just having happy taste buds. I was encouraged to see that our country still has jolly, fun people who love a good story, that root for the underdog and cheer when the little man wins. Of the comments I read and received, 99 percent were positive! The other 1 percent was at least funny.[29]

As we can see, a key reason that he believes that his experience was valuable was due to his engagement with other people. Beyond merely being a patron of the restaurant, within its walls, he felt supported by fellow citizens and surrounded with like-minded, fun people. Similarly, his response suggests that it is not just the fact that some people who dine at the Olive Garden feel connected to other "fans" but also the fact that these other "fans" also eat its "endless" offerings. Therefore, we are *socialized* into becoming "gluttons" because these other patrons serve as reinforcements for our gluttonous behaviors by emboldening us to join them and their voracious appetites. Yet "the Glutton's" rhetoric also has several larger social and political implications.

WIDER IMPLICATIONS OF GLUTTONY ON THE RISE

As we discovered throughout the Olive Garden example, within many of today's food discourses the act of engaging in gluttony often is repositioned as a valuable experience, which allows us to connect with others. Whether it is framed as a competition and "winning," like at the Olive Garden, or as a prize that we have earned through hard work, gluttony and overindulgence are considered as rewards to which we are all entitled. Interestingly, the rewards offered by restaurants like the Olive Garden frequently focus on the *vast quantities* of food to which we are "entitled" rather than offering us gifts, such as providing special dinners for "VIPs," giving us special treatment when dining there, or awarding us an all-expenses-paid trip to Italy, for example. Instead, their rhetoric imperceptibly encourages us to see quantity itself as *the reward.*

At the same time, this reward is framed as never having "enough," such that our desires and pleasures come to be defined not as simple but as gluttonous ones, where we slowly begin to believe that we regularly should be able to engage in the spoils of hyperconsumption without considering the risks. However, for many people, consuming massive quantities of food creates multiple health issues, since we really are not supposed to eat "all you can eat." Similarly, it is not simply about the amount of food that we consume; these meals also often contain high calories. As Cohen and Story claim, even if we are not overeating when dining out, "A review of the calorie content of foods offered by more than 245 restaurant chains and their 30,923 unique menu items found that entrees [alone] averaged 674 calories."[30] These figures suggest that when we dine out, "most meals away from home contain much more than [the] 640 calories" recommended for lunch or dinner by the Institute of Medicine.[31]

Regardless of the potential health risks, if we happen to succumb to "the Glutton's" rhetoric, by partaking in gluttony at the Olive Garden or elsewhere, their discourses often frame these ventures not as being *selfish* but as "self-indulgent." Undertaken within these contexts, this kind of overindulgence also is supposed to be without *guilt.* In other words, if "everyone" is doing it, it cannot be *that* bad. Surrounded by other diners, we may be encouraged to view our excessive eating not as being "gluttonous" because we only ate *two* heaping plates of pasta whereas someone else ate *three* platefuls. In other words, we may compare one level of gluttony to another, but both of these behaviors are still overeating.

Likewise, if we view our consumption in light of "the Glutton's" rhetoric of "endless" portions, it seems like we are eating "even less" than we think, because at some point we will have to cease eating; yet the pasta is "never ending." Since food supplies supposedly are "endless" as well, we convince ourselves that we are not "taking food from someone else's mouth" and none of this food is going to waste. In turn, we justify our actions when we overeat because we assume that we are not the only people who eat excessively. Therefore, we are encouraged to believe that we can engage in gluttony frequently without any consequences.

However, this rhetoric deflects our attention away from our own overindulgence, waste, and the fact that, globally, food is a limited resource. In "Wasted: How America Is Losing up to 40 Percent of Its Food from Farm to Fork to Landfill," Dana Gunders reveals that although food production uses valuable resources in the United States, including "50 percent of U.S. land" and "80 percent of all freshwater consumed in the United States," across America, the amount of food wasted is "the equivalent of $165 billion each year."[32] Furthermore, the author explains, "Reducing food losses by just 15 percent would be enough food to feed more than 25 million Americans every year at a time when one in six Americans lack a secure supply of food to their tables."[33] In other words, hyperconsumption, and its by-product of waste, has a direct impact on both our environment and other people.

I am not suggesting that just because food discourses use highly persuasive appeals means that people automatically are convinced to overeat. Assuredly, there are many people who resist "the Glutton's" temptations. Nor am I implying that everyone's consumption habits are excessive since many people do not gorge themselves when eating out nor do they purchase or waste vast quantities of food. Likewise, there may be other reasons why belonging to the "cult" of gluttony is so appealing for people. Nevertheless, here I have outlined some of the most apparent reasons why this sect frequently seems to attract so many followers.

Moreover, it is not merely that "the Glutton" and its appeals appear in one place, like the Olive Garden's promotions, but also that this rhetoric persistently emerges throughout a multitude of messages about food and eating, which heightens its potential impact. Broadly speaking, these recurrent, public discourses also strongly suggest that this "cult" of gluttony belongs to a much larger category of excess that is rampant within our wider culture. Thus, today many of us are becoming a part of this rising faction of "gluttons," regardless of whether we choose to admit it, because we are all enticed to become gluttonous, to overindulge, to overeat, and to consume excessively through the rhetoric of excess pervading contemporary dining experiences, food media, popular culture, and everyday life.

NOTES

1. Marion Nestle, "Today's 'Eat More' Environment: The Role of the Food Industry," in *The Crisis of 49 Million Hungry Americans and How to Solve It*, ed. Peter Pringle (New York: Public Affairs, 2013), 98–105.

2. Carlnita P. Greene, *Gourmands and Gluttons: The Rhetoric of Food Excess* (New York: Peter Lang, 2015), 24–28.

3. Greene, *Gourmands and Gluttons*, 32–39.

4. Greene, *Gourmands and Gluttons*, 26–28.

5. Greene, *Gourmands and Gluttons*, 36–39.

6. Greene, *Gourmands and Gluttons*, 39–44.

7. Greene, *Gourmands and Gluttons*, 109.

8. Greene, *Gourmands and Gluttons*, 36–39.

9. "Our Brands: Olive Garden Italian Kitchen," Darden, Darden Concepts, Inc., accessed September 17, 2015, https://www.darden.com/restaurants/olive-garden.

10. "About Us," Olive Garden Italian Kitchen, Darden Concepts, Inc., accessed September 17, 2015, http://www.olivegarden.com/about-us.

11. "About Us."

12. Charles Passy, "What Olive Garden's 'Never Ending Pasta Pass' Distracts Patrons from Realizing," *Market Watch*, November 8, 2014, accessed September 17, 2015, http://www.marketwatch.com/story/what-olive-gardens-never-ending-pasta-pass-distracts-eaters-from-realizing-2014-09-09.

13. Bruce Horovitz, "Olive Garden: $100 for 7 Weeks of Pasta," *USA Today*, September 8, 2014, accessed September 17, 2015, http://www.usatoday.com/story/money/business/2014/09/07/olive-garden-never-ending-pasta-casual-dining-restaurants/15139803/; Candice Choi, "Olive Garden Brings Back 'Pasta Pass,'" *AP*, September 16, 2015, accessed September 17, 2015, http://bigstory.ap.org/article/7bc7c0bf02a14b96b00d8fc517dd1940/olive-garden-brings-back-pasta-pass.

14. Horovitz, "Olive Garden: $100 for 7 Weeks of Pasta."

15. Horovitz, "Olive Garden: $100 for 7 Weeks of Pasta."

16. Emily Thomas, "Olive Garden's 'Never Ending Pasta Passes' Sell Out in Hours (Update)," *Huffington Post*, September 8, 2014, accessed September 17, 2015, http://www.huffingtonpost.com/2014/09/08/olive-garden-unlimited-pasta-pass_n_5784604.html.

17. Michal Addady, "Olive Garden's Never Ending Pasta Pass Is Back," *Time*, September 16, 2015, accessed September 17, 2015, http://time.com/4036377/olive-garden-pasta-pass/.

18. Haley Peterson, "Olive Garden's Never Ending Pasta Passes Sold Out in Less than One Second," *Business Insider*, September 17, 2015, accessed September 17, 2015, http://www.businessinsider.com/olive-gardens-never-ending-pasta-passes-sold-out-2015-9. Emphasis added.

19. CNN Wire, "The Olive Garden 'Pasta Pass' Is Back—Here's How You Can Get One," *16 WNEP*, September 17, 2015, accessed September 17, 2015, http://wnep.com/2015/09/17/the-olive-garden-pasta-pass-is-back-heres-how-you-can-get-one/.

20. Benjamin Snyder, "These People Are Angry They Couldn't Get an Olive Garden Pasta Pass," *Fortune*, September 17, 2015, accessed September 17, 2015, http://fortune.com/2015/09/17/olive-garden-pasta-pass-twitter/.

21. Snyder, "These People Are Angry They Couldn't Get an Olive Garden Pasta Pass."

22. "Specials: Never Ending Pasta Pass," Olive Garden Italian Kitchen, Darden Concepts, Inc., last modified April 16, 2015, accessed September 17, 2015, http://www.olivegarden.com/specials/never-ending-pasta-pass.

23. Brad Tuttle, "Olive Garden Never-Ending Pasta Passes Selling for $600+ on eBay," *Money*, September 21, 2015, accessed September 23, 2015, http://time.com/money/4042637/olive-garden-pasta-passes-ebay/. Emphasis Added.

24. Deborah A. Cohen and Mary Story, "Mitigating the Health Risks of Dining Out: The Need for Standardized Portion Sizes in Restaurants," *American Journal of Public Health* 104, no. 4 (2014): 586.

25. "Olive Garden Facebook Page," Olive Garden Italian Kitchen, Darden Concepts, Inc., accessed September 17, 2015, https://www.facebook.com/OliveGarden/.

26. Joanna Rothkopf, "Update: Man Eating Only Olive Garden Achieves His Goal, Eats $1,840 Worth of Food," *Salon*, November 10, 2014, accessed September 17, 2015, http://www.salon.com/2014/11/10/update_man_eating_only_olive_garden_achieves_his_goal_eats_1840_worth_of_food/.

27. George Ritzer, *The McDonaldization of Society*, new century ed. (Thousand Oaks, CA: Pine Forge Press, 2000), 12.

28. Horovitz, "Olive Garden: $100 for 7 Weeks of Pasta."

29. Rothkopf, "Update: Man Eating Only Olive Garden Achieves His Goal."

30. Cohen and Story, "Mitigating the Health Risks of Dining Out," 586.

31. Cohen and Story, "Mitigating the Health Risks of Dining Out," 586.

32. Dana Gunders, "Wasted: How America Is Losing Up to 40 Percent of Its Food from Farm to Fork to Landfill," *NRDC Issue Paper* (2012): 4.

33. Gunders, "Wasted," 4.

BIBLIOGRAPHY

Addady, Michal. "Olive Garden's Never Ending Pasta Pass Is Back." *Time*. September 16, 2015. Accessed September 17, 2015. http://time.com/4036377/olive-garden-pasta-pass/.

Choi, Candice. "Olive Garden Brings Back 'Pasta Pass.'" *AP*. September 16, 2015. Accessed September 17, 2015. http://bigstory.ap.org/article/7bc7c0bf02a14b96b00d8fc517dd1940/olive-garden-brings-back-pasta-pass.

CNN Wire. "The Olive Garden 'Pasta Pass' Is Back—Here's How You Can Get One." *16 WNEP*. September 17, 2015. Accessed September 17, 2015. http://wnep.com/2015/09/17/the-olive-garden-pasta-pass-is-back-heres-how-you-can-get-one.

Cohen, Deborah A., and Mary Story. "Mitigating the Health Risks of Dining Out: The Need for Standardized Portion Sizes in Restaurants." *American Journal of Public Health* 104, no. 4 (2014): 586.

Darden Concepts, Inc. "Our Brands: Olive Garden Italian Kitchen." Accessed September 17, 2015. https://www.darden.com/restaurants/olive-garden.

Greene, Carlnita. *Gourmands and Gluttons: The Rhetoric of Food Excess*. New York: Peter Lang, 2015.

Gunders, Dana. "Wasted: How America Is Losing Up to 40 Percent of Its Food from Farm to Fork to Landfill." *NRDC Issue Paper* (2012): 4.

Horovitz, Bruce. "Olive Garden: $100 for 7 Weeks of Pasta." *USA Today*. September 8, 2014. Accessed September 17, 2015. http://www.usatoday.com/story/money/business/2014/09/07/olive-garden-never-ending-pasta-casual-dining-restaurants/15139803/.

Nestle, Marion. "Today's 'Eat More' Environment: The Role of the Food Industry." In *The Crisis of 49 Million Hungry Americans and How to Solve It*, edited by Peter Pringle, 98–105. New York: Public Affairs, 2013.

Olive Garden Italian Kitchen, Darden Concepts, Inc. "About Us." Last modified April 16, 2015. Accessed September 17, 2015. http://www.olivegarden.com/about-us.

———."Olive Garden Facebook Page." Accessed September 17, 2015. https://www.facebook.com/OliveGarden/.

———."Specials: Never Ending Pasta Pass." Last modified April 16, 2015. Accessed September 17, 2015. http://www.olivegarden.com/specials/never-ending-pasta-pass.

Passy, Charles. "What Olive Garden's 'Never Ending Pasta Pass' Distracts Patrons from Realizing." *Market Watch*. November 8, 2014. Accessed September 17, 2015. http://www.marketwatch.com/story/what-olive-gardens-never-ending-pasta-pass-distracts-eaters-from-realizing-2014-09-09.

Peterson, Haley. "Olive Garden's Never Ending Pasta Passes Sold Out in Less than One Second." *Business Insider*. September 17, 2015. Accessed September 17, 2015. http://www.businessinsider.com/olive-gardens-never-ending-pasta-passes-sold-out-2015-9.

Ritzer, George. *The McDonaldization of Society*. New century ed. Thousand Oaks, CA: Pine Forge Press, 2000.

Rothkopf, Joanna. "Update: Man Eating Only Olive Garden Achieves His Goal, Eats $1,840 Worth of Food." *Salon*. November 10, 2014. http://www.salon.com/2014/11/10/update_man_eating_only_olive_garden_achieves_his_goal_eats_1840_worth_of_food/.

Snyder, Benjamin. "These People Are Angry They Couldn't Get an Olive Garden Pasta Pass." *Fortune*. September 17, 2015. Accessed September 17, 2015. http://fortune.com/2015/09/17/olive-garden-pasta-pass-twitter/.

Thomas, Emily. "Olive Garden's 'Never Ending Pasta Passes' Sell Out in Hours (Update)." *Huffington Post*. September 8, 2014. Accessed September 17, 2015. http://www.huffingtonpost.com/2014/09/08/olive-garden-unlimited-pasta-pass_n_5784604.html.

Tuttle, Brad. "Olive Garden Never-Ending Pasta Passes Selling for $600+ on eBay." *Money*. September 21, 2015. Accessed September 23, 2015. http://time.com/money/4042637/olive-garden-pasta-passes-ebay/.

Chapter Eight

Caving In

The Appeal of the Paleo Diet in the Wake of 9/11

Lenore Bell

In the wake of the September 11 attacks, blame was attributed to a combination of foreign enemies and domestic lapses in national security. However, a small but potent share of the blame was also directed toward the American public, who was caught both off guard and, incidentally, physically out of shape. In her article "The Terror Within: Obesity in Post-9/11 US Life," Charlotte Biltekoff observes the following:

> Rules of conduct concerning food and eating always serve to express social concerns, communicate cultural codes, and construct and maintain both internal and external social boundaries. . . . In post-9/11 American life, the perception of obesity as a national health crisis has led to a thriving national discourse on food rules that at the same time has played a role in structuring the "physical, social, and symbolic world" that Americans now inhabit.[1]

This physically based fear was driven by the particular manner of the attacks. The planes, which crashed into the World Trade Center and the Pentagon, were hijacked by men wielding box cutters and pocketknives. Not only were the airport security measures revealed to be inadequate, but the unsuspecting victims onboard the planes and in the targeted buildings were also caught completely unaware. The frailty of the security protocols was projected onto the body. As Biltekoff notes, one of the concerns that came to the fore was about the high number of potential servicemen who were too obese to face combat. At the surface, this seems like a logistical issue. However, the "barely standing army" became a site for anxieties about individual civilian survival and morality. Biltekoff also mentions that in 2002 the surgeon general felt compelled to warn the public that rising obesity rates could dwarf 9/11 and any other terrorist activity as a threat to American life. In the anxiety about terrorism and obesity, the lines between civilian and soldier became blurred. America as a whole was perceived as having lost its "rugged individuality," instead settling into an excessive, gluttonous lifestyle that left the country vulnerable.

Unsurprisingly, the immediate panic in the wake of 9/11 negatively impacted the American diet. According to Dr. Margaret E. Woltjer:

> Information gleaned from surveys taken after 9/11 indicated that approximately 15% of Americans ate more comfort foods, while an additional 14% reported eating more sweets. Two months after the terrorist attacks, one in ten Americans had gained weight. This example of emotional eating demonstrates the power of stress in altering eating behavior.[2]

Emotional eating in the wake of a crisis is nothing new. However, Woltjer's mention of "comfort foods" is worth examining. While fatty, traditional foods were the immediate post-9/11 meal of choice, I argue that anxieties that set in after the attacks catalyzed the mainstream availability of healthier food options, including grass-fed meat and vegan offerings, which provided a different form of comfort. This comfort was not based on nostalgia but on security and vigilance.

This chapter is about the popularity of paramilitary forms of exercise in conjunction with the paleo diet. The CrossFit/paleo combination emerged as a common diet and exercise pairing in the decade following the attacks. The work of Erving Goffman and, subsequently, Susie Scott provide an illuminating framework for understanding the anxieties and rhetoric behind this crossover.

INTO THE ASYLUM

In his groundbreaking work *Asylums* (1961), sociologist Erving Goffman introduced the concept of the "Total Institution," which is referred to as TI. Inmates eat, sleep, and socialize within the walls of the TI. Participation in a TI is marked by monotony, homogeneity, and the focus on a single goal. The inmates of a TI are often unwilling participants, forced to yield their autonomy. Orphanages, mental hospitals, prisons, and cloisters are all examples of

Total Institutions. In *Total Institutions and Reinvented Identities* (2011), Susie Scott introduces a new concept of the Reinventive Institution, or RI. The inmate of the RI is a willing participant. Scott describes the difference in the following manner:

> An important feature of life within the RI is the participant's understanding and representation of this process to themselves and others. We can contrast this to the moral career of Goffman's TI inmate, who was aware only of being controlled by others, and positioned themselves as victims, secure in their private authenticity. The RI inmate faces a more complex task in having to make sense of their own decision that they are flawed in some way, and that reinvention is needed.[3]

Scott provides examples of the RI: rehabilitation centers, secret societies, performing arts conservatories, and even virtual communities such as online mental health forums. As Scott describes it, "Voluntary members actively seek to cultivate a new social identity, role of status. This is interpreted positively as a process of reinvention, self-improvement or transformation. . . . RIs can be understood as 'institutions without walls,' which members are ostensibly free to leave but choose not to, because of the strength of their commitment."[4]

Scott describes gyms as the type of Reinventive Institutions that are dedicated to transforming the physical appearance in the name of "beauty, fashion and 'healthiness.' . . . These RIs occupy a unique position on the boundary between work and leisure, for although they involve ostensibly relaxing, even self-indulgent activities . . . they simultaneously aim to bring the body into line with culturally normative standards."[5] Dieting is also a part of this process of disciplining the body to perfection, and the process is valued as much as the final result. Bariatric surgery, Scott observes, is often denigrated as "cheating" or a "quick fix," as opposed to the authentic and virtuous diet.

Scott offers the fat camp for adolescents as an example of a health-focused RI. These residential institutions for children and adolescents are designed not just for weight loss but also for personal development:

> There is a distinctly therapeutic, rehabilitative aim to the weight loss camp, with considerable attention paid to boosting the children's self-esteem, improving psychological welfare and addressing emotional reasons behind eating behavior. . . . [R]eferences to "self-monitoring" after each meal suggests that inmates are taught to internalize surveillant gaze upon their attitude to food, in order to reform their thoughts, feelings and behavior.[6]

Some CrossFit participants are like the fat camp participants in wanting to lose a large amount of weight. However, I would argue that CrossFit participants are also trying to gain something: perpetual bodily preparedness for the next terror attack. Scott refers to Foucault when she calls dieting a "technology of infinite discipline."[7] I would argue that post-9/11 discourses of counterterrorism and security are, like dieting, technologies of infinite discipline. In an amorphous war without end, the threat never fully ebbs. The CrossFit/paleo combination is structured to cater to this anxiety.

CROSSFIT

In the fourteen years since the attacks, the American commercial fitness landscape has changed in ways that reflect perceived vulnerabilities, on both national and personal levels. Before the attacks, Tae Bo was one of the most popular forms of commercial fitness. Tae Bo, developed by American trainer Billy Blanks, was derived from elements of Taekwondo and boxing. It was taught in fitness clubs and sold as VHS tapes and DVDs. The exercise gained popularity in the late 1990s and peaked in about 2005, around the time that Blanks had conducted training sessions with troops in Iraq. While it was billed as a martial art, it was not based on sparring. The participant is meant to improve their fitness rather than their self-defense capabilities. According to the Tae Bo website:

> Tae Bo® Fitness' trademark workouts enhance your strength, speed, balance, and mental awareness, by combining aspects of Boxing, Martial Arts, and dance with adrenaline racing musical beats.

As of 2015, Tae Bo has been surpassed in popularity by home DVD programs such as P90X and Insanity, both owned by Beachbody LLC. By contrast, these two franchises promote high-intensity training. Rather than performing a routine, they advocate a randomized method that is meant to increase the body's vigilance for anything. Per Beachbody's website,

> The secret behind the P90X workout system is an advanced training technique called Muscle Confusion™, which accelerates the results process by constantly introducing new moves and routines so your body never plateaus, and you never get bored! Whether you want to get lean, bulk up, or just plain get ripped, there's an endless variety of ways to mix and match the routines to keep you motivated the full 90 days and beyond!

Beachbody LLC claims that its trademarked term, "Muscle Confusion," is a technique backed by "advanced science"; yet it does not cite any specific papers on its website.

This profound shift in emphasis from repetitive strength exercises to intense and randomized moves also can be seen in the rise of CrossFit. Despite the emphasis on flexibility, a crucial part of the CrossFit/paleo institution is contained between four walls: the CrossFit box, or gym. The CrossFit box sets itself apart from the mainstream gym by its design and equipment. In CrossFit parlance, a conventional gym such as Planet Fitness or Virgin Active is pejoratively referred to as a "globo gym," a term taken from the 2004 comedy film *DodgeBall.* The "globo" gym, with its fixed-weight machines and extensive cardio suite, is for fitness dilettantes who must be guided by machines. The CrossFit box, by contrast, is a stark, high-ceilinged room containing free weights, Olympic racks, and things that are often not found in a typical gym. Oftentimes, the CrossFit box is established in a postindustrial location, such as a disused warehouse or factory. In her history of CrossFit, *Learning to Breathe Fire: The Rise of CrossFit and the Primal Future of Fitness* (2014), J. C. Herz explains:

> [W]arehouses, converted light-manufacturing buildings, former auto body workshops. Space needs to be cheap, open to accommodate sparring, and easy to equip with basic training apparatus: mats, weights, punching bags, maybe a drinking fountain. Adding some kettlebells and medicine balls doesn't screw up this kind floor plan.[8]

There are no electronic treadmills, elliptical machines, or fixed-weight machines that mark the traditional modern gym. Instead, CrossFit boxes feature alternative, no-frills tools that are harder to find at a "globo" gym: climbing ropes, tractor tires, monkey bars, prowler sleds, sledgehammers, and plyometric boxes. The reason for this selection is because these tools focus on a wide range of bodyweight movements. CrossFit has a similar goal as Beachbody LLC's "Muscle Confusion." The use of these tools also adds to a hardcore industrial aesthetic that appeals to the customer base. It deliberately counteracts the more luxurious elements that gyms have introduced since the 1980s. Many CrossFit gyms are not even fitted out with showers.

There is, however, one standard piece of equipment that is central to every CrossFit box: the large digital clock on the wall. Everything about CrossFit relies on metrics: weight, distance, and time. Exercises are frequently done "AMRAP" (as many repetitions as possible), completed in the shortest span of time. The main markers of progress in CrossFit are the use of increased weight and speed. Oftentimes, speed and weight take priority over using the strict form.

Every day, a new "WOD" (workout of the day) is posted to CrossFit.com. It could involve running, lifting, plyometric jumps, kettlebell swings, or any range of other activities. There is no pattern, and it is impossible to predict what will come the next day. In other words, it's a guerrilla workout. Over time, the body becomes a "Swiss Army" knife, capable of taking on any task that is thrown its way.

Greg Glassman, the founder and CEO of CrossFit, describes it this way:

> Recognizing that the breadth and depth of a program's stimulus will determine the breadth and depth of the adaptation it elicits, our prescription of functionality and intensity constantly varies. We believe that preparation for random challenges—i.e., unknown and unknowable events—is at odds with fixed, predictable, and routine regimes.[9]

"Unknown and unknowable" is a reference to a famous phrase used in the February 12, 2002, press conference by Donald Rumsfeld. When a reporter asked Rumsfeld about the lack of evidence linking Saddam Hussein with 9/11, Rumsfeld had this to say:

> Reports that say that something hasn't happened are always interesting to me, because as we know, there are known knowns; there are things we know we know. We also know there are known unknowns; that is to say we know there are some things we do not know. But there are also unknown unknowns—the ones we don't know we don't know. And if one looks throughout the history of our country and other free countries, it is the latter category that tend to be the difficult ones.[10]

Rumsfeld was roundly criticized for performing confusing verbal gymnastics in a time of crisis. However, Glassman takes the threat of "unknown and unknowable" events seriously, to the point of basing his fitness empire on that premise. Reebok, CrossFit's corporate sponsor, even features the word *Unknown* on some of its CrossFit apparel. "Unknown and Unknowable" has also become a staple catchphrase of the annual CrossFit Games. Dave Castro, not only an early adopter of the sport but also a former Navy SEAL, designed the programming for the games. In keeping with SEAL training, some of the events take place in the water. Much like daily CrossFit

WODs, elite CrossFit athletes have no idea what they will face at the games, so they must be as generally fit as possible to compete in any circumstances.

John Durant writes extensively of his experience with CrossFit in his book, *The Paleo Manifesto* (2013). Durant is a self-styled "modern caveman" who began his journey to a healthier life in 2006. He founded Paleo NYC, an online meet-up group dedicated to bringing together the city's paleo community. Durant directly address the connection between CrossFit and 9/11 culture:

> Many CrossFitters unironically sport t-shirts with slogans like HEROES DO EXIST. That might sound silly to some, since civilization insulates us from the risks of life, but it didn't sound silly to New Yorkers only a handful of years after 9/11. CrossFit tapped into a deep desire to regain control over their lives, even in small ways—one of the most effective to cope with traumatic events. And more than just coping with the past, working out at CrossFit felt like preparing for the future—the off chance situation might be the difference between being a hero or a burden.[11]

Durant presents us with a stark, apocalyptic binary when it comes to survival, made up of saviors and deadweights. His words emphasize the significance of the September 11 attacks on the American perception of personal safety. While Durant admits that there is only an "off chance" of another 9/11, he embraces the preparation for one as a gamified therapeutic process.

The CrossFit body is not quite weaponized; rather, it is fashioned to survive and rescue others. It is important to note that CrossFit bases its competitive spirit on camaraderie and community, not rivalry. It is about beating one's own personal best rather than another person. Some boxes offer "open gym sessions" for clients to use the space on their own, but every box has a central schedule revolving around performing WODs as a group. This also serves to build community.

CrossFit values a military brand of brotherhood. After Greg Glassman founded CrossFit in 2000, its earliest adopters were emergency services and military personnel. Service members still get discounted memberships at CrossFit boxes. CrossFit.com will frequently post Commemorative Hero WODs, which are named after and dedicated to fallen soldiers. One of the most famous of these WODs is Murph, which is dedicated to Michael Murphy, a Navy SEAL who was killed in Afghanistan. It is performed in a weighted bulletproof vest and consists of a one-mile run, one hundred pull-ups, two hundred pushups, and three hundred squats, followed by another one-mile run. There is also a heavily symbolic 9/11 Memorial WOD performed every September 11. A description of a CrossFit fundraiser captures this military ethos:

> On a cool CrossFit morning, boxes from all over northern Virginia sent athletes. Wounded warriors appeared from CrossFit Rubicon, where guys who've gotten their legs blown off in Afghanistan train to do one-legged deadlifts. These vets, with their high-tech prosthesis and rippling muscles, are the most badass of the badass. Their presence at any CrossFit even renders it instantly legit.[12]

It is telling that the heroes endowing the event with legitimacy are not just veterans but also *amputee* veterans. Their "high-tech" prostheses become trophies. Due to the strenuous nature of the regime, much of CrossFit's culture is about embracing injury, both making light of and valorizing it. Mascots such as Pukie the Clown and Uncle Rhabdo emerged as a response to CrossFit's critics who claimed that the exercise was physically dangerous.

One can see how CrossFit fits Scott's definition of a Reinventive Institution in many ways. Its primary goal is to improve the body through preparing it for further emergencies. By dictating the workouts of the day through the central website, CrossFit is able to enact global uniformity across their gyms. While the CrossFit box holds the community together, the practice of following the paleo diet outside of the box reinforces the sense of connection.

PALEO

The Paleolithic diet (also called the paleo diet) is meant to combat the "disease of civilization." In this instance, the beginning of civilization is understood to be the Agricultural Revolution, circa 7500 BCE. The diet, consisting largely of plants and red meat, claims that modern man's hunter-gatherer ancestors were significantly healthier than modern man due to their simple diet. The diet does not permit wheat, legumes, dairy, or any other food product that only came into wide circulation after the Agricultural Revolution. In one sense, the modern iteration of the paleo diet contrasts from CrossFit's ethos. In the gym, the participant needs to be prepared for any challenge. But when it comes to eating, the participant must exact a high level of control. Meals must be carefully sourced and planned. The point is to block the "unknown and unknowable" from going into the participant's body. As J. C. Herz describes it:

> The key characteristic of the Paleo Diet is its overwhelming emphasis not on what to consume, but on what to reject. In this sense it is like any religious dietary code and draws on the same narrative: In the beginning, we existed in a state of innocent perfection, ideally adapted to our hunter-gatherer environment. And then we tasted sin, in the form of cultivated wheat and beans and vegetables that were bred to be more appetizing than the roots and leaves we'd been gathering from the wild. Poisoned and corrupted, we live in a fallen world. We can never return to our Edenic Past, because nothing available for the modern shopper, even the grass-raised meat and organic vegetables, bears the slightest resemblance to what Paleolithic human beings actually ate. But by rejecting abominable foods, we can purify ourselves. . . . It's not a coincidence that Paleo dieters describe their favored food as "clean food" and the transition to the Paleo Diet as "getting clean."[13]

As one can see, there are many assumptions being made about this diet. First is the idea that having such a diet was a marker of an ideal, "Edenic" past. A muscular body becomes the sign of a perfect world. With its unmistakably biblical overtones, Herz describes the fall from grace as initiated not by an apple but by wheat. It was greed and sloth that lead humanity into agriculture. John Durant has a similar take in *The Paleo Manifesto* (2013). He sums up the transition from the Paleolithic Era to the Agricultural Revolution in the following way: "Life was good. We ate something we shouldn't have. Now life is bad."[14]

One can read Herz's emphasis on rejection over consumption in parallel to other forms of rejection that took place after 9/11. The book *In the Wake of 9/11: The Psychology of Terror* by Tom Pyszczyski, Sheldon Solomon, and Jeff Greenberg, they describe how the everyday lives of Americans were affected by a heightened sense of *mortality salience*, or a strong awareness of one's own death. After 9/11, mortality salience was high in the entire country, despite the fact that the average American is not likely to die in a terror attack. Mortality salience prompts the subject to narrow their worldview. The rejection of abominable foods runs parallel to the rejection of suspicious others.

Paleo's emphasis on rejection satiates two key post-9/11 urges: the first urge is to restrict what enters the body, and the second urge it to eat only from the homeland. While the purchase of "locally grown" food is viewed to be an affectation of the liberal middle class, it has a rustic and somewhat conservative origin. As Gill Seyfrang points out, "Localization can be a reactionary and defensive stance against a perceived threat from globalization and different 'others.'"[15] In some ways, the post-9/11 movement to grow locally resembles the "Victory Garden" movement from the two world wars. Private citizens grew victory gardens in an effort to reduce pressure on wartime food resources. But it also served as a reminder that the American public could live off the land in a time of crisis.

FIGHTING STONE WITH STONE

Many American citizens perceive fundamentalist Islam to be wholly antimodern in its worldview and its methodology. It was not uncommon to hear and see American news outlets describe Al Qaeda and its affiliates as "medieval" and "stone age" in order to express what was perceived as primitive cruelty. In his book *Al Qaeda and What It Means to Be Modern* (2004), John Gray addresses this cliché and argues, "Al Qaeda's peculiar hybrid of theocracy and anarchy is a byproduct of western radical thought."[16] The simple fact that we can criticize ISIS's actions is only because they are recorded and then disseminated through established social media networks.

However, there are many incentives for the West to persist in viewing Al Qaeda as primitive. It simplifies the "Clash of Civilizations" narrative by increasing the gulf between "us" and "them," making it easier to believe that "they hate our freedom." By contrast, the Cold War fear of the Soviet Union stemmed from a fear of secret and advanced Russian science. This time, the fear is contingent on the idea that the enemy has rejected modernity and its values.

Yet, in some ways, Islamic fundamentalism itself had a stake in maintaining its antimodern image. As noted in *The 9/11 Commission Report* (2004), "Seizing on symbols of Islam's past greatness, [bin Laden] promises to restore pride to people who consider themselves victims of successive foreign masters."[17] The September 11 attacks showed that Al Qaeda did not need technology to bring America to its knees. Even bin Laden himself took deliberate measures to distance himself from his wealthy Saudi upbringing.

Opposing sides in the global War on Terror seek to invoke antimodernity in order to simplify and bolster their narrative. One could argue that the paleo diet is another manifestation of this tendency: by glorifying an austere lifestyle, seemingly sacred and ancient, the secular West was able to conjure a tradition even older than Islam. Yet when the "caveman" mascot of the paleo diet is referred to, one cannot help but wonder: Who is the caveman? Is it the cartoon Neanderthal munching berries or bin Laden clutching his radio in the Tora Bora caves of Afghanistan? The many cultural references to the low-tech, primitive nature of the 9/11 attacks served to heighten the sense of American vulnerability. If modern technology can't keep the country safe, then alternatives must be sought. The paleo diet/CrossFit combination, one could argue, is an unconscious attempt to fight stone with stone.

PEOPLE OF THE BOOK

The exact time frame of the Paleolithic Era varies slightly across different diet books and cookbooks. *Nom Nom Paleo* (2013) states, "Agriculture came on the scene a mere 10,000 years ago—a tiny fraction of our evolutionary history."[18] *The Paleo Primer* (2013) doesn't give a time frame but states, "The Paleolithic Era was a time when mankind thrived."[19] *The Paleo Diet* (2002) by Loren Cordain, PhD, places the era as "just 333 generations—and for 2.5 million years before that—every human being on Earth ate this way."[20] The revised edition of the book, released in 2011, acknowledges the rise of CrossFit as instrumental to the success of the book and the diet. Cordain explains some of the improvements between the two editions and inadvertently highlights one of the tensions inherent to advocating a Paleolithic diet. He quotes Boyd Eaton, an early proponent of the paleo diet: "The science behind Paleolithic Nutrition is indisputable; however, we will continually hone the concept as newer information accumulates."[21] While these writers advocate for a diet solidly set in the Stone Age, they allow enough flexibility, for the rules of the diet will change as our understanding of nutrition improves. Cordain describes the leanness and fitness of the caveman as the reader's "birthright."[22] There is a strong, underlying assumption that the diet is compatible with the human genome:

> If you follow the simple nutritional guidelines laid out in this chapter . . . you will lose weight; reduce your risk of heart disease, cancer, diabetes, and other chronic diseases; and feel energized all day long. And unlike with almost every other diet you can think of *you won't feel hungry all the time.* You will feel good on this diet, *because this is the only diet consistent with your genetic makeup.*[23] (Emphasis his)

When it comes to fitness, Cordain advocates cross-training, because "this is the way our Paleolithic ancestors did it."[24] Without openly advocating

CrossFit by name, he subtly hints at its benefits: "The best way to sabotage an aerobic training program is to walk in boring circles around a track or ride a stationary bike in your closet."[25] He then ends his chapter on fitness with a curious imperative:

> Think of exercise as a luxury, a wonderful, opulent pursuit that is not available to all. It is a miraculous elixir that will brighten your spirits, improve your well-being, and make you feel so much better. Exercise will help you complete and maintain your wonderful new Paleo way of life.[26]

Nowhere does *The Paleo Diet* address the factors that prevent people from exercise, be it disability or lack of time and funding. While he acknowledges that processed foods are tempting because they are cheap, there are no suggestions in Cordain's book about how to make the diet work for a person at or below the poverty line. Cordain takes for granted that in a society with a large wealth gap, such as America, exercise is a luxury for many. Both CrossFit box membership fees and the paleo diet come with a high price tag. CrossFit fees can be from $100 to $215 per month, at about three classes a week. The paleo diet, with its requirement of fresh, organic fruit and vegetables alongside grass-fed meat, is also expensive to maintain. Living like a caveman is not a widely accessible endeavor.

Some of the books advocating the paleo diet begin with a conversion narrative. *The Paleo Primer* (2013) by Keris Marsden and Matt Whitmore is one of these. The introduction begins with tales of ailments that plagued the authors before they found the paleo diet. The ailments ranged from polycystic ovary syndrome, irritable bowel syndrome, candida, and fatigue. Then, upon adopting the paleo diet, all of these disorders disappeared. Marsden is a nutritionist and Whitmore is a strength coach, but most of *The Paleo Primer* is devoted to nutrition. However, the duo's website, www.fitterfood.com, pays more attention to exercise. While Whitmore is not CrossFit certified, the exercises he promotes are kettlebell and bodyweight exercises similar to CrossFit.

Marsden and Whitmore have a more tongue-in-cheek attitude to any biblical overtones of the diet: "There is no diet richer in [antioxidants, vitamins, etc.] than the human diet that existed back in the BC era—and by BC, we mean 'Before Crap!'"[27] However, they still strongly believe that the human body is designed for this diet, and that the trappings of modernity cannot help us: "Medicine is not health care. Food is health care. Medicine is sick care."[28]

According to Michelle Tam's account in *Nom Nom Paleo* (2013), her conversion to the diet started after her husband went paleo:

> My husband had joined a local CrossFit gym, where he did high-intensity workouts just three times a week. He ate according to a Paleo template and was in better shape than when he was in college. . . . I went online and read everything I could about the science behind the Paleo framework. I vacuumed up every morsel of information from books and blogs. I quit doing all the crazy cardio and started going to CrossFit classes. I was all-in. I had joined the cult of Paleo. And now, I'm the healthiest I've ever been.[29]

Her story is striking because Tam not only seamlessly elides the world of CrossFit and paleo but also happily goes on to refer to it as a cult. The cheerful, joking referral to the "cultish" nature of both the paleo diet and CrossFit is not uncommon. It stems from the fervor with which new adopters take to their chosen lifestyle. But it also stems from the level of self-surveillance and near total immersion in the lifestyle that takes place. As Herz puts it, "As CrossFitters weave into their kettle-bell-swinging social groups, and try to drag in as many friends and relatives as they can, they've engaged in the same social migrations that happens with radical changes in health habits. . . . It's a good cult."[30]

For those CrossFitters who do not have time to cook locally sourced paleo meals, services such as Kettlebell Kitchen have emerged. This New York City–based company delivers paleo meals to CrossFit boxes. As the website says:

> We believe our Paleo meals provide optimal nutrition without the inflammatory effects of non-Paleo foods like grains, soy and dairy. We only use fresh, local ingredients and the highest quality proteins and vegetables when crafting our meals. And because we're dedicated to providing you with the cleanest fuel possible, they will always be free of artificial ingredients, preservatives and GMOs, and chock full of the good stuff: vitamins, minerals, anti-oxidants, amino acids and essential fatty acids. . . . Thought to optimize human performance, these macronutrient ratios "amplify and accelerate the benefits of the CrossFit regimen," according to Greg Glassman, CrossFit's founder. If you've been looking to give your training the extra edge, this is it.[31]

The reach of services such as Kettlebell Kitchen mark CrossFit as a Reinventive Institution; the paleo diet not only is part of the lifestyle but also can be delivered to the gym and consumed later. While cavemen did not receive their meat and fresh produce at $10 per meal, it is as close as a busy CrossFitter can get.

FEAR RESPONSE

While John Durant argues that priming the body through the CrossFit/paleo combination is a healthy coping mechanism, David J. Morris has a different interpretation of America's post-9/11 cultural and fitness trends:

> The country as a whole continues to exhibit certain aspects of post-traumatic stress, including a compulsion to reenact the events of September 11 in movies and television as well as nurturing obsessions with homeland security and surveillance that, according to military analysts, is out of proportion with the actual threat and smacks of a kind of national hypervigilance. Moreover, the ongoing militarization of American culture—in the form of first-person shooter games, the rise of the Navy SEAL "brand" . . . and martially themed endurance races such as the Tough Mudder series—points to a fixation with the post-9/11 hyper masculinity and ubiquitous violence reminiscent of the disorder.[32]

For Morris, things like CrossFit are symptoms of unresolved trauma. Whether this fitness trend is a helpful way to exorcise trauma or a futile attempt to brace for another national tragedy depends on how much the participant buys into the rhetoric. While these are voluntary activities, the participant may not feel entirely empowered and autonomous. As Scott observes, "An examination of the micro-politics of interactions in each type of RI has revealed that just as much pressure, manipulation and subtle coercion occurs within the democraticized ranks of inmate culture."[33] Since the CrossFit/paleo combination trades on American fears of terrorism, the urge to join may be less voluntary than it appears.

FINAL THOUGHTS

When Goffman referred to food in *Asylums*, it was usually to address the poor quality of institutional rations given to reluctant inmates. Food in the TI, unlike the uniforms and chants, is not a bonding ritual. At best, it is a legally required necessity for keeping the inmates alive. At worst, it becomes a tool of degradation. However, in the Reinventive Institution that Scott describes, food plays a central role of the self-improvement endeavor.

For the CrossFit/paleo combination, participants only consume food onto which they can project positive qualities. The right kinds of food represent purity from chemicals and foreign interference. The right kinds of food are "naturally" American. The right kinds of food are safe. The paleo diet has become, on a subconscious level, a counterterrorism security blanket. While the obesity rate in America remains high, an elite and dedicated number of civilians have convinced themselves that they are honing their bodies out of being burdensome and into being heroic.

NOTES

1. Charlotte Biltekoff, "The Terror Within: Obesity in Post 9/11 U.S. Life," *American Studies* 48, no. 3 (January 2007): 30, accessed October 2, 2015, doi:10.2307/40644148, http://www.jstor.org/stable/40644148.
2. Margaret E. Woltjer, "Relationship of Emotions and Food," *Better Life Unlimited* (July 2006), http://www.betterlifeunlimited.com/healthnews/health_az/issues/relationship_of_emotions_and_food.aspx.
3. Susie Scott, *Total Institutions and Reinvented Identities* (New York: Palgrave Macmillan, 2011), 30.
4. Scott, *Total Institutions and Reinventive Identities*, 3.
5. Scott, *Total Institutions and Reinventive Identities*, 107.
6. Scott, *Total Institutions and Reinventive Identities*, 110.
7. Scott, *Total Institutions and Reinventive Identities*, 109.
8. J. C. Herz, *Learning to Breathe Fire: The Rise of CrossFit and the Primal Future of Fitness* (New York: Crown Publishing Group, 2014), 105.
9. "Understanding CrossFit," *The CrossFit Journal* 26 (April 2007), http://library.crossfit.com/free/pdf/CFJ_56-07_Understanding.pdf.
10. Defense Department Briefing, February 12, 2002, http://www.c-span.org/video/?168646-1/defense-department-briefing.
11. John Durant, *The Paleo Manifesto: Ancient Wisdom for Lifelong Health* (New York: Harmony Books, 2014), 173–74.
12. Herz, *Learning to Breathe Fire*, 304.
13. Herz, *Learning to Breathe Fire*, 202.
14. Durant, *Paleo Manifesto*, 43.
15. Kate Soper, Martin Ryle, and Lyn Thomas, eds., *The Politics and Pleasures of Consuming Differently: Better than Shopping* (New York: Palgrave Macmillan, 2009), 189.
16. John Gray, *Al Qaeda and What It Means to Be Modern* (London: Faber and Faber, 2004), 117.
17. National Commission on Terrorist Attacks, *The 9/11 Commission Report: The Final Report of the National Commission on Terrorist Attacks upon the United States (Authorized Edition)*, ed. Thomas Kean (New York: W. W. Norton, 2004), 48.
18. Michelle Tam and Henry Fong, *Nom Nom Paleo: Food for Humans: Over 100 Nomtastic Recipes!* (New York: Andrews McMeel, 2014), 9.
19. Keris Marsden and Matt Whitmore, *The Paleo Primer: A Jump-Start Guide to Losing Body Fat and Living Primally!* (New York: Primal Nutrition, 2013), 7.

20. Loren Cordain, *The Paleo Diet: Lose Weight and Get Healthy by Eating the Foods You Were Designed to Eat* (Hoboken, NJ: John Wiley & Sons, 2010), 3.
21. Cordain, *The Paleo Diet*, xii.
22. Cordain, *The Paleo Diet*, 7.
23. Cordain, *The Paleo Diet*, 104.
24. Cordain, *The Paleo Diet*, 207.
25. Cordain, *The Paleo Diet*, 206.
26. Cordain, *The Paleo Diet*, 208.
27. Marsden and Whitmore, *The Paleo Primer*, 8.
28. Marsden and Whitmore, *The Paleo Primer*, 9.
29. Tam, *Nom Nom Paleo*, 7–8.
30. Herz, *Learning to Breath Fire*, 237.
31. "Why Paleo?" Kettlebell Kitchen, January 1, 2015, https://kettlebellkitchen.com/why-paleo.php, accessed September 29, 2015.
32. David J. Morris, *The Evil Hours: A Biography of Post-Traumatic Stress Disorder* (New York: Eamon Dolan/Houghton Mifflin Harcourt, 2015), 15.
33. Scott, *Reinventive Institutions*, 238.

BIBLIOGRAPHY

"About Us: Billy Blanks Team Tae Bo Fitness." Accessed October 2, 2015. http://www.taebo.com/index.php?p=page&page_id=about_us.

Biltekoff, Charlotte. "The Terror Within: Obesity in Post 9/11 U.S. Life." *American Studies* 48, no. 3 (January 2007): 29–48. Accessed October 2, 2015. doi:10.2307/40644148. http://www.jstor.org/stable/40644148.

Cordain, Loren. *The Paleo Diet: Lose Weight and Get Healthy by Eating the Foods You Were Designed to Eat*. Hoboken, NJ: John Wiley & Sons, 2010.

Defense Department Briefing. February 12, 2002. Posted October 2, 2015. http://www.c-span.org/video/?168646-1/defense-department-briefing.

Durant, John. *The Paleo Manifesto: Ancient Wisdom for Lifelong Health*. New York: Harmony Books, 2014.

Fainaru-Wada, Mark. "CrossFit's Explosive Growth Fuels Safety Concerns." July 28, 2014. http://espn.go.com/espn/otl/story/_/id/11262964/crossf-explosive-growth-fuels-safety-concerns.

Gilman, Sander L. *Diets and Dieting: A Cultural Encyclopedia*. New York: Routledge, 2009.

Glassman, Greg. "Understanding CrossFit." *The CrossFit Journal* 26 (April 2007). http://library.crossfit.com/free/pdf/CFJ_56-07_Understanding.pdf

Goffman, Erving. *Asylums: Essays on the Social Situation of Mental Patients and Other Inmates*. New York: Bantam Doubleday Dell Publishing Group, 1961.

Gray, John. *Al Qaeda and What It Means to Be Modern*. London: Faber and Faber, 2004.

Herz, J. C. *Learning to Breathe Fire: The Rise of CrossFit and the Primal Future of Fitness*. New York: Crown Publishing Group, 2014.

Marsden, Keris, and Matt Whitmore. *The Paleo Primer: A Jump-Start Guide to Losing Body Fat and Living Primally!* New York: Primal Nutrition, 2013.

May, Elaine Tyler. *Homeward Bound: American Families in the Cold War Era*. New York: Basic Books, 1988, 1990.

Morris, David J. *The Evil Hours: A Biography of Post-Traumatic Stress Disorder*. New York: Eamon Dolan/Houghton Mifflin Harcourt, 2015.

Moskin, Julia. "Bone Broth Evolves from Prehistoric Food to Paleo Drink." *New York Times*, January 6, 2015. http://www.nytimes.com/2015/01/07/dining/bone-broth-evolves-from-prehistoric-food-to-paleo-drink.html?_r=0.

National Commission on Terrorist Attacks. *The 9/11 Commission Report: The Final Report of the National Commission on Terrorist Attacks upon the United States (Authorized Edition)*, edited by Thomas Kean. New York: W. W. Norton, 2004.

Pyszczynski, Thomas A., Sheldon Solomon, and Jeff Greenberg. *In the Wake of 9/11: The Psychology of Terror*. Washington, DC: American Psychological Association, 2002.

Scott, Susie. *Total Institutions and Reinvented Identities*. New York: Palgrave Macmillan, 2011.

Soper, Kate, Martin Ryle, and Lyn Thomas, eds. *The Politics and Pleasures of Consuming Differently: Better than Shopping*. New York: Palgrave Macmillan, 2009.

Tam, Michelle, and Henry Fong. *Nom Nom Paleo: Food for Humans: Over 100 Nomtastic Recipes!* New York: Andrews McMeel, 2014.

Whitmore, Matt. "No Time to Train? No Problem!—Fitter Food." Fitter Food, September 9, 2015. https://www.fitterfood.com/general/no-time-to-train-no-problem-you-just-need-10-minutes/. Accessed February 1, 2016.

"Why Paleo?" Kettlebell Kitchen, January 1, 2015. https://kettlebellkitchen.com/why-paleo.php.

Woltjer, Margaret E. "Health A–Z." July 2006. http://www.betterlifeunlimited.com/healthnews/health_az/issues/relationship_of_emotions_and_food.aspx. Accessed February 3, 2016.

Chapter Nine

"Of Bananas and Cavemen"

Unlikely Similarities between Two Online Food Communities

Amanda Maxfield and Andrea Rissing

This chapter compares two increasingly popular online food communities—the primal diet and fruitarianism. The dietary beliefs of these groups are starkly oppositional: where the primal diet eschews carbohydrates in favor of animal fats and proteins, fruitarians are vegans who believe that a healthy diet consists primarily of carbohydrates sourced from raw fruit. However, we suggest that these differences are largely superficial and belie underlying similarities in each group's logics, tactics, and motivations. First, we argue that the popularity of online food "cults" such as the fruitarians and primal dieters is fundamentally a reaction to contradictory, shifting nutrition science. Second, we suggest that contemporary cultural pressures that moralize health and body size add increased, almost evangelistic, fervor to individuals' pursuit of the "one true diet." Finally, adherents of both diets use evolutionary theory to legitimize their dietary choices and their pursuit of a lean, muscular bodily aesthetic. Both communities believe they draw a degree of moral authority from consuming the most natural and, thus, healthiest diet. Although similar dietary communities existed prior to the Internet, the Internet helps them flourish by facilitating the rapid distribution of nutritional information and opinions. This cultural and technological milieu creates a space in which individuals intensely concerned with the mismatch between what they actually eat and what they *should* eat are drawn to insular, diet-focused communities.

We begin with overviews of the fruitarian and primal diets based on observations drawn from two online discussion forums: 30 Bananas a Day and Mark's Daily Apple, respectively. While forum members do meet and communicate offline, these sites offer insight into their community dynamics. Publicly available, both sites provide an easily accessible home base to anyone with an Internet connection. Each online community clearly delineates approved dietary practices, is run by charismatic leaders, and hosts forums in which members can discuss personal experiences, successes, or struggles. Members can easily exchange advice, swap motivational before and after photos, share recipes, and offer supportive camaraderie. The ways in which community leaders present these diets and the conversations that occur on discussion forums offer a unique avenue via which to understand why individuals are drawn to these food communities and how they situate themselves with respect to the standard American diet.

WHAT DOES GROK EAT FOR DINNER?

Largely an offshoot of Loren Cordain's[1] paleo diet, the Primal Blueprint is based on specific interpretations of Paleolithic humans' dietary and physical habits. Its founder, Mark Sisson, is a former professional marathoner and triathlete who started the website Mark's Daily Apple in 2006 in order to publicize his "Primal Blueprint" for dietary and lifestyle choices. Dietary supplements and Sisson's self-published books are available for purchase through the website, and dietitians, gym trainers, or enthusiasts can pay for access to additional educational materials and modules that, upon completion, certify them as a "Primal Blueprint Expert." Sisson is a celebrity voice within the evolutionary health community with a sizable following; his Twitter feed has more than 95,000 followers, and his site's online forums are home to more than 204,400 members (as of May 2016).

Primal Blueprint followers believe that the healthiest diet derives the majority of its calories from proteins and fats, preferably from animal sources.[2] Adherents argue that these foods not only provide nutrients critical to muscle formation, organ function, balanced hormone levels, and appropriate blood sugar levels but also yield higher satiety than a diet rich in carbohydrates. They suggest that carbohydrate intake, particularly grains, sugars, and starchy vegetables, should be minimized in order to better regulate blood sugar levels. Moreover, followers believe that excess carbohydrate consumption leads to fat accumulation, insulin resistance, and overeating. The Primal

Blueprint views the standard American diet, with its wide base of carbohydrate-heavy grains, as the leading contributor to rising obesity and chronic disease rates. The primal diet does not recommend completely eliminating carbohydrates; rather, generous servings of leafy, low-carb greens are encouraged for their nutrient and fiber content. Smaller quantities of fruit and certain low-glycemic plants, such as wild rice or lentils, are also permitted, especially if one is exercising heavily.

Adherents believe that outdoor physical activity should be a daily occurrence. Occasional short bursts of intense exercise such as sprinting or weightlifting along with adequate sleep are also recommended to best imitate the habits and presumed health of Paleolithic humans.[3] Furthermore, intermittent fasting (IF)—which ranges from skipping a meal to a full day's fast—is promoted among some adherents. Periodic deprivation through IF is understood to allow the body to burn some of its own fat reserves, speeding weight loss and improving LDL cholesterol levels.

The central test of a food's acceptability is a yes or no question: Could our Paleolithic ancestors have eaten it? For this reason, berries are preferred over melons, grass-fed meat over grain fed, and lard over canola oil. The community mascot is an imaginary character named "Grok." Grok hunts or gathers all his own food, leads an active, physically demanding life, and suffers from no chronic diseases. Asking themselves "What would Grok do?" lets people new to the community check in about how well they are staying on plan. Calorie counting is deemphasized; instead, new members are encouraged to get in touch with their appetite cues and to eat until satiated. Trusting one's own bodily signals is posited as the most natural way to make food choices and, when followed alongside the Primal Blueprint's general tenets, should result in fat loss and overall improved health.

Notably, the primal diet suggests that for long-term maintenance, followers should aim to eat strictly "primally" at least 80 percent of the time.[4] The other 20 percent can be used more flexibly, allowing for borderline foods like dark chocolate, and to enable desirable lifestyle choices such as occasionally eating at restaurants or sharing food with nonprimal friends. This facilitates long-term maintenance and makes the diet accessible to more people.

While the primal approach is broadly similar to Cordain's original Paleolithic diet, differences do exist between the two. For example, dairy products occupy a gray space in both diets, but the primal diet is generally more permissive of dairy consumption, particularly pastured dairy in raw or fermented forms. More significantly, the primal approach places additional importance on non-food-related recommendations. Sunlight, certain forms of exercise, and sufficient nightly sleep are all emphasized. In this sense, the primal diet can be considered a lifestyle guide as much as a list of nutritional rules.

30 BANANAS A DAY KEEP THE DOCTOR AWAY

Fruitarianism is a subset of raw veganism, and many adherents refer to their specific diet as high-carb, low-fat raw veganism (HCLFRV).[5] Although there are multiple varieties of fruitarianism, this chapter focuses on the viewpoints popular within the 30 Bananas a Day community and promoted by the website's founders, Leanne "Freelee" Ratcliffe, also known as "the Banana Girl," and Harley "Durianrider" Johnstone. Freelee and Harley both run a variety of social media accounts, including on YouTube, Instagram, Facebook, and Twitter, as well as their own personal blogs. On 30 Bananas a Day alone there are over 30,600 current members, while Freelee and Harley's main YouTube channels each have more than 130 million views (as of May 2016). Through these media outlets, Harley and Freelee sell their own ebooks, logo-bearing merchandise, and an iPhone application.

Like raw vegans, fruitarians eschew animal products and generally avoid cooked foods. Some raw food proponents argue that high temperatures destroy the beneficial enzymes, vitamins, and minerals present in raw plants.[6] Others suggest that cooked foods contain chemical by-products that are toxic to the body.[7] However, even though raw vegans may eat plant-based fats and proteins such as those found in avocados, nuts, and sprouted seeds or legumes, many fruitarians explicitly avoid consuming so-called overt fats and protein.[8]

Instead, many fruitarians follow a version of the 80/10/10 plan outlined by Douglas Graham[9] and lean heavily on research findings popularized in *The China Study*,[10] which claims correlations between meat eating, cancer, and a variety of chronic diseases. The 80/10/10 diet recommends that 80 percent of an individual's daily caloric intake should come from carbohydrates, 10 percent from proteins, and 10 percent from fats.[11] Moreover, according to fruitarianism, eating a diet that consists primarily or exclusively of raw fruits will de facto ensure sufficient protein and fat intake.[12] For example, a large, raw banana provides about 1.5 grams of protein and a little less than 0.5 grams of fat.[13] In fruitarian reckoning, the only protein-deficient person is a starving person.[14] Moreover, based largely on *The China Study*, many fruitarians further argue that eating too much protein actually increases one's risk for chronic diseases, particularly cancer.[15]

Instead, heavy carbohydrate consumption, especially from the sugars found in raw fruits, is believed to be key to weight loss and good health. Many fruitarians encourage relatively high caloric intakes, hovering around 2,500- and 3,000-calorie daily minimums for men and women, respectively. A key fruitarian tenet is the harmfulness of calorie restriction. When new diet converts express concerns with their bodies' responses to the HCLFRV meal plan, veteran community members frequently suggest insufficient calorie consumption as the primary culprit. In community parlance, individuals are starving and "undercarbed" if they eat less than the 2,500–3,000 calories proscribed. Low carbohydrate consumption is seen as a path to depression, fatigue, and weight gain.[16]

Additional practices popular in the community include eating large quantities of a single fruit at each meal, a so-called mono meal, avoiding fruit mixing and consuming many of the day's calories in semi-liquefied, smoothie form. Mono mealing can continue for weeks at a time. For example, eating only bananas for an extended period constitutes going to "Banana Island."[17] About thirty bananas a day achieves fruitarians' three-thousand-calorie-per-day recommendation, and this practice lends its name to the 30 Bananas a Day brand. Guidelines about fruit mixing are meant to promote digestion and prevent stomach bloat, which underlies much of the logic behind mono meals. For example, acidic fruits like pineapple or citrus should not be consumed in the same meal as sweet fruits like bananas. Finally, smoothies are a popular way to consume the large quantities of bulky foods included in the fruitarian diet.[18]

It is worth noting, however, that not all communities here glossed as fruitarian follow identical dietary rules. Fairly virulent in-fighting has occurred over the relative importance of various dietary guidelines. One school of thought argues that maintaining a fully raw diet, rather than high carbohydrate consumption, is the most critical rule. If necessary, carbohydrate consumption may be sacrificed to stay fully raw. Alternatively, some individuals elect to eat raw nuts or avocados as occasional treats.[19]

In contrast, the second school of thought holds that cooked food is, in fact, acceptable—*if* it remains high carbohydrate, low fat, and vegan. Usually called "Raw till 4" (4:00 p.m.), this approach is a newer, more flexible take on the fruitarian diet, which allows cooked starches in the evening.[20] Generally, this equates to foods such as potatoes and rice. "Raw till 4" increases fruitarianism's appeal to a wider base of potential adherents. The community leaders who run the 30 Bananas a Day forums subscribe to the latter view.[21] Ultimately, however, the more fine-grained disagreements between fruitarian subfactions do not detract from the larger observations this chapter makes regarding fruitarian and primal diet communities.

THE STANDARD AMERICAN DIET WILL PROBABLY KILL YOU

The standard American diet (SAD) is characterized by high intakes of fatty meats and refined carbohydrates as well as added sugars, fats, and sodium. Such a diet has been variously linked with an increased risk of obesity, diabetes, cardiovascular disease, and stroke.[22] Yet, despite increasing concern over the health consequences of a standard American diet, available nutritional information on preferable alternatives is notoriously unclear. Scientific and popular experts alike acknowledge that healthy eating advice ranges from complex to contradictory. Marion Nestle describes how, for many people, choosing what to eat for their daily meals feels like walking through a "minefield."[23] As more nutrition studies are conducted, new discoveries are made and old knowledge is challenged, leaving many consumers feeling simultaneously bombarded by information and lost when it comes to actual decision making.

In 1984, *Time* magazine published a story on the impacts that saturated fat and cholesterol had on the dangerously high rates of heart disease in America; the iconic cover portrayed a frowning face of fried eggs and bacon. Thirty years later, saturated fat was again featured on *Time*'s cover, but now as an appealing curlicue of golden butter. The story had changed, *Time* reported, and when Americans reduced fat, they swapped in carbs. The result? Although overall heart disease rates dropped, cardiovascular disease remained the leading cause of death in the United States.[24] Meanwhile, diabetes rates skyrocketed. People who spent the 1990s and early 2000s believing that low-fat yogurt and fat-free cookies would keep them healthy were suddenly confronted with a nutritional about-face.

The lack of consensus on saturated fat exemplifies the confusion that confronts people trying to identify and follow mainstream nutritional advice. Is coffee healthy or dangerous, or does it depend on the dose? Is fish a vital source of omega-3s or a treacherous source of mercury? Are calorie-free sweeteners a boon or a carcinogen? Such back and forth in conventional nutrition science can frustrate consumers looking for simple, affordable advice on what they should feed their families. Ethical and environmental concerns only exacerbate the confusion.

Popular media's treatment of diet-related disease further aggravates public anxiety about healthy eating; get it exactly right, they warn, or else. Panic-driven metaphors make frequent reference to a "diabetes time bomb," the "war on obesity," and "epidemics" of cardiovascular disease, cancer, and stroke. These metaphors have been abundantly effective at ratcheting up public concern. Although it is now nearly impossible to avoid viral content about the so-called battle against obesity, it was not until the early 2000s that popular media took notice of the expansion in Western waistlines, which first experienced a marked uptick in the 1980s.[25] In the early 2000s only 2–3 percent of Americans believed that obesity was a major health concern. Now, however, 67 percent believe that obesity is a critical issue, and 90 percent think that most Americans are overweight.[26]

These metaphors work in part because they touch a moral nerve, tapping into notions of responsibility—that being healthy is an individual duty.[27] Internalizing these messages, individuals focus their energies toward constant self-discipline of behavior and body. Today, this frequently takes the form of stringent attention to one's exercise habits, weight, and dietary choices.

According to such a moral system, only lazy or ignorant individuals are unhealthy and overweight. This drives people to seek out new knowledge and technologies for regulating health and body size. Previously, most people encountered nutrition information via the education system, federal programs, or paid television and print advertisements for diet-related supplements and schemes. However, since the late twentieth century, the Internet has served as an increasingly important source of lay information. Through blog posts, videos, and social forums, people can quickly generate, acquire, and share new ideas about healthy eating. Coupled with the advent of electronic tools for nutrition tracking like MyFitnessPal and CRON-O-Meter, the Internet now makes it easier than ever for like-minded eaters to find and hold each other accountable. However, while the Internet facilitates information sharing, access to so much easily searchable and widely reported nutrition data may, paradoxically, increase confusion.

Against this background—constantly shifting nutritional advice and the belief that health is a personal responsibility in which most individuals are failing—a space is created in which online food "cults" emerge. Online forums offering clearly articulated doctrines coupled with supportive communities are especially well positioned to thrive. As different as the fruitarian and primal tenets are, we suggest that both are symptomatic of the current state of nutritional science and wider cultural discourse about health.

DO YOUR RESEARCH

It would be difficult to imagine two sets of dietary advice more fundamentally in disagreement with each other than the primal diet, with its heavy emphasis on animal fats and proteins, and the raw fruitarian diet, with its embrace of veganism and sugary fruits. And yet these two drastically different approaches to healthy eating emerged in response to the same widespread dissatisfaction with mainstream dietary advice and the moralizing pressure to be healthy. They promise nearly identical end results for followers, and they engage with the evolutionary record in remarkably similar ways. In the remainder of this chapter, we explicate their parallel logics, tactics, and motivations.

In recognition of the difficult-to-navigate landscape of nutrition advice, many popular writers have sought to simplify healthy eating. Specifically, voices such as Mark Bittman, Michael Pollan, Walter Willett, Alice Waters, and others advocate for a more holistic approach to healthy eating. Emphasizing whole foods, cooking from scratch, and the importance of fresh fruits and vegetables, these "new mainstream" food experts argue that eating healthfully need not be nerve-racking. However, although these writers fault the classic USDA food pyramid for tacitly condoning processed foods by, for example, not differentiating between flavored and plain yogurt, they nonetheless reify its foundations by never seriously questioning the role of any macronutrient.

In contrast, primal and fruitarian communities encourage followers to eliminate, almost entirely, certain macronutrients from their plates. Fruitarians, with their more limited diet, are more extreme in this regard, as they refuse to eat not only animal fats and proteins but also plant foods high in those macronutrients. In their view, "fat makes you fat," and the human body's need for amino and fatty acids can be met simply through consuming ripe fruit and the occasional leafy vegetable.[28] The primal diet is less radical in that it allows for some carbohydrates, but followers are quite limited in the suggested sources for these carbohydrates. Leafy greens are acceptable, even celebrated, but all grains and starchy vegetables are strongly discouraged.

Some members drop carbohydrate intake so low that they enter ketosis in order to lose weight.[29]

As dissimilar as their specific diets are, the underlying logic of both fruitarianism and the primal diet reveals a shared distrust of not only conventional dietary standards but also the very position that mainstream nutritional science holds in society. When met with research or guidelines that contradict their views, each groups' respective members employ parallel tactics to discredit those sources. Members quickly point out methodological problems, such as sample size and the unreliability of nutritional self-reporting, or question funding sources. Fruitarians, for example, readily dismiss research funded by meat and dairy organizations, and individuals often post such studies specifically to solicit help in "debunking" them. When primal dieters encounter research that finds negative health effects associated with high-protein, low-carbohydrate diets, community members suggest that study participants consumed soybeans or processed meat, not the "right" kind of protein. Importantly, however, the mistrust that these communities hold toward mainstream nutritional science does not result in the wholesale rejection of peer-reviewed research. Rather, both groups rely heavily on favorable scientific evidence and frequently ask for advice on how to use science to convince nonadherents.[30]

Fruitarians and primal dieters' distrust of standard dietary guidelines merges with concerns about health as individual responsibility in divisive ways. Since each community believes that its diet represents the single best approach to eating, individuals who do not follow those proscriptions are necessarily also failing in their moral duty to safeguard health. Community members characterize nonadherents as mindless consumers who eat whatever they find in grocery stores, believe food labels without hesitation, and fail to question federal dietary guidelines. Interestingly, a great deal of criticism is also aimed specifically at opposing dietary communities. This jeering is particularly virulent at 30 Bananas a Day, which likely reflects fruitarians' position as a more marginalized dietary community than the comparatively mainstream Paleolithic and primal diets.[31]

WE EVOLVED TO BE FIT

Both communities rely on similar logics even as they arrive at markedly different conclusions. Specifically, followers of both diets delicately balance two related concepts as explanation for the superiority of their preferred diet.

First, members from each of these communities believe that their diet approximates how humans evolved to eat. This belief further assumes that following humankind's ancestral diet will necessarily result in optimum health for contemporary eaters. Second, each community believes that the lithe, muscular bodies its successful followers cultivate are evidence for the naturalness of their diet. As "natural" and "evolved" are equated with healthy, members further assume that a lean physique indicates well-being, while failing to achieve this body type suggests personal failure.

The primal diet begins with the assumption that most people living in high-income countries have abandoned the dietary habits of hunter-gatherers. Primal Blueprint adherents trace the origins of this shift back around ten thousand years to the Neolithic Revolution, when humans began to practice a more settled, agricultural lifestyle. They suggest that this shift heralded harmful changes to human lifestyles, including increased sedentism, a decline in dietary diversity, and greater reliance on cultivated grains. Primal dieters hold that the human genome has not caught up to these comparatively new diet and activity patterns. The standard American diet is even further removed from the conditions characterizing much of human evolution, and primal dieters blame this mismatch for increased chronic disease, obesity, and mortality rates.[32]

Fruitarians also rely on evolution to justify their diet's healthfulness but throw the dietary target several million years further in the past. For fruitarians, the most appropriate diet is the one practiced by humanity's closest living relatives: the great apes. According to fruitarians, the genetic and anatomical similarities between humans and apes demonstrate that we are, above all, frugivores. For example, fruitarians argue that human teeth are most similar to those of frugivorous mammals, as we lack large canines and exhibit molars useful for processing plant material. Similar conclusions are drawn via comparisons between humans, frugivores, and carnivores with respect to the presence or absence of particular salivary enzymes, intestine length, and facial structure. Although Paleolithic Grok may have eaten meat, fruitarians argue that human physiology still reflects an earlier, superior frugivory. Moreover, they believe that insufficient time has elapsed for humans to adequately adapt to any other diet, thus explaining the contemporary rise in chronic disease rates.[33]

Conceptually and discursively, both fruitarians and primal dieters conflate health and physique such that attaining the desired body type is *itself* considered confirmation of their diet's healthfulness. However, that bodily aesthetic is invariably the slender-yet-muscular build generally favored by contemporary Westerners.[34] Yet, throughout much of human history, the preference for lean bodies was likely anything but universal; rather, ethnographic research details the diversity of body-type preferences across cultures.[35] Indeed, many of the cultural groups assumed to practice a diet closest to the idealized consumption patterns of our human ancestors may very well have favored a physique different from those idealized by the online dietary communities in question. Thus, the outcome of the assumed evolutionarily best and universally appropriate diet promoted by each group is a culturally and historically specific beauty ideal.

Primal dieters usually assume that the healthiest bodies will be lean and muscular. The primal and CrossFit communities often overlap, and the forums at Mark's Daily Apple have an entire subsection devoted to fitness, where members compare the efficacy of different Paleolithic-inspired exercises. Community members regularly post before and after photographs as they lose weight and gain muscle definition. Fellow community members celebrate these photographs as evidence that the primal diet makes people healthier. The desire to "look good naked" is an oft-cited goal among forum members. People who are thin but do not adhere to primal principles are labeled "skinny fat"—that is, they look good in clothes but not naked, lack muscle definition, and (according to community logic) are probably at high risk of chronic disease. Slight differences exist in ideal body types for men and women, as community members frequently discuss how female physiology evolved to need a higher body fat percentage than men. On the whole, however, the primal community prefers and pursues a muscular, slim bodily aesthetic.[36]

Similarly, fruitarians at 30 Bananas a Day emphasize their diet's ability to help adherents "get lean." Leaders' lithe physiques are *the* key marketing strategy used in the community's online dietary evangelism. Freelee and Harley share images of their markedly thin, defined bodies, and several discussion threads on 30 Bananas a Day are devoted to sharing members' before and after pictures. Although new fruitarians sometimes complain about a lack of energy and mood swings after switching to a HCLFRV diet, perhaps the most common complaint is weight gain. In response, more established members advise that initial increases in weight are temporary while the body "detoxes" from the standard American diet. If individuals will just push through, they promise, weight loss will invariably result. In addition, fruitarians attribute weight gain or weight loss stagnation during 80/10/10 to insufficient caloric intake. They argue that the body needs carbohydrate-sourced calories to effectively burn fat. If an individual's carbohydrate consumption is inadequate, a larger waistline can be expected. Yet if fruitarianism is the healthiest diet, and if physique reflects health, then how does one explain skinny, fit nonvegans? How does one reconcile a fruitarian diet as best for health and physique when primal dieters employ similar, figure-focused evangelizing tactics and boast equally large numbers of weight-loss success stories? To explain this, fruitarians assume that individuals who achieve the idealized body type via alternative means teeter on the edge of cataclysmic failure (e.g., heart attack) and face long-term health problems.

This is not to say that online food communities ignore physical, emotional, or mental health. Both primal and fruitarian communities repeatedly emphasize that their diets are one part of a whole lifestyle approach to health. Getting plenty of sunlight, reducing stress, and remaining active are critical components of both plans. Moreover, in addition to figure-focused success stories, each diet attracts individuals through the plethora of testimonials about overcoming various health problems, from mental health and eating disorders to gastrointestinal issues and skin concerns.[37]

The fruitarian and primal diet communities discussed here have developed as parallel responses to contemporary cultural pressures. These pressures include discourse linking individual moral responsibility to health, media-fueled public anxiety regarding diet-related illness, and an ever-shifting landscape of official nutritional advice. The virtue that individuals feel in achieving the slim physique currently popular in Western contexts merges with the satisfaction they derive from following the diet humans evolved to consume. Together, these underlying beliefs lead adherents to feel that they have (re)discovered the "one food truth." Moreover, the presumed simplicity, constancy, and naturalness of eating the diet humans were designed to eat offers followers an empowering alternative to mainstream dietary advice. While radically different dietary rules prevent them from sharing a meal, these communities ultimately travel the same path.

NOTES

1. Loren Cordain, *The Paleo Diet: Lose Weight and Get Healthy by Eating the Foods You Were Designed to Eat*, 2nd ed. (Hoboken, NJ: John Wiley & Sons, 2011).

2. Mark Sisson, "Introducing the New Primal Blueprint Food Pyramid," Mark's Daily Apple, November 3, 2011, http://www.marksdailyapple.com/introducing-the-new-primal-blueprint-food-pyramid/#axzz3m1cShXqQ.

3. Mark Sisson, "Definitive Guide: The Primal Blueprint," Mark's Daily Apple, June 4, 2008, http://www.marksdailyapple.com/definitive-guide-primal-blueprint/.

4. Mark Sisson, "Remember the 80-20 Principle," Mark's Daily Apple, September 15, 2010, http://www.marksdailyapple.com/remember-the-80-20-principle/.

5. www.30bananasaday.com, accessed October 1, 2015.

6. Gabriel Cousens, *Rainbow Green Live-Food Cuisine* (Berkeley: North Atlantic Books, 2003).

7. Douglas Graham, *The 80/10/10 Diet: Balancing Your Health, Your Weight, and Your Life One Luscious Bite at a Time* (Key Largo: FoodNSport Press, 2006).

8. www.30bananasaday.com, accessed October 1, 2015.

9. www.30bananasaday.com, accessed October 1, 2015.

10. T. Colin Campbell, *The China Study: The Most Comprehensive Study of Nutrition Ever Conducted and the Startling Implications for Diet, Weight Loss and Long-Term Health* (Dallas: BenBella Books, 2004).

11. Graham, *The 80/10/10 Diet.*

12. www.30bananasaday.com, accessed October 1, 2015.

13. "USDA National Nutrient Database for Standard Reference, Release 28," United States Department of Agriculture, Agricultural Research Service, Nutrient Data Laboratory, http://www.ars.usda.gov/nea/bhnrc/ndl, accessed September 2015.

14. www.30bananasaday.com, accessed October 1, 2015.

15. Campbell, *The China Study.*

16. www.30bananasaday.com, accessed October 1, 2015.

17. Leanne Ratcliffe, *Raw Till 4 Diet—Banana Girl Cleanse*, self-published ebook, 2016.

18. www.30bananasaday.com, accessed October 1, 2015.

19. www.30bananasaday.com, accessed October 1, 2015.

20. Ratcliffe, *Raw Till 4 Diet.*

21. www.30bananasaday.com, accessed October 1, 2015.

22. David Grotto and Elisa Zied, "The Standard American Diet and Its Relationship to the Health Status of Americans," *Nutrition in Clinical Practice* 25, no. 6 (2010): 603–12.

23. Marion Nestle, *What to Eat* (New York: North Point Press, 2006), 4.

24. Bryan Walsh, "Don't Blame Fat," *Time*, June 23, 2014.

25. Colleen L. Barry, Victoria L. Brescoll, Kelly D. Brownell, and Mark Schlesinger, "Obesity Metaphors: How Beliefs about the Causes of Obesity Affect Support for Public Policy," *Milbank Quarterly* 87, no. 1 (2009): 7–47.

26. Barry et al., "Obesity Metaphors."

27. Jan Wright, "Biopower, Biopedagogies and the Obesity Epidemic," in *Biopolitics and the "Obesity Epidemic": Governing Bodies*, ed. Jan Wright and Valerie Harwood (New York: Routledge, 2009), 1–14; Michel Foucault, *Discipline and Punish: The Birth of the Prison* (New York: Vintage Books, 1977).

28. www.30bananasaday.com, accessed October 1, 2015.

29. http://www.marksdailyapple.com/forum, accessed October 1, 2015.

30. www.30bananasaday.com, accessed October 1, 2015; http://www.marksdailyapple.com/forum, accessed October 1, 2015.

31. www.30bananasaday.com, accessed October 1, 2015.

32. http://www.marksdailyapple.com/forum, accessed October 1, 2015.

33. www.30bananasaday.com, accessed October 1, 2015.

34. www.30bananasaday.com, accessed October 1, 2015; http://www.marksdailyapple.com/forum, accessed October 1, 2015.

35. Elisa Sobo, "The Sweetness of Fat: Health, Procreation, and Sociability in Rural Jamaica," in *Many Mirrors: Body Image and Social Meaning*, ed. Nicole Sault (Brunswick, NJ: Rutgers University Press, 1994), 132–54; Rebecca Popenoe, *Feeding Desire: Fatness, Beauty and Sexuality among a Saharan People* (New York: Routledge, 2004); Alexandra A. Brewis, Amber Wutich, Ashlan Falletta-Cowden, and Isa Rodriguez-Soto, "Body Norms and Fat Stigma in Global Perspective," *Current Anthropology* 52, no. 2 (2011): 269–76.

36. http://www.marksdailyapple.com/forum, accessed October 1, 2015.

37. www.30bananasaday.com, accessed October 1, 2015.

BIBLIOGRAPHY

30 Bananas a Day. http://www.30bananasaday.com.

Barry, Colleen L., Victoria L. Brescoll, Kelly D. Brownell, and Mark Schlesinger. "Obesity Metaphors: How Beliefs about the Causes of Obesity Affect Support for Public Policy." *Milbank Quarterly* 87, no. 1 (2009): 7–47.

Brewis, Alexandra A., Amber Wutich, Ashlan Falletta-Cowden, and Isa Rodriguez-Soto. "Body Norms and Fat Stigma in Global Perspective." *Current Anthropology* 52, no. 2 (2011): 269–76.

Campbell, T. Colin. *The China Study: The Most Comprehensive Study of Nutrition Ever Conducted and the Startling Implications for Diet, Weight Loss and Long-Term Health*. Dallas: BenBella Books, 2004.

Cordain, Loren. *The Paleo Diet: Lose Weight and Get Healthy by Eating the Foods You Were Designed to Eat*. 2nd ed. Hoboken, NJ: John Wiley & Sons, 2011.

Cousens, Gabriel. *Rainbow Green Live-Food Cuisine*. Berkeley: North Atlantic Books, 2003.

Foucault, Michel. *Discipline and Punish: The Birth of the Prison*. New York: Vintage Books, 1977.

Graham, Douglas. *The 80/10/10 Diet: Balancing Your Health, Your Weight, and Your Life One Luscious Bite at a Time*. Key Largo: FoodNSport Press, 2006.

Grotto, David, and Elisa Zied. "The Standard American Diet and Its Relationship to the Health Status of Americans." *Nutrition in Clinical Practice* 25, no. 6 (2010): 603–12.

Nestle, Marion. *What to Eat*. New York: North Point Press, 2006.

Popenoe, Rebecca. *Feeding Desire: Fatness, Beauty and Sexuality among a Saharan People*. New York: Routledge, 2004.

Ratcliffe, Leanne. *Raw Till 4 Diet—Banana Girl Cleanse*. Self-published ebook, 2016.

Sisson, Mark. "Definitive Guide: The Primal Blueprint." Mark's Daily Apple, June 4, 2008. http://www.marksdailyapple.com/definitive-guide-primal-blueprint.

Sisson, Mark. "Introducing the New Primal Blueprint Food Pyramid." Mark's Daily Apple, November 3, 2011. http://www.marksdailyapple.com/introducing-the-new-primal-blueprint-food-pyramid/#axzz3m1cShXqQ.

Sisson, Mark. "Remember the 80-20 Principle." Mark's Daily Apple, September 5, 2010. http://www.marksdailyapple.com/remember-the-80-20-principle.

Sobo, Elisa. "The Sweetness of Fat: Health, Procreation, and Sociability in Rural Jamaica." In *Many Mirrors: Body Image and Social Meaning*, edited by Nicole Sault, 132–54. Brunswick, NJ: Rutgers University Press, 1994.

United States Department of Agriculture. Agricultural Research Service, Nutrient Data Laboratory. "USDA National Nutrient Database for Standard Reference, Release 28." September 2015. http://www.ars.usda.gov/nea/bhnrc/ndl.

Walsh, Bryan. "Don't Blame Fat." *Time*, June 23, 2014.

Wright, Jan. "Biopower, Biopedagogies and the Obesity Epidemic." In *Biopolitics and the "Obesity Epidemic": Governing Bodies*, edited by Jan Wright and Valerie Harwood, 1–14. New York: Routledge, 2009.

Chapter Ten

Eschew Your Food

Foodies, Healthism, and the Elective Restrictive Diet

Michele Scott

Socially acceptable instances of food restriction are not a modern invention, evidenced in the writings of Plato and the food diaries of Renaissance-era artist Pontormo.[1] Since these ancient examples, various conceptualizations of health have solidified the connection between morality,[2] health, and the physical body.[3] What seems to be a more recent phenomenon is the food cult: an identity-based association with particular patterns of eating that, despite no ties to any specific religion, are met with similar fervor.

For the purposes of this chapter, I discuss a specific type of "food cult" that I call the "elective restrictive diet" (ERD) and define it as restrictive patterns of eating for reasons other than allergy or direct medical necessity. More specifically, I discuss vegan diets, or those forgoing all animal byproducts, including meat, dairy, eggs, and sometimes honey. I do so in contrast with the Paleolithic (paleo) diet, which shuns all grains, legumes, dairy, and processed foods in favor of lean protein, vegetables, and "good" fats. Though these restrictions are often related to health by their followers, they are not motivated by a direct allergy to specific foods. Because veganism and paleo appear diametrically opposed themselves, comparing these food cults sharpens patterns in unique and useful ways. Specifically, I analyze components of each related to foodies and healthism, and subsequently, links between diet, identity, and neoliberal ideals.

Understanding foodies, healthism, and neoliberalism helps tease out common threads within the contradictory impulses between vegan and paleo diets, including dieters' motivations and justifications as well as the social construction of the diets themselves. Broadly speaking, this allows a richer understanding of the way that neoliberal discourse and policy are affecting the lived experience of individuals. Scholars in a variety of subfields extol the salience of eating practices and food to discussions of culture,[4] politics, economics, place,[5] ideology, emotion, sexuality, eroticism, taste, gender,[6] class, social movements, social justice, family, history, tradition, ethnicity, race, nationalism,[7] tradition, innovation, and development.[8] In turn, social scientists understand restrictive eating patterns in terms of risk society, morality, healthism, mental health,[9] neoliberalism, traditional femininity,[10] Western standards of beauty, processes of civilization, propriety, good taste, piety,[11] religiosity,[12] and identity work, especially those related to gender and class.[13]

It is important to note in each of these cases that restriction is also a sign of morality, goodness, worth, and proper performance. Directly related to religion or not, members of food cults mobilize religious language to justify their practices and habits that might otherwise imply disordered eating. The way we talk about food shows that food shapes the stories about our lives just as much as it shapes the lives themselves, but I argue that the way we talk about what we refuse to eat tells similar stories. More specifically, I argue that the pursuit of godliness and goodness through restriction can be increasingly understood through the lens of the food cult—in this case, the particular iteration I call the "elective restrictive diet."

FOODIES: JUSTIFYING AND ENCOURAGING OBSESSION

Individuals with religious obsession to food can be understood as foodies, whether it be through an impetus to "be modern: worship food"[14] or devotion to the "gospel[s] of food."[15] Many foodies self-identify as such, citing intellectual, physical, sensual, and obsessive relationships to what they eat. Such individuals mark milestones from vacations[16] to birthdays through memorable encounters with cuisine[17] and cultivate new relationships through sharing meals.[18] Even homes show evidence of how foodies construct their lives differently, boasting larger kitchens, more appliances, and, in an extreme case, a special kitchen solely for sausage making.[19] Whether it be producing, consuming, or analyzing food, these processes are vital to the foodie experience of ordinary life and the consequential understanding of the self. Even places change with enough exposure to the foodie gaze.[20]

Food, then, must be entertaining and intellectually stimulating, but with particular focus on qualities of exoticism and authenticity. Foodies create moral dichotomies based on such criteria,[21] with the same enthusiasm that fuels food trends like fondue, cupcakes, and a curious obsession with bacon.[22] Ultimately, whether called "foodies," "tastemakers," or "food adventurers," importance lies in the evaluation of food on moral terms, and a subsequent obsession with whatever is deemed "good."

However, food also exists in political contexts, with the increasing momentum of the alternative food movement a key example. As demonstrated in the push for organics, GMO (genetically modified organism) labeling,[23] local purchasing, and "Slow Food,"[24] eating can be a stage for social justice and social action.[25] One battle cry commonly associated with these movements ("Vote with your dollar!") emphasizes good citizenship through proper consumption and links an ability to make personal choices that will elicit structural change. Critics of the alternative food movement observe that these changes rarely materialize, and market-based solutions cannot fix the market itself.[26] For foodies, good choices indicate an intellectual understanding of complex yet vague issues like sustainability, genetic engineering, fair trade, and organic processes, and are, when merged with tenets of the alternative food movement, infused with genuine belief in the power of choice to elicit social change.[27] To this end, alternative food movements can be more accurately understood as consumerism steeped in liberating rhetoric and occasional philanthropy.[28]

Though many experts deny that market mechanics achieve social justice,[29] for the argument in this chapter, it is equally important to understand that foodies often perceive alternative markets with genuine confidence that is inextricable from their understandings of themselves as upstanding, ethical citizens. Criticism, however, points directly at this mentality, noting that attaching identity and morality to eating habits prevents honest and objective evaluation of alternative food movements and programming.[30] With foodways framed both ethically and politically, food choices become a road diverged. One path is ethical, one is not; one inspires self-satisfaction, the other inspires guilt. Desire to improve the food system drives these impulses, but there is a twin desire to elevate the self into a more thoughtful, moral consumer and citizen.[31] I argue that food cults in general are worthy of similar critique, and especially the elective restrictive diet and its borrowing of religious rhetoric and operationalization of moralistic metaphors.

HEALTHISM AND THE MORALIZATION OF CHOICE

The term *healthism* describes an intense moralization of personal health, with particular focus on personal choice and responsibility.[32] Constant personal surveillance is requisite, demanded in order to achieve ever-increasing degrees of healthiness.[33] The advent of "m-health," or mobile health, increases the ability to quantify the body, and the pervasiveness of such devices increases the pressure to the participant.[34] The result is a consumer-patient, who must practice self-care through self-monitoring, self-surveillance, and self-discipline. The body mass index (BMI) requires special attention, as thinness is conflated with heath, allowing body size to become an observable indicator of moral superiority via good health. Thus, restriction becomes the focus of intellectual effort devoted to food choices, requiring religious commitment and sophisticated awareness of what should, or should not, be consumed.[35] Interestingly, some consider preoccupation with health and diet to be a food trend, with critics particularly attentive to how science is manipulated in service of certain restrictive diets.

Perhaps unsurprisingly, the religious ethos related to health extends into more deliberate religious rhetoric. Criticism specifically focuses on the diet industry and the use of such language to symbolically attach goodness, moral superiority, and self-worth to a bodily aesthetic—namely, one that is thin.[36] These rhetorical tactics offer thinness as a "form of salvation" and are subsequently achieved through ritual and rules more commonly associated with Christianity. Specifically, "dietary theology" marries the "moral logic" of religion that associates restriction and piety to conceptual understandings of health. Moralizing positive health outcomes, attaching health to thinness, and demanding perpetual pursuit of better health are all underwritten by deliberately religious language and a complex theology regarding diet.

Moral and religious overtones, coupled with individual achievement as a core value, make healthism a compelling ethos, but they also position individuals against a deliberate "other" in those who are unhealthy, with their poor personal choices and missteps earning varying degrees of disapproval and disgust.[37] The quantified self in particular is a key element in the medicalization of obesity and its framing as an "epidemic," via the BMI as gospel in the measurement and assessment of health. Subsequently, thinness is the gold star and reward to the individual that achieves good health.[38]

If the theoretical picture of healthism involves individualism and moralization, the practical manifestations include reducing nutrition to nutrients and health to quantifiable biomarkers. Without context, however, blood sugar, cholesterol levels, BMI, and even the human genome say little about health.[39] In more extreme cases, nutritional rhetoric makes claims about food's ability to cure and prevent disease.[40] The danger of this situation lies not only in forgoing more aggressive (but tested) treatments but also in the "orthorexic society"[41] that is pathologically obsessed with health. Again, joy associated with eating is obscured by an understanding of food only as it relates to the body, reinforcing bodily aesthetic as a primary idol.

All of these processes occur within the larger discussion of healthism, attaching personal choice to intrinsic morality, emphasizing health as a consummate indicator of strength of character and personal morality. Once again, the citizen is rebranded as a consumer, and health care is available for purchase in the market. Individualism is a crucial ideology in this model, as the assumed system relies on self-preservation and the pursuit of personal goodness to yield social good.[42] The health of the collective, then, improves only when each individual makes choices for themselves that result in good health. Because health and thinness are so inextricably linked,[43] much of this individualization translates to the consideration of how food choices affect the physical body. Evidenced by an aesthetic of the physical body, the assumption remains that few forces outside of personal choice matter, and food continues to be a significant path to self-improvement. Thus, fat bodies are built from the accumulation of poor choices; skinny bodies require commitment to good choices.[44]

Feminist critiques call attention to the "embodied neoliberalism" found in the framing of restriction as a positive and proactive choice and the self-imposed diet restrictions. Even further, tensions exist within the individual, who is caught between personal discipline and an alleged freedom of consumer choice when making decisions about what and, more important, what not to eat. The "do diet" imprisons women in their own bodies by constructing boundaries between good and bad, thin and fat, edible and not, while simultaneously appointing women as wardens.[45] In sum, healthism serves to rationalize, justify, and even glorify dietary restrictions by creating an ideology that values piety and religious fervor regarding health and positions an idealized body as a divine reward. Within this ideology, the ability to restrict food intake becomes a badge of honor.

NEOLIBERALISM: THE TIE THAT BINDS

Neoliberalism is part ideology, part political project, and is characterized by supporters as a powerful form of capitalism through free markets, and by its critics as the systematic redistribution of wealth to elites.[46] Examples from global food policies over the last several decades help untangle the complexities of how related policies have shaped individual lives, from global food insecurity to the more pointed food crisis in 2007. The alternative food movement discussed in relation to foodies, then, is in many ways a reaction to neoliberalism, globalization, and the damage the food systems have suffered as a result of deregulation. The flaws in alternative food movements demonstrate the distinction between the neoliberal *ideology* and *project*, with elements of the project deliberately forsaken, even as the ideology remains. Relentless faith in markets, affirmed through focus on the individual's duty to perform correctly within the market, is a key tenant in the guiding ethos of alternative food. So even though the market mechanics may operate somewhat differently, the market remains, relying on social norms, moral values, and emotional manipulation to recruit support, and it shifts burdens to citizens as consumers.[47]

Though these policies began in the 1930s, neoliberalism as we know it today gained most of its momentum in the era of Ronald Reagan and Margaret Thatcher, when arguments that unrestricted markets were more effective and efficient. Since then, the health care system has changed dramatically. Messages about the role of the state in relation to individuals and their health have changed as well. Privatizing and commodifying care makes health. In practice, neoliberal health policies use language that justifies for-profit models and competitiveness by citing state-based inefficiencies, escalating costs, and the inevitability of a declining welfare state.[48] Once again, the citizen is rebranded as a consumer, and health care is commodified, available exclusively in the market. Thus, health care in a free-market system relies on self-indulgent pursuits of personal goodness to accumulate and yield social good.[49] Collective entities are improved when, and only when, each individual makes choices for themselves that result in good health. Recalling ties between health and thinness, much of this individualization translates to consideration of how food choices affect the physical body. With the assumption that few forces outside of personal choice matter, food remains a significant path to self-improvement, evidenced by an aesthetic of the physical body. Alternatively stated, neoliberal health policy works to burden the individual with their health outcomes by privatizing and deregulating care in favor of free-market policies.

These "embodied" ideologies, specifically those related to neoliberalism, underwrite and reinforce values of foodies and healthism alike. In theory, neoliberalism is related to the privatization of health care, prioritization of free markets, and the politicization of individual choice. In practice, the impetus to "vote with your dollar" and the idea that health is a personal responsibility are quintessential examples of how neoliberalism plays out in everyday life. Moralization of food comes from both sides: from the foodie, who demands democracy through exoticism and authenticity, and the healthism devotee, who eats to fulfill a moral imperative of health. In sum, the neoliberal ideology moralizes personal choice as righteous obligation. Foodies and healthism can be understood as simultaneously derivative of and contributing to neoliberal governance and policy, especially as related to bodily health and diet. As neoliberalism tightens its grasp on identities, understandings of food,[50] health, and the relationship between the two become increasingly individualistic.[51]

At the intersection of foodie-ism and healthism, catalyzed by these highly individualistic values, lies a specific type of food cult, the elective restrictive diet (ERD), veganism and paleo being two key examples. These diets incorporate the foodie's political and social attachment to food but also glorify the pervasive restriction and moralization seen in healthism. Ideology is the common denominator, with its messages about individualism, personal choice, and emphasis on the citizen-consumer providing structure for the more specific information about the diets, and why they qualify as healthy.

Importantly, neoliberal policies were necessary in priming society for foodies and for healthism, as they shift responsibility for public issues like health, food security, food safety, and workers' rights onto the shoulders of the individual, emphasizing the significance of personal choice. More specifically, both foodies and healthism can be reframed as practical applications of the neoliberal politicization of individual choice and together inspire religious devotion to restrictive diets: the food cults we can understand as "elective restrictive diets."

ERDs: FOOD CULTS FOR THE HEALTH OBSESSED

The expectation would be to find no foodies in the realm of the ERD. Because restriction is more commonly understood as a part of healthism, mealtimes are assumed to simply deliver the appropriate balance of nutrients in the name of health and performance. But instead of finding tensions between culinary omnivorism and restriction, there seems to be deliberate embracing of both foodie ideologies and healthism among those following an ERD. Despite inherent contradictions, many individuals who seem to embody the ideals of healthism self-identify as foodies. This phenomenon is observable in the online presence of veganism and paleo, specifically in the realm of food blogs. Vegan[52] and paleo[53] bloggers both unapologetically claim to be foodies, with the word recurring mundanely in the text of individual posts but also deliberately in blog titles and descriptions. Placing flavor, culture, and pleasure at the forefront of discussions about food, even in conversations about restriction, works to overcome objections that restriction is inherently disordered and that the ERD is a positive manifestation of a range of personal values and interests. Elements of religion shine through in three major ways.

In further embrace of the foodie identity, both vegan and paleo eaters emphasize food choices that fit into "authentic" and "exotic" frames, but each choice is simultaneously framed with health benefits. Both diets claim that their culinary ethos is more natural, historically accurate, and, importantly, superior to other diets because it represents authentic eating. For vegans, the diet is more "natural" because consuming animal protein requires manipulative cooking processes in order to yield a product safe for consumption, whereas fruits, vegetables, and grains are safe to eat in their natural state.[54] Additionally, supporters of veganism cite physiological evidence such as tooth shape and size, fingernails, jaw structure, stomach acidity, and even length of the intestinal track as more similar to herbivores in nature than carnivores.[55]

Conversely, followers of the paleo diet cite physiological, historical, anthropological, cultural, and philosophical reasons for why their diet is a more authentic way for humans to eat, indicting modern agriculture and food science for an array of contemporary health concerns like obesity, heart disease, diabetes, and depression.[56] Prehistoric man's "ancient wisdom"[57] to avoid grains, sugar, and additives add credence to further observations that early farmers were shorter than "cave men," had poorer dental health, and experienced disease epidemics that were unknown in generations past.[58] To this end, "authenticity" in the ERD world implies a way of eating that is authentically *human*, and thus healthier, as it does not compete with "natural" processes in the body. Like many religions, it highlights the errors of modern living and encourages a type of purity through returning to what humans were created to be.

Exerting influence from the other side of foodie-ism is exoticism, which manifests differently in ERDs than in the lives of the more typical foodie. The more "cultish" aspects of the ERD—namely, severe restriction—are at odds with the omnivorous ethos of the foodie and the pursuit of the exotic. So foodies inside the cult of the ERD perform both roles simultaneously by seeking out odd, unique, and hard-to-find foods that aid in the perpetual pursuit of better health. This can include foods that are unusual, as well as foods that are prepared and consumed in atypical ways or that require exceptional effort to obtain.

For vegans, among these specialized foods are spirulina and chlorella powders. Both are species of algae that contain a plant-based source of protein, amino acids, a host of B vitamins, and other micronutrients. Spirulina and chlorella are touted as "nutrient-dense" foods and can be supplemented via tablet or powder. Often, vegans suggest adding the half-teaspoon dose to smoothies to cover up the potent flavor and smell; it is not consumed for its contribution to flavor profile, but rather for its health value.[59] Increasingly, spirulina and chlorella are available at health food stores and natural groceries, with online retailers filling gaps, but their acquisition is unlikely to be accidental. The deliberate effort required to obtain spirulina and chlorella demonstrates their exotic nature, and their contribution to health justifies it.

Paleo dieters, with their emphasis on animal protein, commonly recommend including organ meats in the diet on a regular basis. Beef tongue, liver, heart, cheek, and kidney meat are all among suggested superfoods. While some related dishes, like liver pate, have been consumed as delicacies historically, most are not a part of the standard American diet. Devoted paleo eaters refer to organ meats as "adventurous" cuts that are either an acquired taste or something to be consumed in spite of whatever aversions may arise.[60] Here, the adventurous spirit of the foodie is implored to encourage consumption of the unpalatable. For both vegans and paleo eaters, it becomes clear that "exoticism" means sourcing better health via unlikely, atypical, or hard-to-find food items. Much like a religious pilgrimage, the quest for exotic means of improving health becomes a rite of passage for members of food cults within the ERD frame.

Vague promises of "better" health are offered by vegans and paleo eaters alike, with increased energy, sharper focus, improved athletic performance, and better sleep among more frequent claims,[61] while specific claims evoke healthism's fixation on physical biomarkers. According to certain sources for both diets, blood pressure can be lowered, blood sugar regulated, weight loss achieved, and life spans lengthened. Even further, ERDs are sometimes presented as cures for conditions as serious as cancer, autoimmune diseases, multiple sclerosis, diabetes, and depression. Obsession with food is justified, if not demanded, and restrictive efforts can be imagined with the same taken-for-grantedness as brushing your teeth. Elective restrictive diets offer the individual a chance to be "born again" in terms of personal health, freed from the grips of illness and physical imperfection alike.

YOU ARE WHAT YOU (DON'T) EAT

The paleo diet and the vegan diet are often assumed to be diametrically opposed personal ethos. However, when both are understood as iterations of the larger categories of elective restrictive diets and "food cults," similarities emerge. It becomes evident that the food involved is far less important than how choices about food are constructed and, in turn, how the self is constructed in light of those choices. In ERDs, food is worthy of consumption if it embodies twin roles: the foodie's obsession with food and healthism's demand for nutritional integrity. If those following either diet can effectively demonstrate dedication to restriction, the neoliberal ideology providing frameworks of individual achievement and personal responsibility rewards them with moral standing comparable to that seen with religious piety.

In the United States today, there are currently more households that identify as "gluten-free" than as kosher.[62] Anecdotal evidence is certain, but nevertheless it is an indicator that primary ideologies in Americans are shifting to a new "religion." As neoliberal ideology becomes ever more present in social discourse, individuals increasingly embody and internalize relationships between their personal choices, their self-worth, and the outcomes of their lives. Though ideological obsession with diet and restriction of food in pursuit of morality are not symptoms of modernity, I argue that the elevation of such practices to "food cult" status is a result of how internalized these ideologies have become. Elective restrictive diets are, in many ways, severe versions of self-surveillance. They require significant effort but simultaneously simplify the process by eliminating offenders and justifying restriction. Like religion, neoliberalism is an ideology, internalized by the individual in similar ways. The food cult is simply one operationalization of this more general concept.

NOTES

1. P. K. Skiadas and J. G. Lascaratos, "Dietetics in Ancient Greek Philosophy," *European Journal of Clinical Nutrition* 55 (2001): 532–37; Ken Albala, *Eating Right in the Renaissance* (Berkeley: University of California Press, 2002).

2. Charlotte Biltekoff, *Eating Right in America* (Durham, NC: Duke University Press, 2013).

3. Abigail C. Saguy, *What's Wrong with Fat?* (Oxford: Oxford University Press, 2013).

4. Albala, *Eating Right in the Renaissance*.

5. Josée Johnston, Alexandra Rodney, and Michelle Szabo, "Place, Ethics, and Everyday Eating: A Tale of Two Neighbourhoods," *Sociology* 46 (2012): 1091–108.

6. Deborah Lupton, *Food, the Body and the Self* (Thousand Oaks, CA: Sage, 1996).

7. Lucy Long, "Culinary Tourism: A Folklorist Perspective on Eating and Otherness," in *Culinary Tourism*, edited by Lucy Long (Lexington: University Press of Kentucky, 2004).

8. Priscilla Parkhurst Ferguson, *Word of Mouth* (Oakland: University of California Press, 2014).

9. C. Rangle, S. Dukeshire, and L. MacDonald, "Diet and Anxiety," *Appetite* 58 (2012): 124–32.

10. Kate Cairns and Josée Johnston, "Choosing Health," *Theory and Society* 44 (2015): 153–75.

11. Emily J. H. Contois, "Guilt-Free and Sinfully Delicious," *Fat Studies* 4 (2015): 112–26.

12. Miri Rotkovitz, "'Kosher Treif,' and the Observant American Jew," in *Culinary Tourism*, edited by Lucy Long (Lexington: University Press of Kentucky, 2004).

13. Kandi Stinson, *Women and Dieting Culture* (New Brunswick, NJ: Rutgers University Press, 2001).

14. Ann Barr and Paul Levy, *The Official Foodie Handbook* (London: Ebury Press, 1984).

15. Barry Glassner, *The Gospel of Food* (New York: Harper Perennial, 2007).

16. Donald Getz, Tommy Andersson, Richard Robinson, and Sanja Vujicic, *Foodies and Food Tourism* (Oxford: Goodfellow, 2014).

17. Long, "Culinary Tourism."

18. Josée Johnston and Shyon Baumann, *Foodies* (Florence, KY: Routledge, 2009).

19. Katy McLaughlin, "Foodie Cities," *Wall Street Journal*, September 11, 2014.

20. Amy Hanser and Zachary Hyde, "Foodies Remaking Cities," *Contexts* 13 (2014): 44–49.

21. Glassner, *The Gospel of Food*.

22. David Sax, *The Tastemakers* (New York: PublicAffairs, 2014).

23. Julie Guthman, "The Polanyian Way?" *Antipode* 39 (2007): 456–78; Craig Dublin Macmillan, "Genetically Modified Foods, Personal Values, Perceptions of Morality, and the Effects of Self-Confrontation on That Stability of Personal Values" (PhD diss., Washington State University, 2012).

24. Carlo Petrini, *Slow Food: The Case for Taste* (New York: Columbia University Press, 2001).

25. Kristen Lyons, Tabatha Wallington, and Geoffrey Lawrence, *Food Security, Nutrition and Sustainability* (London: Earthscan, 2009).

26. Daniel Jaffee and Philip Howard, "Corporate Cooptation of Organic and Fair Trade Standards," *Agriculture and Human Values* 27 (2010): 387–99.

27. Jafee and Howard, "Corporate Cooptation."

28. Josée Johnston, "The Citizen-Consumer Hybrid," *Theory and Society* 37 (2008): 229–70; Laura DeLind, "Are Local Food and the Local Food Movement Taking Us Where We Want to Go?" *Agriculture and Human Values* 28 (2011): 273–83.

29. C. Hinrichs, "Embeddedness and Local Food Systems," *Journal of Rural Studies* 16 (2000): 295–303; Guthman, "The Polanyian Way?"; Jafee and Howard, "Corporate Cooptation"; DeLind, "Local Food."

30. DeLind, "Local Food."

31. Julie Guthman, "Neoliberalism and the Making of Food Politics in California," *Geoforum* 39 (2008): 1171–83; Johnston, "The Citizen-Consumer Hybrid."

32. B. Crawford, "Healthism," *International Journal of Health Services* 10 (1980): 365–88; Julie Guthman, *Weighing In* (Berkeley: University of California Press, 2011), 57–59.

33. Deborah Lupton, *Imperative of Health* (London: Sage, 1995).

34. Deborah Lupton, "M-Health and Health Promotion," *Social Theory & Health* 10 (2012): 229–44.

35. Guthman, *Weighing In*; Contois, "Guilt-Free and Sinfully Delicious."

36. Contois, "Guilt-Free and Sinfully Delicious."

37. Guthman, *Weighing In*; Deborah Lupton, "The Pedagogy of Disgust," *Critical Public Health* 25 (2014): 4–14.

38. Guthman, *Weighing In*; Saguy, *What's Wrong with Fat?*; Biltekoff, *Eating Right in America*.

39. Gyorgy Scrinis, "On the Ideology of Nutritionism," *Gastronomica* (2008): 39–48; Jacqueline Savard, "Personalised Medicine," *Journal of Bioethical Inquiry* 10 (2013): 197–203.

40. Lyons, Wallington, and Lawrence, *Food Security*; Michaela DeSoucey and David Schleifer, "Technique and Technology in the Kitchen," *Studies in Law, Politics, and Society* 51 (2010): 185–218.

41. Rangle, Dukeshire, and MacDonald, "Diet and Anxiety."

42. Sue McGregor, "Neoliberalism and Health Care," *International Journal of Consumer Studies* 25 (2001): 82–89; James McCarthy and Scott Prudham, "Neoliberal Nature and the Nature of Neoliberalism," *Geoforum* 35 (2004): 275–83.

43. Susan Bordo, "Feminism, Foucault and the Politics of the Body," in *Up Against Foucault: Explorations of Some Tensions between Foucault and Feminism*, edited by Caroline Ramazanoglu (London: Routledge, 1993).

44. Julie Guthman and Melanie DuPuis, "Embodying Neoliberalism," *Environment and Planning D: Society and Space* 24, no. 3 (2006): 427–48; Saguy, *What's Wrong with Fat?*

45. Cairns and Johnston, "Choosing Health."

46. David Harvey, *A Brief History of Neoliberalism* (London: Oxford University Press, 2007).

47. Harvey, *A Brief History of Neoliberalism*; Martha Crowley and Randy Hodson, "Neoliberalism at Work," *Social Currents* 1 (2014).

48. McGregor, "Neoliberalism and Health Care."

49. McCarthy and Prudham, "Neoliberal Nature and the Nature of Neoliberalism."

50. Guthman, "Neoliberalism and the Making of Food Politics"; Johnston, "The Citizen-Consumer Hybrid."

51. Julianne Cheek, "Healthism: A New Conservatism?" *Qualitative Health Research* 18 (2008): 974–82; Guthman and DuPuis, "Embodying Neoliberalism."

52. Jay Astafa, "About," *The Vegan Foodie* (blog); Kele Webner, "About," *Vegan Foodies* (blog).

53. Juli Bauer, "About Me—Juli," *PaleOMG* (blog); Emily Busenitz, "30 Things about Me," *Practical Paleo* (blog); Jenny Castaneda, "About," *Paleo Foodie Kitchen* (blog).

54. Kimberly Snyder, *The Beauty Detox Solution* (Don Mills, Ontario: Harlequin, 2011); Brennan Braizer, *Thrive* (Toronto: Penguin Group, 2007).

55. PETA, "The Natural Human Diet," http://www.peta.org/living/food/natural-human-diet.

56. Robb Wolf, *The Paleo Solution* (Auberry: Victory Belt Publishers, 2010); Melissa and Dallas Hartwig, *It Starts with Food* (Auberry: Victory Belt Publishers, 2012).

57. John Durant, *The Paleo Manifesto* (New York: Penguin Random House, 2013).

58. Elizabeth Kolbert, "Stone Soup," *New Yorker*, July 28, 2014.

59. Snyder, *The Beauty Detox Solution*; Braizer, *Thrive*.

60. Chris Kresser, "How to Eat More Organ Meats," *Chris Kresser—Let's Take Back Your Health* (blog).

61. Braizer, *Thrive*; David Asprey, *The Bulletproof Diet* (Emmaus: Rodale, 2014).

62. Michael Schulson, "Diet Fads Are Destroying Us," *Salon*, May 3, 2015.

BIBLIOGRAPHY

Albala, Ken. *Eating Right in the Renaissance.* Berkeley: University of California Press, 2002.

Asprey, David. *The Bulletproof Diet*. Emmaus: Rodale, 2014.

Astafa, Jay. "About." *The Vegan Foodie* (blog), 2012. http://theveganfoodie.wordpress.com/.

Barr, Ann, and Paul Levy. *The Official Foodie Handbook.* London: Ebury Press, 1984.

Bauer, Juli. "About Me—Juli." *PaleOMG* (blog), 2014. http://paleomg.com/about-me/.

Biltekoff, Charlotte. *Eating Right in America: The Cultural Politics of Food and Health.* Durham, NC: Duke University Press, 2013.

Bordo, Susan. "Feminism, Foucault and the Politics of the Body." In *Up Against Foucault: Explorations of Some Tensions between Foucault and Feminism*, edited by Caroline Ramazanoglu. London: Routledge, 1993.

Braizer, Brennan. *Thrive: The Vegan Nutrition Guide to Optimal Performance in Sports and Life*. Toronto: Penguin Group, 2007.

Busenitz, Emily. "30 Things about Me." *Practical Paleo* (blog), 2014. http://practicalpaleo.blogspot.com/2013/06/30-things-about-me.html.

Cairns, Kate, and Josée Johnston. "Choosing Health: Embodied Neoliberalism, Postfeminism, and the 'Do-Diet.'" *Theory and Society* 44, no. 2 (2015): 153–75.

Castaneda, Jenny. "About." *Paleo Foodie Kitchen* (blog), 2014. http://paleofoodiekitchen.com.

Cheek, Julianne. "Healthism: A New Conservatism?" *Qualitative Health Research* 18, no. 7 (2008): 974–82.

Contois, Emily J. H. "Guilt-Free and Sinfully Delicious: A Contemporary Theology of Weight Loss Dieting." *Fat Studies* 4, no. 2 (2015): 112–26.

Crawford, B. "Healthism and the Medicalization of Everyday Life." *International Journal of Health Services* 10, no. 3 (1980): 365–88.

Crowley, Martha, and Randy Hodson. "Neoliberalism at Work." *Social Currents* 1 (2014): 91–108.

DeLind, Laura. "Are Local Food and the Local Food Movement Taking Us Where We Want to Go? Or Are We Hitching Our Wagons to the Wrong Stars?" *Agriculture and Human Values* 28, no. 2 (2011): 273–83.

DeSoucey, Michaela, and David Schleifer, "Technique and Technology in the Kitchen: Comparing Resistance to Municipal Trans Fat and Foie Gras Bans." *Studies in Law, Politics, and Society* 51 (2010): 185–218.

Durant, John. *The Paleo Manifesto*. New York: Penguin Random House, 2013.

Ferguson, Priscilla Parkhurst. *Word of Mouth: What We Talk about When We Talk about Food.* Oakland: University of California Press, 2014.

Getz, Donald, Tommy Andersson, Richard Robinson, and Sanja Vujicic. *Foodies and Food Tourism*. Oxford: Goodfellow, 2014.

Glassner, Barry. *The Gospel of Food: Why We Should Stop Worrying and Enjoy What We Eat.* New York: Harper Perennial, 2007.

Guthman, Julie. "Neoliberalism and the Making of Food Politics in California." *Geoforum* 39, no. 3 (2008): 1171–83.

Guthman, Julie. "The Polanyian Way? Voluntary Food Labels as Neoliberal Governance." *Antipode* 39, no. 3 (2007): 456–78.

Guthman, Julie. *Weighing In: Obesity, Food Justice, and the Limits of Capitalism.* Berkeley: University of California Press, 2011.

Guthman, Julie, and Melanie DuPuis. "Embodying Neoliberalism: Economy, Culture, and the Politics of Fat." *Environment and Planning D: Society and Space* 24, no. 3 (2006): 427–48.

Hanser, Amy, and Zachary Hyde. "Foodies Remaking Cities." *Contexts* 13, no. 3 (August 1, 2014): 44–49.

Hartwig, Melissa, and Dallas Hartwig. *It Starts with Food.* Auberry: Victory Belt Publishers, 2012.

Harvey, David. *A Brief History of Neoliberalism*. London: Oxford University Press, 2007.

Hinrichs, C. C. "Embeddedness and Local Food Systems: Notes on Two Types of Direct Agricultural Market." *Journal of Rural Studies* 16, no. 3 (2000): 295–303.

Jaffee, Daniel, and Philip Howard. "Corporate Cooptation of Organic and Fair Trade Standards." *Agriculture and Human Values* 27, no. 4 (2010): 387–99.

Johnston, Josée. "The Citizen-Consumer Hybrid: Ideological Tensions and the Case of Whole Foods Market." *Theory and Society* 37, no. 3 (2008): 229–70.

Johnston, Josée, and Shyon Baumann. *Foodies: Democracy and Distinction in the Gourmet Foodscape.* Florence, KY: Routledge, 2009.

Johnston, Josée, Alexandra Rodney, and Michelle Szabo. "Place, Ethics, and Everyday Eating: A Tale of Two Neighbourhoods." *Sociology* 46, no. 6 (2012): 1091–108.

Kolbert, Elizabeth. "Stone Soup." *New Yorker*, July 28, 2014. http://www.newyorker.com/magazine/2014/07/28/stone-soup.

Kresser, Chris. "How to Eat More Organ Meats." *Chris Kresser—Let's Take Back Your Health.* August 2, 2013, http://chriskresser.com/?s=organ+meat.

Long, Lucy. "Culinary Tourism: A Folklorist Perspective on Eating and Otherness." In *Culinary Tourism*, edited by Lucy Long. Lexington: University Press of Kentucky, 2004.

Lupton, Deborah. *Food, the Body and the Self.* Thousand Oaks, CA: Sage, 1996.

Lupton, Deborah. *The Imperative of Health.* London: Sage, 1995.

Lupton, Deborah. "M-Health and Health Promotion: The Digital Cyborg and Surveillance Society." *Social Theory & Health* 10, no. 3 (2012): 229–44.

Lupton, Deborah. "The Pedagogy of Disgust: The Ethical, Moral and Political Implications of Using Disgust in Public Health Campaigns." *Critical Public Health* 25, no. 1 (2014): 4–14.

Lyons, Kristen, Tabatha Wallington, and Geoffrey Lawrence. *Food Security, Nutrition and Sustainability*. London: Earthscan, 2009.

Macmillan, Craig Dublin. "Genetically Modified Foods, Personal Values, Perceptions of Morality, and the Effects of Self-Confrontation on That Stability of Personal Values." PhD dissertation, Washington State University, 2012. https://research.wsulibs.wsu.edu/xmlui/bitstream/handle/2376/4072/Macmillan_wsu_0251E_10366.pdf?sequence=1.

McCarthy, James, and Scott Prudham. "Neoliberal Nature and the Nature of Neoliberalism." *Geoforum* 35, no. 3 (2004): 275–83.

McGregor, Sue. "Neoliberalism and Health Care." *International Journal of Consumer Studies* 25, no. 2 (2001): 82–89.

McLaughlin, Katy. "Foodie Cities: Real Estate for the Restaurant Set." *Wall Street Journal*, September 11, 2014. http://www.wsj.com/articles/foodie-cities-real-estate-for-the-restaurant-set-1410452222.

PETA. "The Natural Human Diet." http://www.peta.org/living/food/natural-human-diet/.

Petrini, Carlo. *Slow Food: The Case for Taste*. New York: Columbia University Press, 2001.

Rangle, C., S. Dukeshire, and L. MacDonald. "Diet and Anxiety: An Exploration into the Orthorexic Society." *Appetite* 8, no. 1 (2012): 124–32.

Rotkovitz, Miri. "'Kosher Treif,' and the Observant American Jew." In *Culinary Tourism*, edited by Lucy Long. Lexington: University Press of Kentucky, 2004.

Saguy, Abigail C. *What's Wrong with Fat?* Oxford: Oxford University Press, 2013.

Savard, Jacqueline. "Personalised Medicine: A Critique on the Future of Health Care." *Journal of Bioethical Inquiry* 10, no. 2 (2013): 197–203.

Sax, David. *The Tastemakers: Why We're Crazy for Cupcakes but Fed Up with Fondue*. New York: PublicAffairs, 2014.

Schulson, Michael. "Diet Fads Are Destroying Us: Paleo, Gluten-Free and the Lies We Tell Ourselves." *Salon*, May 3, 2015. http://www.salon.com/2015/05/03/diet_fads_are_destroying_us_paleo_gluten_free_and_the_lies_we_tell_ourselves_partner/.

Scrinis, Gyorgy. 2008. "On the Ideology of Nutritionism." *Gastronomica* (2008): 39–48.

Skiadas, P. K., and J. G. Lascaratos. "Dietetics in Ancient Greek Philosophy: Plato's Concepts of Healthy Diet." *European Journal of Clinical Nutrition* 55, no. 7 (2001): 532–37.

Snyder, Kimberly. *The Beauty Detox Solution.* Don Mills, Ontario: Harlequin, 2011.

Stinson, Kandi. *Women and Dieting Culture.* New Brunswick, NJ: Rutgers University Press, 2001.

Webner, Kele. "About." *Vegan Foodies*, 2014. http://theveganfoodies.tumblr.com/about.

Wolf, Robb. *The Paleo Solution: The Original Human Diet.* Auberry: Victory Belt Publishers, 2010.

Chapter Eleven

Breaking Bread

The Clashing Cults of Sourdough and Gluten-Free

L. Sasha Gora

Painted in 1657 to 1658, Johannes Vermeer's *The Milkmaid* is a highlight in Amsterdam's Rijksmuseum. With soft lighting and a pale background, the painting captures a woman pouring milk from a jug. It is a familiar image; yet something is missing. The table is less cluttered, the basket in front of the jug empty. Featured alongside the original, this is the breadless version, exhibited in the Gluten Free Museum.[1] Created by artist Arthur Coulet, this online collection reimagines iconic artworks by the likes of Caravaggio, Wayne Thiebaud, and Édouard Manet without gluten—hence without wheat. When reporting on the popularity of the website, the BBC first wondered if it was poking fun at how popular gluten-free diets have become, but Coulet says, "This is a serious matter. That's why I've decided to bring lightness and pleasure with art."[2]

The Gluten Free Museum captures the tension between the historical significance of wheat and that today, among certain groups, it seems to be losing its importance. Nonetheless, bread occupies a holy position in food history and has many cults. From Ethiopian *injera* to Afghanistan's *nan-i-Afghan* and from French baguette to San Francisco sourdough, the concept of bread is nearly universal. Wheat provides more nourishment than any other food and 20 percent of the world's calories.[3] Furthermore, no other food better represents the whole as more than the sum of its parts than bread. Water provides moisture; it binds the flour to become dough. Flour provides protein and substance. Two things inedible alone, salt and flour, along with water—which will quench our thirst, but never our hunger—become a meal.

This chapter contrasts the revival of baking with sourdough and a variety of wheat and grains in Europe and North America to the development of gluten-free lifestyles—both arguably food cults in their own rights that are positioned around bread but with polarizing views. How can looking at the sourdough movement affect how we see the development of gluten-free lifestyles? And vice versa? By discussing these two positions in tandem, this chapter provides a deeper understanding of contemporary appreciation and anxiety around bread and what this reveals about a general understanding of food, culture, and choice.

WHERE THE WILD THINGS GROW: SOURDOUGH AND INDUSTRIAL BREAD

Aaron Bobrow-Strain, food politics professor, writes about American, industrial bread in *White Bread: A Social History of the Store-Bought Loaf.* In the preface he brings up the difficulties in researching something as ordinary as bread:

> As important as it has been . . . bread is not something that typically gets written about in diaries, described in letters, or remembered in oral histories. As social reformer Eleanor Bang reflected in 1951: "Bread? Of course. There it is for breakfast, for lunch, for dinner in a rhythm as regular as the ticking of our electric clocks—so regular we'd notice it only if it stopped."[4]

Despite Bobrow-Strain's claim, there has been much scholarship on the history of bread. Nonetheless, it is fruitful to keep in mind the implications of bread being such a given it escapes notice. Like Vermeer's *The Milkmaid,* one only notices bread once it is missing.

Broken apart, sourdough suggests dough gone sour. However, it is a technique for making bread with natural yeast as opposed to a type of bread. It is made with flour, salt, water, and time. Natural yeast has been used in ancient food practices, and its use can be traced back to ancient Egypt.[5] The word *yeast* comes from an Indo-European root, *yes*, which means "to bubble or foam." To bake a loaf of sourdough is a performance in three acts. The first is to develop a culture that becomes a starter, or, as the French call it, *le chef*[6] (made from flour, water, and sometimes a spoonful of yogurt or fresh fruit to help hurry things along); the second is to manage that starter by feeding it and thus administering to its bacteria and wild yeasts. The third act is to shape the dough and bake it into bread. Adam Gopnik describes the character of dough: "Bread dough isn't like dinner food, which usually rests inert under the knife and waits for you to do something to it: bread dough sits there, respiring and rising, thinking things over."[7] It breathes, bubbles, and foams.

Natural leaven remained the standard until bakers switched to commercial baker's yeast. Contrasting the two, Malin Elmlid writes, "Commercial yeast was developed to give the baker the ability to command the dough and to take control of the process. A sourdough process demands more of you as a baker."[8] Commercial yeast is more reliable, hence why it became the norm for industrial baking. Chad Robertson in *Tartine Bread* shares the recipe for his bakery's Basic Country Bread. With fifteen pages of instructions, thirteen pages of step-by-step photos, and ten pages that go into further details, the recipe, using a natural leaven, is not for those concerned with convenience.

No longer made with natural yeast and by hand, bread became a processed food. Emine Saner describes industrialized bread making. To make bread quickly on an industrial scale, an important step is skipped: fermentation. However, fermentation breaks down proteins, making it easier to digest. Bakers in France stopped using natural leaven in the 1930s.[9] Then the more yeast one would add, the faster the bread would rise and the sooner it could be baked. Dough was now aerated instead of fermented. This also meant bread would go stale faster. To prevent this, preservatives had to be added.

Flour is the single most important ingredient in bread, as it is most responsible for how the loaf tastes. Amanda Benson identifies three distinct, yet entwined, industries that make up the flour industry: farming, milling, and baking.[10] This leads her to ask how power is distributed among them. She argues industrialization has affected who has the most influence. Previously, it was the farmers, as they determined the type of wheat grown, taking into consideration which species were most compatible with the weather or could best withstand local bugs. With industrialization, millers and bakers gained more influence and could determine the types of wheat. With this shift in power came a shift in flour.

In "The Food Industry and New Preservation Techniques," Giorgio Pedrocco writes, "In the first half of the nineteenth century, mills were transformed by a series of innovations increasing the quantity and quality of the flour that could be obtained from grain."[11] Steel rollers came into use, replacing the traditional way of grinding wheat on stones. The wheat grain has three parts: germ, bran, and endosperm. White flour only uses the latter, unlike whole-wheat flour. This means a field of wheat yields more whole-wheat flour than white flour, as white flour has a higher extraction rate since other parts of the grain are tossed aside. This is why historically white flour was more expensive than whole wheat, but because of mechanization and industrialization, white flour became cheaper to produce. The *New Yorker* describes this shift:

> Steel was fast, efficient, and easy to maintain, and it permitted millers to discard the germ and the bran in the wheat kernel and then rapidly process the starchy endosperm. . . . Almost nobody seemed to notice, or care, that by tossing out the rest of the kernel industrial bakers were stripping bread of its vitamins, its fiber, and most of its healthy fats.[12]

White flour no longer was a luxury but instead the norm. Industrialization changed both the flour with which bread was baked and the process with which dough was made. It introduced a difference between commercial, factory-made bread and handmade "artisan" bread.

SOURDOUGH REVIVAL

Fashions in food change over time. Bread is no exception. During World War II due to shortages in flour, bakers added fillers such as potatoes and even sawdust to stretch out dough.[13] After the war, whole-wheat bread thus carried negative associations. White baguettes instead were preferred. When researching the revival of sourdough, one name comes up again and again: Poilâne. Founded in 1932 by Pierre Poilâne in Paris, his granddaughter Apollonia Poilâne now runs the business, but it was his son, Lionel, whose name became synonymous with reviving the quality of French bread. Lauren Collins writes:

> Poilâne almost single-handedly saved sourdough from obscurity, reviving its reputation as the true French bread. . . . The Paris-based food writer Alexander Lobrano told me, "When French baking was in great danger, seriously and perhaps permanently damaged by industrialization, Poilâne was among the first, and surely the most important, to blow the whistle."[14]

Referred to as *miche*, *pain au levain*, or *pain Poilâne*, the bread responsible for this revival is a four-pound wheel of sourdough. Grossing $18 million a year, today the bakery, with several locations, "produces about three per cent of all the bread sold in Paris."[15] Lionel Poilâne also influenced a new generation of bakers, including Chad Robertson, who opened the acclaimed bakery Tartine in San Francisco in 2002. Robertson tells a similar story: in the late 1970s Lionel Poilâne sparked this revival, thus marking "the beginning of a shift in taste back toward traditional country breads."[16] The artisan bread revival then arrived in the United States in the 1980s.

In *The Bread Exchange*, Elmlid describes the sourdough trend in Sweden as first beginning to take root around 2005.[17] What could be described as the sourdough scene has made its presence felt in the Swedish capital, and now there are even sourdough hotels.[18] For example, at Urban Deli and RA Chocolat at Arlanda Airport, bread-baking enthusiasts pay a fee for their sourdough to be watered and fed while away from home.

There is also an increasing interest in heritage wheats and grains. Cookbooks reflect a period's tastes, trends, priorities, and concerns. Because of the vast range in techniques and ingredients, they may not always accurately reflect what people are cooking and baking at home. However, they do relay interests and ambitions. Tartine's latest cookbook *Tartine Book No. 3: Modern, Ancient, Classic, Whole* (2013) demonstrates an interest in baking bread with a larger variety of grains and wheats. It includes recipes with kamut, semolina, rye, spelt, and emmer/einkorn.

Confronting and challenging the grain industry in the United States is the subject of the 2015 documentary *The Grain Divide*. It makes the claim "the farm to table movement forgot our most basic food"[19] and features the voices of food professionals passionate about wheat, including Chad Robertson, Michael Pollan, and chef Dan Barber. It charts the change in the production of wheat in the United States from 1880, when roughly twenty-four thousand commercial mills spread across the country, to 2014, when there were only two hundred. Four companies now control 80 percent of the market. If some of those in the film discuss what the industry has become, Dr. Stephen Jones is working on reengineering what it could be. Jones has a PhD in genetics and is a wheat breeder directing the Bread Lab at Washington State University. "Our philosophy is that wheat has to work for the farmer: something with low input, that they won't have to fertilize, and something that they won't have to spray with pesticides, whether they're organic or not," he tells Elyssa Goldberg in an interview with *Bon Appétit*.[20] "What we develop and bring in will yield enough that the price point can come down so that there's access for most, if not all, people. It has to yield enough so that it's not $20 to buy it," he continues.[21] In other words, the Bread Lab is challenging the notion that different varieties of wheat (and hence quality bread) need to be expensive. We often talk about "wheat" and not "wheats." However, at the Svalbard Global Seed Vault in Norway, set up in 2008, there are more than 150,000 different varieties of wheat, making it the caregiver of a "living history of grain."[22] The aim of the research at the Bread Lab is diversification, which challenges the monocrop standards of industrial agriculture.[23] In short, contemporary interests in sourdough are fueled by a desire for better flour, bread, and even a better agricultural system. Previously the trend in baking was to add flavor to white flour. Now the trend is to use different grains to create flavor.

THE WEIGHT OF WHEAT: GOING GLUTEN-FREE

Gluten is a curious thing. It has attracted a lot of attention, concern, and confusion. In "Gluten-Free Eating Appears to Be Here to Stay," Kim Severson writes that comedian Jimmy Kimmel "spoofed the diet by filming health-conscious, gluten-free Southern Californians who were stumped when asked to describe what gluten is. The video has been viewed more than 2.5 million times on YouTube."[24] More than a year later the number of views has increased, and so have questions concerning gluten. Michael Specter gives a sound explanation of gluten in the *New Yorker*:

> Gluten, one of the most heavily consumed proteins on earth, is created when two molecules, glutenin and gliadin, come into contact and form a bond. When bakers knead dough, that bond creates an elastic membrane, which is what gives bread its chewy texture and permits pizza chefs to toss and twirl the dough into the air. Gluten also traps carbon dioxide, which, as it ferments, adds volume to the loaf.[25]

It is what makes dough bounce back when poked. It is found not only in wheat but also in other grains such as barley and rye, but for people with celiac disease, it makes them sick.

Celiac disease means "sickness of the belly" in Greek.[26] Dr. Samuel Gee gave the first comprehensive description of the condition in 1887. Although he never determined its cause, he believed it could be cured by diet; however, his recommended diet included bread.[27] It was not until 1941 that Dutch physician Willem Dicke published a report recommending a wheat-free diet.[28] It was then British physician Margot Shiner who, in 1956, realized it was gluten that "altered the intestinal mucosa in coeliac patients."[29] Other than avoiding gluten, there is no cure.

For those with celiac disease, gluten is dangerous as it has severe health implications, but for those without it, things become more complicated. MUNCHIES reports, "According to the University of Chicago Celiac Disease Center, about one out of 133—or just under 1 percent—of the population suffers from celiac disease, a four-fold increase in the past 50 years. (Eighty percent or more don't know that they have it.)"[30] This explains why some people must avoid gluten, but not why people without celiac disease choose to do so. MUNCHIES continues: "An additional 1.6 million Americans, and possibly more, are on a gluten-free diet despite lack of diagnosis."[31] Since for those with celiac disease eating a gluten-free diet was a cure for their ailments, the hope was that it would be a cure for others too. Beyond blaming gluten, there are other theories about why people are experiencing sensitivity, including one related to FODMAPs (a group of carbohydrates found in foods other than just grains).[32] However, at least for now MUNCHIES seems to be right in claiming, "*Gluten*. Like its predecessor, 'carbs,' the word has practically become public enemy number one."[33]

What is the difference between being allergic to gluten versus being sensitive to it? Viv Groskop addresses this question in "Do We Worry Too Much about What We Eat?"

> An allergy is an immediate reaction that occurs directly after consuming a food, even in tiny amounts, and can require urgent medical attention. Allergy is an immune system reaction and can cause swelling, vomiting and, in extreme cases, anaphylactic shock. . . . Intolerance (or sensitivity) usually takes longer to show up in the body and is affected by volume: you might be able to consume small amounts of that food and be fine. Intolerance is likely to have less serious physical effects.[34]

For some not eating gluten is a medical requirement, and for others it is a lifestyle choice. This also leads to the gluten-free paradox, which Ellen McCarthy mentions in "Gluten-Free Option Hard to Stomach as Intolerance of Fad Diet Grows in the US": people without celiac disease eat a gluten-free diet; yet people with celiac disease continue to eat gluten, as they have not been diagnosed.[35]

If the name *Poilâne* comes up again and again when reading about sourdough, then there are two names, tied to two books, that are infamous in connection with the gluten-free lifestyle: William Davis's bestseller *Wheat*

Belly: Lose the Wheat, Lose the Weight, and Find Your Way Back to Health (2011) and David Perlmutter's *Grain Brain: The Surprising Truth about Wheat, Carbs, and Sugar—Your Brain's Silent Killers* (2013). As Specter wrote in 2014:

> Until about a decade ago, the other ninety-nine per cent of Americans rarely seemed to give gluten much thought. But, led by people like William Davis, a cardiologist whose book *Wheat Belly* created an empire founded on the conviction that gluten is a poison, the protein has become a culinary villain.[36]

Davis blames everything from schizophrenia to asthma on whole grains. Perlmutter considers gluten sensitivity to be a threat to humanity.[37]

Specter's accusations bring back to mind the claim that gluten has become public enemy number one. Both books are also discussed at length in *The Gluten Lie: And Other Myths about What You Eat* by Alan Levinovitz. As a scholar of religion specializing in classical Chinese thought, Levinovitz is not who one would expect to write a book about food trends, as science and religion are thought to be separate explanatory systems. Yet he argues that "the appeal of dietary fads had to do with myths, not facts."[38] Diets and lifestyles are emotional as they are expressions of who one wants to be and how one wants to live.

Regarding the popularity of a gluten-free lifestyle, Levinovitz uses myth as a way of explaining how readers can be coaxed into being gullible. "The first sentences of Davis's and Perlmutter's introductions are eerily similar. . . . Each reinforces the lie that the past was better—safer, healthier—than the present," Levinovitz argues.[39] "Meanwhile, diet gurus saw an opportunity to repackage the long-popular low carb Atkins diet using new myths and a new villain."[40] *Dangerous Grains* by Dr. James Braly and Ron Hoggan, published in 2002, was the "first book-length argument against eating gluten-containing grains" (though it is not mentioned in either *Grain Brain* or *Wheat Belly*).[41]

What comes from going gluten-free when there is no medical need? MUNCHIES reports on a study from Australia's the George Institute for Global Health, which tested whether there are health benefits for those without celiac disease to give up gluten. In a statement, Dr. Jason Wu, who led the study, says about gluten-free options, "The foods can be significantly more expensive and are very trendy to eat, but we discovered a negligible difference when looking at their overall nutrition."[42] For example, a gluten-free version of pasta or crackers contained less protein than their conventional counterparts, "but sugar and sodium levels were almost totally consistent."[43] The biggest difference was the price.

Health sells. The *New York Times* reports the low-carb trend peaked in 2004 "as a $2.7 billion business in the United States" and that it got to the point that McDonald's was even considering launching a bunless burger.[44] Gluten-free is now a big business. The *Guardian* reports, "In 2012 'free-from' sales (of gluten- or wheat-free foods) were valued at £228m, an increase of 25% in a year." This number seems be increasing, and the market in Britain for gluten-free is expected to grow to £561 million by 2017.[45] In the United States, the industry is expected to "exceed fifteen billion dollars by 2016, twice the amount of five years earlier."[46]

HEALTH, POWER, AND CHOICE

The implication of the expression-turned-mantra "you are what you eat" is that we can control our bodies, appearances, health, and future through what we eat and what we do not. Fueling the decision to reject gluten when one has no medical reason to do so, similar to what is fueling the decision to cut your sourdough at home instead of buying sliced, factory-made bread, is the desire to take control over food, to have a sense of choice. Jeffrey Steingarten writes:

> There is no society that encourages gluttony, and there never has been. Until recently, few people had enough money to be gluttons. And those who did were held back by law, religion, custom, or scarcity. None of these hinder us today. We are all in grave danger of running amok. We desperately need something to restrain us. That's why we invented the nutrition fads and fears of the past 20 years.[47]

Diets and lifestyles provide a way to navigate the overwhelming choice of what to eat and how much.

In *You Aren't What You Eat: Fed Up with Gastroculture*, Steven Poole brings up when health-conscious eating gets out of hand: "It is called 'orthorexia.' From the Greek *orthos* (straight or correct), orothorexia means an obsession with eating correctly, according to some understanding of what the healthiest diet is."[48] This employs a binary understanding of food, which operates within the extremes of either good or bad food. This relates to Roland Barthes's writing about "nutritional consciousness" in "Towards a

Psychosociology of Contemporary Food Culture," which is worth quoting at length:

> Food is henceforth *thought out*, not by specialists, but by the entire public, even if this thinking is done within a framework of highly mythical notions. . . . Modern nutritional science . . . is not bound to any moral values, such as asceticism, wisdom, or purity, but on the contrary to values of *power*. (original italics)[49]

Value is differentiated from power. Value is tied up in a system, a way of structuring life that goes back to Steingarten's idea that a value system (or a shortage) works in restricting what people eat and how much. Furthermore, Barthes's mention of myth recalls the parallels Levinovitz draws between myths and diets. Eating becomes a way of gaining physical power and exercising emotional power.

CONCLUSION

As terms like *breadwinner* and *daily bread* or referring to money as *dough* illustrate, even the English language has been shaped by bread and its influence on society and culture. "The Latin word *companion* means literally 'a person with whom we share bread.'"[50] Bread is deeply engrained in Western culture.

By discussing sourdough and gluten-free cults, this chapter reveals the common root behind both. It has surveyed the development of industrial bread (including both wheat and white bread). Artisan bakers, the sourdough revival, and a renewed interest in a richer variety of wheats and grains are challenging industrial, standardized bread. The gluten-free diet, with its health implications for some and its significance as a lifestyle choice for others, similarly challenges the industrial production of wheat. Having to give up gluten for medical reasons does not necessarily imply one has to give up bread. For example, King Arthur Flour has a recipe for a gluten-free sourdough starter that includes the company's Gluten-Free Multi-Purpose Flour, Ancient Grains Flour Blend, Florapan French Sourdough Starter, and cool water.[51] After all, the sourdough and gluten-free movements are both reactions to the industrialization and mechanization of bread.

Food is cultural. It relates to myths, power, control, and personal choice. Whether one is part of the artisan-bread-buying slice or avoids glutens out of choice, both positions express a desire to gain control, navigate, and make sense of a complex food system.

NOTES

1. Gluten Free Museum, http://glutenimage.tumblr.com, accessed August 8, 2015.
2. BBC, "What Does Classic Art Look Like without the Gluten?" April 20, 2015, http://www.bbc.com/news/blogs-trending-32348847, accessed August 22, 2015.
3. Michael Specter, "Against the Grain: Should You Go Gluten-Free?" *New Yorker*, November 3, 2014, http://www.newyorker.com/magazine/2014/11/03/grain, accessed November 27, 2014.
4. Aaron Bobrow-Strain, *White Bread: A Social History of the Store-Bought Loaf* (Boston: Beacon Press, 2012), ix.
5. Edda Bresciani, "Food Culture in Ancient Egypt," in *Food: A Culinary History from Antiquity to the Present*, ed. Jean-Louis Flandrin and Massimo Montanari (New York: Penguin, 1999), 39.
6. Jeffrey Steingarten, *The Man Who Ate Everything* (New York: Vintage Books, 1998), 20.
7. Adam Gopnik, "Bread and Women: Two Muses, One Loaf," *New Yorker*, November 4, 2013, http://www.newyorker.com/magazine/2013/11/04/bread-and-women, accessed September 10, 2015.
8. Malin Elmlid, *The Bread Exchange* (San Francisco: Chronicle Books, 2014), 39.
9. Chad Robertson, *Tartine Bread* (San Francisco: Chronicle Books, 2010), 15.
10. Amanda Benson, "The Rise and Fall of Bread in America" (honors thesis, Johnson & Wales University, 2013), http://scholarsarchive.jwu.edu/student_scholarship/11.
11. Giorgio Pedrcocco, "The Food Industry and New Preservation Techniques," in *Food: A Culinary History from Antiquity to the Present*, ed. Jean-Louis Flandrin and Massimo Montanari (New York: Penguin, 1999), 483.
12. Specter, "Against the Grain: Should You Go Gluten-Free?"
13. Lauren Collins, "Bread Winner: A Daughter Upholds the Traditions of France's Premier Baking Dynasty," *New Yorker*, December 3, 2012, http://www.newyorker.com/magazine/2012/12/03/bread-winner, accessed August 28, 2015.
14. Collins, "Bread Winner."
15. Collins, "Bread Winner."
16. Chad Robertson, *Tartine Book No. 3: Modern Ancient Classic Whole* (San Francisco: Chronicle Books, 2013), 12–13.
17. Elmlid, *The Bread Exchange*, 39.
18. Camila-Catalina Fernandez, "There Is Now a Hotel for Bread Dough in Sweden," *MUNCHIES: Food by Vice*, September 9, 2015, https://munchies.vice.com/articles/there-is-now-a-hotel-for-bread-dough-in-sweden, accessed September 10, 2015.
19. *The Grain Divide*, http://thegraindivide.com/, accessed September 5, 2015.
20. Elyssa Goldberg, "The Bread Lab Wants to Change the Way We Eat Wheat," *Bon Appétit*, May 18, 2015, http://www.bonappetit.com/entertaining-style/trends-news/article/bread-lab, accessed September 26, 2015.
21. Goldberg, "The Bread Lab Wants to Change the Way We Eat Wheat."
22. BBC, "Food Programme: The Grain Divide," *BBC Radio 4*, February 2, 105, 15:30, http://www.bbc.co.uk/programmes/b050yh95, accessed September 27, 2015.

23. Goldberg, "The Bread Lab Wants to Change the Way We Eat Wheat."

24. Kim Severson, "Gluten-Free Eating Appears to Be Here to Stay," *New York Times*, June 16, 2014, http://www.nytimes.com/2014/06/18/dining/gluten-free-eating-appears-to-be-here-to-stay.html?_r=3, accessed August 22, 2015.

25. Specter, "Against the Grain: Should You Go Gluten-Free?"

26. Alan Levinovitz, *The Gluten Lie: And Other Myths about What You Eat* (New York: Regan Arts, 2015), 34.

27. Levinovitz, *The Gluten Lie*, 34.

28. Levinovitz, *The Gluten Lie*, 35.

29. Levinovitz, *The Gluten Lie*, 35–36.

30. MUNCHIES, "Can Scientists Really Take the Gluten Out of Our Wheat?" *MUNCHIES: Food by VICE*, March 23, 2015, http://munchies.vice.com/articles/can-scientists-really-take-the-gluten-out-of-our-wheat, accessed July 9, 2015.

31. MUNCHIES, "Can Scientists Really Take the Gluten Out of Our Wheat?"

32. Emine Saner, "Gluten-Free: Health Fad or Life-Saving Diet?" *The Guardian*, February 25, 2015, http://www.theguardian.com/lifeandstyle/2015/feb/25/gluten-free-diet-life-saving-fad, accessed August 22, 2015.

33. MUNCHIES, "Can Scientists Really Take the Gluten Out of Our Wheat?"

34. Viv Groskop, "Do We Worry Too Much about What We Eat?" *The Guardian*, April 19, 2015, http://www.theguardian.com/lifeandstyle/2015/apr/19/do-we-worry-too-much-about-what-we-eat-allergies-food-intolerance-gluten-free-diets, accessed August 5, 2015.

35. Ellen McCarthy, "Gluten-Free Option Hard to Stomach as Intolerance of Fad Diets Grows in the US," *The Guardian*, July 12, 2014, http://www.theguardian.com/lifeandstyle/2014/jul/12/gluten-free-diet-nutrition-fad, accessed August 4, 2015.

36. Specter, "Against the Grain: Should You Go Gluten-Free?"

37. Specter, "Against the Grain: Should You Go Gluten-Free?"

38. Levinovitz, *The Gluten Lie*, 13.

39. Levinovitz, *The Gluten Lie*, 27.

40. Levinovitz, *The Gluten Lie*, 44.

41. Levinovitz, *The Gluten Lie*, 42.

42. MUNCHIES, "Even Doctors Are Saying You Should Stop Buying Gluten-Free Food for No Reason," *MUNCHIES: Food by VICE*, July 8, 2015, http://munchies.vice.com/articles/even-doctors-say-you-should-stop-buying-gluten-free-food-for-no-reason, accessed July 9, 2015.

43. MUNCHIES, "Even Doctors Are Saying You Should Stop Buying Gluten-Free Food for No Reason."

44. Severson, "Gluten-Free Eating Appears to Be Here to Stay."

45. Linda Geddes, "Leave It Out: Are Food Intolerances Fact or Fad?" *The Guardian*, August 16, 2015, http://www.theguardian.com/society/2015/aug/16/leave-it-out-are-food-intolerances-fact-or-fad-gluten-dairy-free-from-coeliac, accessed August 17, 2015.

46. Specter, "Against the Grain: Should You Go Gluten-Free?"

47. Jeffrey Steingarten, *It Must've Been Something I Ate* (London: Review, 2002), 6.

48. Steven Poole, *You Aren't What You Eat: Fed Up with Gastroculture* (London: Union Books, 2012), 10–11.

49. Roland Barthes, "Towards a Psychosociology of Contemporary Food Consumption," in *Food and Culture*, 2nd ed., ed. Carole Counihan and Penny Van Esterik (Routledge: New York and London, 2008), 33.

50. Margaret Visser, *The Rituals of Dinner: The Origins, Evolution, Eccentricities and Meaning of Table Manners* (Toronto: HarperCollins, 1991), 3.

51. “Gluten-Free Sourdough Starter Recipe,” King Arthur Flour, August 11, 2012, http://www.kingarthurflour.com/recipes/gluten-free-sourdough-starter-recipe, accessed September 27, 2015.

BIBLIOGRAPHY

Barthes, Roland. “Towards a Psychosociology of Contemporary Food Consumption.” In *Food and Culture*, 2nd ed., edited by Carole Counihan and Penny Van Esterik, 28–35. New York and London: Routledge, 2008.

BBC. “Food Programme: The Grain Divide.” *BBC Radio 4*, February 2, 2015, 15:30. http://www.bbc.co.uk/programmes/b050yh95. Accessed September 27, 2015.

BBC. “What Does Classic Art Look Like without the Gluten?” April 20, 2015. http://www.bbc.com/news/blogs-trending-32348847. Accessed August 22, 2015.

Benson, Amanda, “The Rise and Fall of Bread in America.” Honors thesis, Johnson & Wales University, 2013. http://scholarsarchive.jwu.edu/student_scholarship/11.

Bobrow-Strain, Aaron. *White Bread: A Social History of the Store-Bought Loaf.* Boston: Beacon Press, 2012.

Bresciani, Edda. “Food Culture in Ancient Egypt.” In *Food: A Culinary History from Antiquity to the Present*, edited by Jean-Louis Flandrin and Massimo Montanari, 38–45. New York: Penguin, 1999.

Collins, Lauren. “Bread Winner: A Daughter Upholds the Traditions of France’s Premier Baking Dynasty.” *New Yorker*, December 3, 2012. http://www.newyorker.com/magazine/2012/12/03/bread-winner. Accessed August 28, 2015.

Elmlid, Malin. *The Bread Exchange*. San Francisco: Chronicle Books, 2014.

Fernandez, Camila-Catalina. “There Is Now a Hotel for Bread Dough in Sweden.” *MUNCHIES: Food by Vice*, September 9, 2015. https://munchies.vice.com/articles/there-is-now-a-hotel-for-bread-dough-in-sweden. Accessed September 10, 2015.

Geddes, Linda. “Leave It Out: Are Food Intolerances Fact or Fad?” *The Guardian*, August 16, 2015. http://www.theguardian.com/society/2015/aug/16/leave-it-out-are-food-intolerances-fact-or-fad-gluten-dairy-free-from-coeliac. Accessed August 17, 2015.

Gluten Free Museum. http://glutenimage.tumblr.com. Accessed August 8, 2015.

Goldberg, Elyssa. “The Bread Lab Wants to Change the Way We Eat Wheat.” *Bon Appétit*, May 18, 2015. http://www.bonappetit.com/entertaining-style/trends-news/article/bread-lab. Accessed September 26, 2015.

Gopnik, Adam. “Bread and Women: Two Muses, One Loaf.” *New Yorker*, November 4, 2013. http://www.newyorker.com/magazine/2013/11/04/bread-and-women. Accessed September 10, 2015.

The Grain Divide. http://thegraindivide.com/. Accessed September 5, 2015.

Groskop, Viv. “Do We Worry Too Much about What We Eat?” *The Guardian*, April 19, 2015. http://www.theguardian.com/lifeandstyle/2015/apr/19/do-we-worry-too-much-about-what-we-eat-allergies-food-intolerance-gluten-free-diets. Accessed August 5, 2015.

King Arthur Flour. “Gluten-Free Sourdough Starter Recipe.” August 11, 2012. http://www.kingarthurflour.com/recipes/gluten-free-sourdough-starter-recipe. Accessed September 27, 2015.

Levinovitz, Alan. *The Gluten Lie: And Other Myths about What You Eat.* New York: Regan Arts, 2015.

McCarthy, Ellen. "Gluten-Free Option Hard to Stomach as Intolerance of Fad Diets Grows in the US." *The Guardian*, July 12, 2014. http://www.theguardian.com/lifeandstyle/2014/jul/12/gluten-free-diet-nutrition-fad. Accessed August 4, 2015.

MUNCHIES. "Can Scientists Really Take the Gluten Out of Our Wheat?" *MUNCHIES: Food by VICE*, March 23, 2015. http://munchies.vice.com/articles/can-scientists-really-take-the-gluten-out-of-our-wheat. Accessed July 9, 2015.

MUNCHIES. "Even Doctors Are Saying You Should Stop Buying Gluten-Free Food for No Reason." *MUNCHIES: Food by VICE*, July 8, 2015. http://munchies.vice.com/articles/even-doctors-say-you-should-stop-buying-gluten-free-food-for-no-reason. Accessed July 9, 2015.

Pedrocco, Giorgio. "The Food Industry and New Preservation Techniques." In *Food: A Culinary History from Antiquity to the Present*, edited by Jean-Louis Flandrin and Massimo Montanari, 481–91. New York: Penguin, 1999.

Poole, Steven. *You Aren't What You Eat: Fed Up with Gastroculture.* London: Union Books, 2012.

Robertson, Chad. *Tartine Bread.* San Francisco: Chronicle Books, 2010.

Robertson, Chad. *Tartine Book No. 3: Modern Ancient Classic Whole*. San Francisco: Chronicle Books, 2013.

Saner, Emine. "Gluten-Free: Health Fad or Life-Saving Diet?" *The Guardian*, February 25, 2015. http://www.theguardian.com/lifeandstyle/2015/feb/25/gluten-free-diet-life-saving-fad. Accessed August 22, 2015.

Severson, Kim. "Gluten-Free Eating Appears to Be Here to Stay." *New York Times*, June 16, 2014. http://www.nytimes.com/2014/06/18/dining/gluten-free-eating-appears-to-be-here-to-stay.html?_r=3. Accessed August 22, 2015.

Specter, Michael. "Against the Grain: Should You Go Gluten-Free?" *New Yorker*, November 3, 2014. http://www.newyorker.com/magazine/2014/11/03/grain. Accessed November 27, 2014.

Steingarten, Jeffrey. *It Must've Been Something I Ate*. London: Review, 2002.

Steingarten, Jeffrey. *The Man Who Ate Everything: And Other Gastronomic Feats, Disputes, and Pleasurable Pursuits*. New York: Vintage Books, 1998.

Visser, Margaret. *The Rituals of Dinner: The Origins, Evolution, Eccentricities and Meaning of Table Manners.* Toronto: HarperCollins, 1991.

Chapter Twelve

The Gluten-Free Cult

A World without Wheat

Jennifer Martin

Gluten, that devious protein lurking in wheat, has been the cause of much anguish among those who medically are condemned to avoid wheat or suffer dire health repercussions. The card-carrying members of the Gluten-Free Cult are diagnosed with either celiac disease or non-celiac gluten intolerance. Sufferers of both conditions must adhere to the same treatment plan, a lifelong avoidance of wheat, rye, and barley (yes, this means no beer). There is no medicine or treatment available to these sufferers other than strict avoidance of wheat and its cousins. The penalties for falling off the gluten-free wagon are insidious and varied. Exposure to gluten for this group can result in immediate and severe stomach distress—sometimes diagnosed as irritable bowel syndrome—extreme migraine headaches, skin rashes, and loss of energy and brain function, to name a few. Sometimes gluten can trigger a host of autoimmune diseases, including autoimmune thyroid disease and rheumatoid arthritis. This group of medical sufferers forms the inner circle of the Gluten-Free Cult. The seriousness of the effects of gluten on these eaters is often in direct conflict with the perceived frivolity and lack of true commitment to the diet of those outside the inner circle who claim a gluten-free diet. This tension over authentic membership to the gluten-free community is complicated further by the other types of eaters drawn to the gluten-free diet.

The medical sufferers are not the only eaters that benefit from gluten avoidance. Many parents of children suffering from autism, attention deficit disorder (ADD), and attention deficit/hyperactivity disorder (ADHD) claim that maintaining a strict gluten-free diet for their children results in a lessening of the symptoms of autism, ADD, and ADHD. This group forms a secondary membership to the group. While the children following the diet are not placing their health at risk by slipping up and downing a piece of pizza at a friend's birthday party, they suffer the consequences in a different and sometimes equally frustrating manner.

All of this seemed like very eccentric and sometimes socially ridiculous posturing to the wheat eaters of the world until celebrities and the American media became involved. Then what was a quiet and somewhat strange little medically aligned cult exploded into the stuff of television personalities and tennis stars. All of a sudden everyone wanted to brag that they ate gluten-free and rushed to join the Gluten-Free Cult. However, the card-carrying members of the cult, whose very health depends on the strict avoidance of gluten, have a very uneasy union with the new hordes, the hobbyists, begging for membership. Can a person truly be a member of the community if he eats gluten-free one day and gorges on Krispy Kreme doughnuts the next? Those at the core of the gluten-free eaters, those whose membership is necessitated by health issues over which they have no control, give an emphatic "no" to the hobbyist Krispy Kreme doughnut eater.

You might assume, unlike some of the notorious cults making the news with their violence, that the interior mentality of this group of eaters is perhaps mundane and peaceful. However, all bets of harmony are off when a hobbyist sharing a table with a medically required gluten-free eater at the only restaurant in a hundred miles that serves gluten-free bread (and it's warm, soft, and delicious bread served with salted organic butter) reaches her glutenated hands into the specially prepared gluten-free bread basket for the last gluten-free roll in the restaurant—and in one hundred miles—while taking bites of real pizza and pasta from everyone at the table. You have never witnessed anger and disappointment so personal and poignant as that displayed by the now breadless gluten-free eater. These medically required gluten-free eaters are the core of this community that possesses many cult-like tendencies because the avoidance of gluten becomes the central defining motif of their lives. The need to stay strictly gluten-free directs where, what, and sometimes with whom they may eat. Food becomes a forum to ferret out true membership to the Gluten-Free Cult.

THE CARD-CARRYING MEMBERS OF THE GLUTEN-FREE CULT

Membership into the inner sanctum of the medically required members is a long and harrowing initiation process that typically begins with years of painful and sometimes disabling illness. In the United States, celiac disease and non-celiac gluten intolerance is typically merely a footnote in the education of traditional medical doctors. In a capitalist society, where medical schools and research are typically funded by large pharmaceutical companies and a government that subsidizes the wheat crop, there is little to be gained in a diagnosis of celiac disease or non-celiac gluten intolerance since the only treatment plan for these conditions is lifelong and strict abstinence from all things gluten.[1] There is no expensive pharmaceutical that magically allows the afflicted to eat platefuls of fried chicken and gravy with no ill effects, so there is no money to be made by the ruling class of the medical industry, the pharmaceutical companies. However, if such a pill were developed, doctors would be lobbied by the pharmaceutical companies to diagnose and treat celiac disease and non-celiac gluten sensitivity with new enthusiasm, as evidenced by other diseases such as diabetes and hypertension that could be controlled completely by diet in some cases but are typically controlled by long-term use of pharmaceuticals.

So it sounds fairly easy, and, really, what would be the fuss over avoiding something as simple sounding as gluten? Wheat is a member of the grass family—a part of the monocot branch, to be exact. It rests on a branch of the monocots with its close cousins, rye and barley. Gluten is the storage protein that makes up 10–15 percent of wheat. Genetically, the protein in rye and barley is similar enough to the wheat protein to cause issues for those sensitive to gluten.[2] Certainly, it is simple enough to avoid the obvious culprits—bread, pasta, and beer—but things are a bit more complicated than this cursory look. The problem is that wheat is a cheap binder, and, as a result, it is in everything from yogurt, salad dressing, and soy sauce to lotion, shampoo, and lipstick. Thus, a large part of the initiation and membership to the gluten-free society is the ability to plow through the myriad of labels on food and personal care products to determine which are safe and which could potentially poison your body.

However, reaching the point of realizing gluten is at the root of suffering can take years for a patient with celiac disease. Peter H. R. Green, MD, the director of the Celiac Disease Center at Columbia University, and Rory Jones in *Celiac Disease: A Hidden Epidemic* report, "In the United States today, *the average time to diagnosis of celiac disease is currently nine years. . . .* Patients normally see numerous physicians and specialists for symptoms that are misdiagnosed, do not respond to drug therapy, or are treated without concern for their underlying cause."[3] This long initiation time to membership is due not only to the lack of education in the medical field about the disease and the many forms it may take but also to the many confusing symptoms spurred by intolerance to gluten. Dr. Rodney Ford, a pediatrician in New Zealand, associate professor at the Christchurch School of Medicine, University of Otago, fellow of the Royal Australasian College of Physicians, and advocate of nutritional health, reports in *The Gluten Syndrome: Is Wheat Causing You Harm?* that epilepsy, ataxia, depression, mood disorders, defects in tooth enamel, irritable bowel syndrome, liver disease, type 1 diabetes, infertility in men and women, thyroid disorders, anemia, eczema, psoriasis, and alopecia areata can all result from sensitivity to gluten.[4] With this wide array of symptoms, doctors find it easier to treat the symptoms of these diseases instead of discovering and treating the cause. This helps explain the long, sometimes frustrating and painful initiation time into the Gluten-Free Cult. James Braly, MD (California physician practicing integrative medicine), and Ron Hoggan, MA (patient advocate), in *Dangerous Grains* add, "The connection between autoimmune disease and gluten grains is supported by evidence that is clear and compelling. . . . The risk of the many autoimmune disorders common in celiac disease increases with the length of time a celiac consumes gluten."[5] This adds urgency to Green and Jones's findings that the average time to diagnosis is nine years.

In her irreverent look at the problems gluten can wreak on the body, April Peveteaux in *Gluten Is My Bitch: Rants, Recipes, and Ridiculousness for the Gluten-Free* calls her first chapter "What to Do When You're Crapping Your Pants." She begins by saying, "Whatever your gluten situation, you're here [reading her book] because there is pooping, or perhaps, retching involved. If you're super lucky you'll also have a little itchiness, a bit of achiness, or all around crankiness."[6] Beyond dealing with the betrayal of their bodies, the gluten intolerant must also discuss the taboo of bowel habits with at least a medical provider. Danna Korn, in her self-help book *Wheat-Free, Worry-Free: The Art of Happy, Healthy, Gluten-Free Living*, acknowledges this additional initiation rite through the title of her chapter on bowel issues: "Talking to Your Doctor: Discussing Diarrhea and Other Fates Worse than Death."[7] Korn describes the experience at the doctor's office: "Feeling awkward and humiliated, and wishing you could trade places with someone in the middle of an IRS audit, you attempt to sound nonchalant as you force yourself to discuss your most intimate and disgusting bodily functions or lack thereof."[8] Not only are the digestive experiences for the gluten adverse horrible, but, in order to receive help, the patient must also break through the taboo of discussing diarrhea. The core members of the gluten-free community have suffered. They have had weird stomach issues featuring explosive diarrhea one day and painful constipation the next. Their brains have been fogged from continual gluten poisoning to the point that they wonder if they are still sane or if their IQs have been adversely affected. Their moods can swing from joy to despair in a matter of minutes. Their hair can fall out, and their bodies can be covered in horrible, itchy rashes. Some endure this abuse for nine or more years. This process to diagnosis can leave the core of the cult a bit testy about their position and a bit impatient with interlopers attempting to claim the community as their own, particularly when there's only one homemade gluten-free cookie left in the gluten-free cookie jar and a wheat eater has greedily snatched that cookie and claimed it for his own.

The final rite of initiation to the group of gluten-free eaters is screening through a blood test followed by a biopsy. If the blood test should indicate a possibility of celiac disease, it is followed by an endoscopic biopsy of the small intestine to confirm damage of the villi from gluten. If the biopsy is positive, then a diagnosis of celiac disease is made. Even this process is fraught with complications. If a patient has tried a gluten-free diet prior to diagnosis and the diet worked to alleviate their symptoms, then the process of diagnosis will be inconclusive. The only means to achieve a definitive diagnosis would be for the patient to consume gluten for one to three months in large quantities (the equivalent of four slices of bread daily) in order to redamage the villi so the gastroenterologist, the gatekeeper of the inner core of the group, can determine the validity of the patient's membership.[9]

The innermost core of the gluten-free community has suffered and ultimately had pieces of their intestines clipped out of their bodies after a sometimes-painful gluten challenge to gain their positions inside the group. In the hierarchy of societal organization, these are the privileged class. The gluten intolerant possess less clout than the other medically enforced brethren since their suffering did not culminate in a biopsy and celiac disease diagnosis. The gluten intolerant lack the "disease" designator. They also lack the designator of "food allergy" that most Americans at least superficially understand. They suffer both inside the gluten-free community and outside of it since the term *intolerance* does not carry the same weight as *disease* or *allergy*. In *The Gluten Connection: How Gluten Sensitivity May Be Sabotaging Your Health—and What You Can Do to Take Control NOW*, Shari Lieberman, a sometimes-controversial clinical nutritionist closely aligned with the health-food industry, describes the medical implications of this perceived second-class citizen to the gluten-free community, averring, "If you are gluten sensitive, your digestive system does not have the ability to break gluten down into soluble proteins (amino acids). Consequently, whenever you eat wheat, barley, or rye in *any* form and *any* amount (not necessarily a big slice of bread or cake!), your body reacts to the gluten because it interprets the gluten to be an antigen. The gluten fails to be broken down and passes into the bloodstream."[10] Once in the bloodstream, the body attacks the undigested gluten particles, causing inflammation and potentially triggering a host of autoimmune issues. The cure is a lifelong avoidance of gluten, identical to the treatment plan of the inner core suffering from celiac disease.

There has also been a link explored between autism, ADD, and ADHD and gluten. Many parents of children who engage in negative behavior stemming from autism, ADD, and ADHD claim to have seen improvements in their children when these children follow a gluten-free diet. There is debate as to whether there is a direct link between celiac disease and these groups, but scientists are exploring possible links between gluten sensitivity and the negative behaviors of autism, ADD, and ADHD, supporting the anecdotal evidence supplied by parents.[11] These children who follow the diet, not because of the adverse health effects that gluten causes in their bodies but because of the adverse mental effects that generate difficult behavior, create a bridge between the medically required gluten-free eaters and the hobbyists.

THE HOBBYISTS: HOW THE OUTER FRINGE OF THE GLUTEN-FREE CULT FORMED

Sometimes discussed with scorn and sometimes lauded as heroes among the inner core of the gluten-free community, the hobbyists come to the group and attempt to gain admittance to the club, bypassing all the rites of initiation caused from years of suffering undiagnosed symptoms that call into question their true allegiance to a gluten-free life. The hobbyist could stuff his face with Chicago-style pizza from Uno Pizzeria and wake up feeling fine the next day. This same action could leave the inner-core member sick, exhausted, and bedridden for weeks. The hobbyists have a different set of motivators to follow (sometimes sporadically) this difficult and expensive diet.

Many hobbyists are sympathetic followers. Within this subset, most have a gluten-free eater from the inner core in their household. Instead of preparing separate meals, the sympathetic eater chooses to eat gluten-free, at least at home. This cuts down on the labor in the kitchen and also can maintain the household kitchen as a gluten-free space, ensuring the safety of the medically mandated gluten-free eater at home from cross-contamination from errant gluten crumbs. This hobbyist has allegiance to their loved one and not necessarily to the cult. A lunch break at work might find him at Firehouse Subs eating his fill of freshly baked, glutenated bread.

Gluten can do funny things to the body of the medically necessitated gluten-free eater. Observers of those in the gluten-free community sometimes equate a gluten-free diet to almost instant weight loss. This is not tough to explain. When you instantly eliminate most of the grocery store from your diet, particularly the prepackaged, processed snack foods—think Little Debbie and Twinkies here—because it is all laced with a hearty dose of gluten, it is not difficult to shed some pounds. However, what most of the inner core knows and understands is that processed gluten-free foods are laced with added sugar and calories to generate taste, and Reese's Peanut Butter Cups, Snickers, and M&Ms are naturally gluten-free. Therefore, once the inner-core members learn what they can eat, their weight typically stabilizes. It is the dramatic initial weight loss that brings some hobbyists to the party. They envy the size-four-dress body without understanding the long years of bowel trouble that led to the body shape. This appropriation of a culture without the understanding of the trials of membership creates friction between the inner core and the weight-loss hobbyists.

Then there is Novak Djokovic, world-class tennis player and winner of the 2015 Wimbledon and Australian Open Championships and, as of July 2015, ranked number one in the world. Djokovic is the leading example of a performance-driven gluten-free eater and a bridge between the hobbyists and the inner core. Despite his talent and work ethic, Djokovic was inconsistent on the court, featuring a pre-2010 career fraught with on-court collapses and retirement from tournaments. Serbian doctor Igor Cetojevic, who was watching Djokovic's breakdown in his Australian Open quarter-final match, proposed a new solution, a gluten-free diet. Cetojevic believed Djokovic to be gluten intolerant.[12] After collapsing on the court in 2010, Djokovic returned to become the highest ranked male tennis player in the world, a success he attributes to his diet and that is detailed in his book, *Serve to Win*. Djokovic's success has inspired other performance-minded athletes, especially weekend warriors, to join the league of hobbyists and follow a gluten-free diet to sports glory. These athletes do not pursue an inquiry into their own health to determine whether a gluten-free diet is necessary. Instead, they believe that gluten-free is the magic bullet that sent Djokovic (ignoring Djokovic's talent and dedication to perfection as well as his unique medical situation) to the top of the tennis world.

Really, what good is a cult unless a lot of celebrities are clawing their way to get in with the cool kids? Celebrities such as Miley Cyrus and Lady Gaga have squeezed their way into the fringe of the non-wheat-eating community with their gluten-free weight-loss plans, but they will never be taken seriously by the inner core of gluten-free eaters since they can binge on gluten-free cookies one day and fine French dining featuring sauces begun with a roux of wheat and butter the next. Keith Olbermann, a political commentator, has publicly announced that he has celiac disease. Chelsea Clinton reports gluten sensitivity and had a much-touted gluten-free wedding cake at her 2010 nuptials. Elisabeth Hasselbeck, one-time co-host of *The View*, shared her experience with celiac disease in her book *The G-Free Diet*.[13] While Olbermann, Clinton, and Hasselbeck are all inner-core members of this community of eaters, their celebrity has inspired a swell in gluten-free hobbyists.

In *Digestive Wellness*, a June 2015 supplement to *USA Today*, Jennifer Esposito is featured on the cover as she "opens up about her road to diagnosis and learning to manage digestive wellness in a new way."[14] Esposito tells of a lifetime of "anxiety attacks, stomach issues, [and] sinus infections. 'I just learned to live with it and accept it, going through my life thinking that symptoms like these were normal.'"[15] Her diagnosis of celiac disease and the life-changing improvement in her health has turned her into a public and vocal advocate for the gluten-free community. In 2012, she opened a Manhattan restaurant featuring a gluten-free kitchen called Jennifer's Way Bakery. As these celebrities flock to the cult for both medical reasons and body-image reasons, they bring with them a horde of fad followers who wish to emulate their idols. This has expanded the group of hobbyists that toy with the gluten-free diet and sometimes frustrates the initiated members of the inner circle.

LIFE IN THE GLUTEN-FREE CULT

While outside celebrities attempt to merge their stardom with a gluten-free life, there are also internal celebrities sprung from their role inside the Gluten-Free Cult. The ability of the group to create its own rock stars demonstrates its rising power. In the area of gluten-free research is Alessio Fasano, author of *Gluten Freedom: The Nation's Leading Expert Offers the Essential Guide to a Healthy, Gluten-Free Lifestyle*. Fasano, chief of the division of Pediatric Gastroenterology and Nutrition at Massachusetts General Hospital and director of the Center for Celiac Research, authored the 2003 study that showed the rate of celiac disease at 1 in 133 Americans. He has become the face and voice of research in the areas of celiac disease and gluten intolerance, with hundreds of interviews in media such as the *New York Times*, National Public Radio, and CNN.[16]

In the search for real-life advice and experience in navigating the gluten-free world, many newbies to the group turn to the Web and bloggers to help them adjust to their new world order. Blogger Shauna James Ahern developed a large enough following to launch her career as an author and food writer. Her initial book, *Gluten-Free Girl: How I Found Food That Loves Me Back . . . & How You Can Too*, was such a success that she has followed with two additional titles. Danielle Walker, the founder of againstallgrain.com, blogged that food became the answer to her chronic suffering from an autoimmune disease. Her recipes are grain-free, gluten-free, free of refined sugars, and low in dairy. Her blog led to the successful publication of four cookbooks.[17]

Danna Korn, known as the Gluten-Free Guru, also rose to stardom within the Gluten-Free Cult. Korn has been active in the gluten-free community since 1991 when her son was diagnosed with celiac disease. That year, she founded R.O.C.K. (Raising Our Celiac Kids), a support group for families with gluten-free children. She is also the founder of Gluten Freedom, offering consulting to food companies and others providing services to the gluten-free community. Her bubbly personality and deep knowledge of all things gluten-free has fueled her rise within this group of eaters as the media darling sought by the likes of *People* magazine and ABC's *20/20* for interviews. She is the author of three books, including the well-known primer *Living Gluten-Free for Dummies*.[18]

Even the world of celebrity chefs has been the breeding ground for new gluten-free celebrities. Emeril Lagasse's daughters both follow strict gluten-free diets. Jilly has celiac disease, while her sister, Jessie, is gluten intolerant. Jessie says that they understand the frustration of navigating the gluten-free food world and wanted to produce a book of recipes that would reassure the community that there is plenty of good gluten-free food out there. Their rise to stardom among gluten-free eaters has been aided by their famous last name. Their father has supported their projects by writing ten recipes for their first book, *The Gluten-Free Table*, and five for their 2014 cookbook, *The Lagasse Girls' Big Flavor, Bold Taste and No Gluten.*[19]

Religious cults create exclusive environments for their members, and the Gluten-Free Cult has followed suit. The GF & AF (gluten-free and allergen-friendly) Expo hails itself as the largest gluten-free event in the United States, with conventions in eleven cities in 2015. These conferences, which are similar in set-up to other gluten-free conferences, feature gluten-free vendors offering free samples, books, and magazines, as well as sessions featuring some of the gluten-free stars of the lecture circuit.[20] The expos create a space to celebrate liberation from wheat. Likewise, there are many gluten-free travel destinations offering this same form of sanctuary. Chicken Paradise, a small, exclusive bed and breakfast in San Antonio, Texas, offers "the only bed and breakfast with a gluten-free kitchen in San Antonio, and is the only bed and breakfast that is a participant in the Gluten-Free Restaurant Awareness Program, administered by the Gluten Intolerance Group of North America."[21] Lesley Hock, a travel agent from Boston, has built her business around finding and booking gluten-free vacations for clients. She believes demand for this type of travel will expand as more people are being tested and diagnosed.[22] The National Foundation for Celiac Awareness in 2015 listed eighteen summer camps for children and teens featuring gluten-free foods with names like Camp Gluten-Free, Gluten-Free Fun Camp, and the Great Gluten Escape Camp. All promise a safe haven from the threat of gluten.[23]

Perhaps the most sacred of grounds for the Gluten-Free Community are the dedicated gluten-free restaurants and bakeries that have sprung up across the United States. Shine Restaurant & Gathering Place in Boulder, Colorado, touts a 100 percent gluten-free kitchen featuring such delicacies as gluten-free macaroni and cheese, hamburgers with homemade gluten-free buns, and house-baked gluten-free rolls. The restaurant is committed to "maintain[ing] a 100% gluten-free and GMO-free kitchen, and accommodating food allergies and sensitivities, because everyone should be able to eat a beautiful meal without fear of discomfort or judgment."[24] Dempsey Bakery in Little Rock,

Arkansas, maintains a 100 percent gluten-, wheat-, soy-, and nut-fee kitchen. TAPAteria in Colorado Springs offers a huge menu of tapas in a 100 percent gluten-free environment, while just down the street, Outside the Breadbox features gluten-free breads, sweets, and crackers baked in a 100 percent gluten-free kitchen. Mariposa Baking Company in Oakland, California, offers a variety of gluten-free breads and sweets as well as lunches at its 100 percent gluten-free facility founded in 2004. Everybody Eats in Brooklyn, New York, also founded in 2004, offers an array of gluten-free breads and sweets in a 100 percent gluten-free kitchen that are shipped all over the country. With its focus on taste and texture, the bakery offers one of the best-quality gluten-free French loaves on the market. Anheuser-Busch introduced Redbridge, a gluten-free sorghum-based beer in 2006. Since then, many microbrews have brought gluten-free beers to the market. The Gluten-Free Cult has gained enough membership and clout to demand sanctuary from wheat and receive it.

THE INNER CORE AND THE HOBBYISTS: AN UNEASY PARTNERSHIP

The medically driven gluten-free eaters tend to have a love-hate relationship with the hobbyists. The tension is a result of the danger that the hobbyists bring to the inner-core gluten-free consumer. Many restaurants that are not dedicated gluten-free facilities still cater to gluten-free eaters. They offer gluten-free options and safe spaces in their kitchens away from anything prepared with wheat to avoid unintentional cross-contamination that could leave a member of the inner core ill for weeks. Even an errant breadcrumb or a knife used to cut a sandwich for another customer and then a baked potato for the gluten-free eater could cause reactions for the inner-core eaters. Therefore, restaurants go to great trouble in their kitchens to clean workspaces, change gloves, use clean utensils and pans, use separate toasters, and (sometimes) even use separate plates to avoid confusion at the table. This special treatment takes important time and staffing in the fast-paced world of restaurant kitchens, but it is essential to the health of the medically driven gluten-free eater. All this is terrific until a hobbyist walks in and makes the same demands of the kitchen. Meanwhile, the hot bread that the waiter leaves on the table for the rest of the dining party wafts its way to the hungry hobbyist's nose, and in no time flat he is snarfing down that gluten-filled deliciousness and is caught in the act by the confused waiter, who has just asked the kitchen to perform wild feats of safety for the guy who says he is gluten-free and is now shoving bread into his mouth back at the table. This same waiter, armed with the fury of the kitchen, is less likely to take his next gluten-free customer seriously. He believes that people who claim to be gluten-free are obviously not harmed by a little gluten, as evidenced by the bread-eating hobbyist. Thus begins the vicious cycle of restaurants relaxing their gluten-free standards and endangering the health of the inner core of the Gluten-Free Cult.

Not only do the hobbyists confuse restaurants about the gravity of medically required gluten-free eating, but they also confuse the public. Hobbyists have a special skill of talking boorishly for hours about their diet; however, since their health does not necessarily depend upon the diet, their information is not always as carefully considered and based on research as that of the inner core. Their friends and colleagues who have listened to this talk endlessly and witnessed the dining habits of the hobbyists that include a small piece of glutenated pizza here and a cinnamon roll there have been taught through this example that it is not necessary to be gluten-free all the time and that all gluten-free eaters can have gluten when it pleases them without harmful effects. Once the cult outsiders form these attitudes, it becomes difficult and dangerous for the inner core to experience food with friends and family unless the gluten-free eater prepares the meal herself.

The news media have also fallen prey to the work of the hobbyists. *Healthline* in April 2015 featured the headline, "Is Non-Celiac Gluten Sensitivity a Real Thing?" *Forbes* in May 2014 said, "Gluten Intolerance May Not Exist." In April 2015, *Huffington Post* echoed this headline, "Is Non-Celiac Gluten Sensitivity a Real Thing?" and *Scientific American* asked, "Is Non-Celiac Gluten Sensitivity for Real?" Shauna Ahern reacted to the spate of headlines in her May 27, 2014, blog in *Gluten-Free Girl* with "Not Again." In this blog she explores a study performed in at Monash University in Australia on thirty-seven patients with diagnosed irritable bowel syndrome (IBS) that spawned the flood of headlines such as those above. She notes the problems with the study and responses to it by leading researchers such as Dr. Alessio Fasano, who argued that the study was flawed because it only included patients with IBS.[25] The fad status of the diet generated by the hobbyists has conditioned the press to cling to any derogatory information about medically necessitated gluten-free lifestyles without fully examining the validity of the information they are covering. Once again, this irresponsibility by the hobbyists regarding a very serious dietary issue for many

Americans has provided the fuel for the press to attack the Gluten-Free Cult and lower its credibility in the eyes of the media consumers.

However, the inner core also benefits from the addition of the hobbyists to the community. There is consumer power in numbers. With more people interested in purchasing gluten-free foods, not only are more foods widely available, but they also taste better. Gluten-free foods that had been relegated to health food stores, specialty stores, and mail order have made their way to Kroger, Publix, and King Soopers. There are more choices then ever before, and the gluten-free shopper does not have to work as hard to find the food he needs by traveling to multiple stores. A plethora of more affordable and better-tasting gluten-free food is now on the shelves of most general grocery stores.

In addition to the placement of gluten-free items in mainstream groceries, the mainstream food companies are delving into gluten-free production. Tyson did an initial rollout of gluten-free fried chicken nuggets in May 2013 followed by a national rollout a few months later. In December 2013, Pillsbury released a gluten-free pie crust, chocolate chip cookie dough, pizza dough, and flour. Specialty food companies have also entered the gluten-free market. In 2012, specialty retailer Williams-Sonoma began selling Cup4Cup gluten-free flour and mixes developed by Chef Lena Kwak under the mentorship of Chef Thomas Keller, owner of the French Laundry in Yountville, California. These high-end mixes taste delicious, and with the Cup4Cup flour, regular bread and dessert recipes can be used without alteration to make them gluten-free. In our market-driven economy, these products could only exist with enough interest and buying power to make them profitable. Without the hobbyists, the inner core might still be driving across town to the small health food store to peruse its meager and sometimes dismal gluten-free offerings.

Perhaps the biggest innovation for the cult has been the Food Allergen Labeling and Consumer Protection Act of 2004, which went into effect in 2006 and made reading labels even easier since any of the eight major food allergens, including wheat, must be clearly listed on the label if the product contains them. In August 2014 the gluten-free label rule took effect so that a packaged food can only contain a gluten-free label if it contains less than twenty parts per million of gluten. This clarity in food labels only came about due to increased pressure on lawmakers to create the requirements. The combined efforts of the entire community of gluten-free eaters led to this important victory that makes shopping less complicated and the purchased food less likely to poison the inner circle of eaters with gluten.

THE FORECAST FOR THE GLUTEN-FREE CULT

There is no cure for celiac disease or diagnosed gluten intolerance. There are dreams among the inner core of days filled with endless consumption of glutenated delights, but science has yet to render a magic pill that erases the harm gluten can cause to the afflicted. Even if researchers succeed in creating such a pill, it is likely that many members of the community will prefer their new and healthy eating habits instead of access to the processed foods this pill would allow. Therefore, the heart of the Gluten-Free Cult will not become just a passing fad. In fact, as doctors are more aware of celiac disease and gluten intolerance, diagnoses will be more widespread, expanding the size of the inner core of medically necessitated gluten avoiders. Those whose health and well-being depend upon strict avoidance of gluten will maintain the group as the hobbyists who have rushed to the latest diet craze will move to the next "get-thin-quick gimmick," leaving the gluten-free eaters at peace to dine on their plentiful, new, and improved (thanks to the help of the hobbyists) gluten-free bread, pizza, pasta, cookies, and crackers.

NOTES

1. For an overview of the wheat crop and the subsidies offered to farmers, see "Wheat Policy," *United States Department of Agriculture/Economic Research Service*, June 2015, http://www.ers.usda.gov/topics/crops/wheat/policy.aspx, accessed July 13, 2015.

2. Peter H. R. Green and Rory Jones, *Celiac Disease: A Hidden Epidemic* (New York: Collins, 2006), 22–23.

3. Green and Jones, *Celiac Disease*, 4 (emphasis in original).

4. Dr. Rodney Ford, *The Gluten Syndrome: Is Wheat Causing You Harm?* (Christchurch, New Zealand: RRS Global Ltd., 2007), 78–79.

5. James Braly and Ron Hoggan, *Dangerous Grains* (New York: Avery, 2002), 118–19.

6. April Peveteaux, *Gluten Is My Bitch: Rants, Recipes, and Ridiculousness for the Gluten-Free* (New York: Stewart, Tabori & Chang, 2015), 15.

7. Danna Korn, *Wheat-Free, Worry-Free: The Art of Happy, Healthy, Gluten-Free Living* (Carlsbad, CA: Hay House, Inc., 2002), vi.

8. Korn, *Wheat-Free, Worry-Free*, 89.

9. "Diagnosing Celiac Disease," Celiac Disease Foundation, http://celiac.org/celiac-disease/diagnosing-celiac-disease/, accessed July 13, 2015.

10. Shari Lieberman, with Linda Segall, *The Gluten Connection: How Gluten Sensitivity May Be Sabotaging Your Health—and What You Can Do to Take Control NOW* (New York: Rodale, 2007), 14.

11. Anecdotal information from parents with children experiencing autism, ADHD, and ADD supports behavioral improvement from a gluten-free and sometimes casein-free (the protein in milk) diet. Scientists are still exploring the causation creating these results. Discussions engaging these issues can be found in Helmut Niederhofer, "Association of Attention-Deficit/Hyperactivity Disorder and Celiac Disease: A Brief Report," *U.S. National Library of Medicine/National Institutes of Health*, 2011, http://www.ncbi.nlm.nih.gov/pmc/articles/PMC3184556/, accessed July 14, 2015, and "Autism Study Finds No Link to Celiac Disease: Gluten Reactivity Real," *Autism Speaks*, September 25, 2013, https://www.autismspeaks.org/science/science-news/autism-study-finds-no-link-celiac-disease-gluten-reactivity-real, accessed July 14, 2015.

12. Hannah Britt, "Novak Djokovic: Going Gluten-Free Was a Real Game Changer," *Express: Home of the Daily and Sunday Express*, September 11, 2013, http://www.express.co.uk/life-style/health/428272/Novak-Djokovic-Going-gluten-free-was-a-real-game-changer, accessed July 14, 2015.

13. "Celebs Who Go Gluten-Free," *ABC News*, http://abcnews.go.com/Health/Allergies/photos/celebs-gluten-free-17828847/image-17828956, accessed July 14, 2015.

14. I-Hsien Sherwood, "Decades to Diagnosis: Jennifer Esposito's Long Battle," *Mediaplanet for USA Today*, June 2015, cover.

15. Sherwood, "Decades to Diagnosis," 6.

16. "Alessio Fasano, MD," *MassGeneral Hospital for Children*, 2015, http://www.massgeneral.org/children/doctors/doctor.aspx?id=19184, accessed July 14, 2015.

17. Danielle Walker, *Against All Grain*, http://againstallgrain.com/about-me/, accessed July 14, 2015.

18. "Danna Korn," *Gluten Free Café*, Hain Celestial Group, Inc., 2010, http://www.myglutenfreecafe.com/about_danna.html, accessed July 14, 2015.

19. Mary MacVean, "Emeril Lagasse's Daughters Are Out with a New Gluten-Free Cookbook," *Los Angeles Times*, November 13, 2014, http://www.latimes.com/food/dailydish/la-dd-lagasse-daughters-gluten-free-cookbook-20141111-story.html, accessed July 14, 2015.

20. "GF & AF Expo," *Gluten Free Classes, LLC*, 2014, accessed July 14, 2015, http://gfafexpo.com, accessed July 14, 2015.

21. *Chicken Paradise: A Country B&B in the Heart of San Antonio*, http://www.chickenparadise.com. Accessed July 14, 2015.

22. Lilit Marcus, "Gluten-Free Travel Is a Thing (and Yes, You Can Still Visit Italy)," *Conde Nast Traveler*, December 8, 2014, http://www.cntraveler.com/stories/2014-12-08/gluten-free-travel-agent-lesley-hock-celiac-disease, accessed July 15, 2015.

23. "Gluten-Free Friendly Camps for Kids and Teens," National Foundation for Celiac Awareness, July 2015, http://www.celiaccentral.org/kids/gluten-free-camps/list/, accessed July 15, 2015.

24. "The Food," *Shine Restaurant & Gathering Place*, 2014, http://www.shineboulder.com/food/, accessed July 15, 2015.

25. Shauna James Ahern, "Not Again," *Playing with Our Food: Gluten-Free-Girl and the Chef*, May 27, 2014, http://glutenfreegirl.com/2014/05/gluten-sensitivity-is-real/, accessed July 15, 2015.

BIBLIOGRAPHY

Ahern, Shauna James. "Not Again." *Playing with Our Food: Gluten-Free-Girl and the Chef*, May 27, 2014. http://glutenfreegirl.com/2014/05/gluten-sensitivity-is-real/. Accessed July 15, 2015.

"Alessio Fasano, MD." *MassGeneral Hospital for Children*, 2015. http://www.massgeneral.org/children/doctors/doctor.aspx?id=19184. Accessed July 14, 2015.

"Autism Study Finds No Link to Celiac Disease: Gluten Reactivity Real." *Autism Speaks*, September 25, 2013. https://www.autismspeaks.org/science/science-news/autism-study-finds-no-link-celiac-disease-gluten-reactivity-real. Accessed July 14, 2015.

Braly, James, and Ron Hoggan. *Dangerous Grains*. New York: Avery, 2002.

Britt, Hannah. "Novak Djokovic: Going Gluten-Free Was a Real Game Changer." *Express: Home of the Daily and Sunday Express*, September 11, 2013. Accessed July 14, 2015.

"Celebs Who Go Gluten-Free." *ABC News*. http://abcnews.go.com/Health/Allergies/photos/celebs-gluten-free-17828847/image-17828956. Accessed July 14, 2015.

Chicken Paradise: A Country B&B in the Heart of San Antonio. http://www.chickenparadise.com. Accessed July 14, 2015.

"Danna Korn." *Gluten Free Café*. Hain Celestial Group, Inc., 2010. http://www.myglutenfreecafe.com/about_danna.html. Accessed July 14, 2015.

"Diagnosing Celiac Disease." Celiac Disease Foundation. http://celiac.org/celiac-disease/diagnosing-celiac-disease/. Accessed July 13, 2015.

"The Food." *Shine Restaurant & Gathering Place*, 2014. http://www.shineboulder.com/food/. Accessed July 15, 2015.

Ford, Rodney. *The Gluten Syndrome: Is Wheat Causing You Harm?* Christchurch, New Zealand: RRS Global Ltd., 2007.

"GF & AF Expo." *Gluten Free Classes, LLC*, 2014. http://gfafexpo.com. Accessed July 14, 2015.

"Gluten-Free Friendly Camps for Kids and Teens." National Foundation for Celiac Awareness, July 2015. http://www.celiaccentral.org/kids/gluten-free-camps/list/. Accessed July 15, 2015.

Green, Peter H. R., and Rory Jones. *Celiac Disease: A Hidden Epidemic*. New York: Collins, 2006.

Korn, Danna. *Wheat-Free, Worry-Free: The Art of Happy, Healthy, Gluten-Free Living*. Carlsbad, CA: Hay House, Inc., 2002.

Lieberman, Shari, with Linda Segall. *The Gluten Connection: How Gluten Sensitivity May Be Sabotaging Your Health—and What You Can Do to Take Control NOW*. New York: Rodale, 2007.

MacVean, Mary. "Emeril Lagasse's Daughters Are Out with a New Gluten-Free Cookbook." *Los Angeles Times*, November 13, 2014. http://www.latimes.com/food/dailydish/la-dd-lagasse-daughters-gluten-free-cookbook-20141111-story.html. Accessed July 14, 2015.

Marcus, Lilit. "Gluten-Free Travel Is a Thing (and Yes, You Can Still Visit Italy)." *Conde Nast Traveler*, December 8, 2014. http://www.cntraveler.com/stories/2014-12-08/gluten-free-travel-agent-lesley-hock-celiac-disease. Accessed July 15, 2015.

Niederhofer, Helmut. "Association of Attention-Deficit/Hyperactivity Disorder and Celiac Disease: A Brief Report." *U.S. National Library of Medicine/National Institutes of Health*, 2011. Accessed July 14, 2015.

Preveteaux, April. *Gluten Is My Bitch: Rants, Recipes, and Ridiculousness for the Gluten-Free*. New York: Steward, Tabori & Chang, 2015.

Sherwood, I-Hsien. “Decades to Diagnosis: Jennifer Esposito’s Long Battle.” *Mediaplanet for USA Today*, June 2015.

Walker, Danielle. *Against All Grain*. http://againstallgrain.com/about-me/. Accessed July 14, 2015.

“Wheat Policy.” *United States Department of Agriculture/Economic Service*, June 2015. http://www.ers.usda.gov/topics/crops/wheat/policy.aspx. Accessed July 13, 2015.

Chapter Thirteen

Erasure of Indigenous Food Memories and (Re-)Imaginations

Preety Gadhoke and Barrett P. Brenton

On independent, temporally staggered, yet somehow parallel paths, our collective ethnographic fieldwork has taken us over the years across the tall and short grasses of the central and eastern plains through the dry dessert plateaus of the Southwest, culminating into a recent, joint venture into the lush, high jungle of the Ecuadorian Amazon with a special opportunity to work with indigenous Shuar communities. As space folds and time curves, Barry and I have both worked with American Indian communities for our dissertation work in the 1990s and 2010s, respectively. Within the indigenous context, I have worked with Ojibwa, Potawatomi, Navajo, and Pueblo communities, and Barry has worked with Hopi communities for our respective dissertations. My experiences have spanned Anishinaabe harvest feasts, powwows, drum ceremonies and rituals, and chronic disease prevention health programs in tribal schools and communities in the Midwest to Pueblo community gardening and school programs in the Southwest. Barry's experiences have encompassed ritual dance performances, feast celebrations, and farming among the Hopi to powwows and tribal casinos from California to Connecticut. Being the two anthropologists and faculty at St. John's University who possessed the rare commonality of working with American Indians brought with it ongoing conversations about indigeneity, food, culture, and health. It is through these conversations over nearly three years that our growing interest in writing a piece on indigenous food cults came about. As part of this edited volume on food cults, we discuss our experiences in the field, primarily focusing upon the North American Indian context.

In this chapter, we argue that indigenous underlying foodways and related belief systems are actively redefined and realized by communities as products of their own organic experience of multiple waves of traumatic losses and the resulting embodiment of social devastations. While we take a critical medical anthropological perspective, our discussion in this chapter focuses on the importance of meaning-making and terminology usage by American Indian communities for their foodways, foods, and identity.

DEFINING AND DEFYING THE "NORMATIVE"

Even with the vast diversity and array of dietary traditions of the 567 American Indian tribes now officially recognized by the U.S. federal government,[1] these communities face the ongoing challenge of living with the dissonance of the normative *etic* or outsider's perspective on what constitutes "healthy" diets, food, and eating in conjunction with each community's own trajectories of modernization.

This normative process of assimilation has even defined what culturally constitutes a tribe. A report by the U.S. Department of the Interior's Bureau of Indian Affairs (BIA) noted that since 1978, 237 tribes have petitioned, mostly unsuccessfully, for federal recognition, including 65 state-recognized tribes, making them even more marginalized.[2] The development of a structure of dietary colonization that has sought to homogenize the "American" diet has a long tradition that integrates a complex merging of historical movements in nutrition science, public health, and the corporate food industry.

Discordance with the resulting hegemonic control over the relationship between diet and health has led to the classification of nonconforming traditions as being peripheral traditions in need of intervention. Terms such as *food quackery*, *fads*, and *cults* are often used as labels to identify groups or individuals who make counterclaims to established mainstream dietary standards. We do not dismiss the potential concerns and harm to public health for nutrition claims based more on profiteering than scientific merit.[3] However, what about the case of traditions that are rooted in cultures that far precede current "modern" diet and health orthodoxy, the case of indigenous systems of diet and health in particular? Rather than being de facto dismissive of those practices as nonconformist, we call for an evidence-based validation of those traditions.

The modern emergence of the field of nutritional science in the United States around the turn of the twentieth century was spearheaded by the work of Wilbur O. Atwater. His research on the principles of nutrition is credited with using the scientific method to develop dietary guidelines to improve health and well-being.[4] During this time and before the passage of the U.S. Pure Food and Drug Act of 1906, diet and health claims were widely speculative and anecdotal rather than being truly evidence based. While the act only mildly curbed food faddism and subsequent legislation was needed, work by Atwater and others began to establish a greater understanding of nutritional requirements, food composition, food consumption by the population, and the effects of socioeconomic factors on food choice.[5] It also greatly influenced the development of standardized dietary guidelines for healthy eating by the United States Department of Agriculture (USDA) throughout the twentieth century.

While we do not dispute here the physiological fundamentals of nutrition and metabolism at the foundation of these recommendations, we do argue that the recommended dietary inputs to meet those needs were part of a larger normative movement to homogenize the "American" diet for the sake of food safety, security, social order, and commerce. It supported a reductionist framework of "nutritionism" that was more focused on nutricentric dietary guidelines and disease preventative nutrients[6] rather than on a more holistic view of food as being something greater than the sum of its nutrient parts.[7] This approach also became a driving force behind the commoditization of food by lobbying corporate interests in the food manufacturing industry.

These formulations heavily influenced the types of food being promoted through home economics education at Indian boarding schools on and off the reservation. This was enforced through the assimilation work of U.S. government field agents on the reservation in terms of the types of diets and methods of food production and preparation that were being prescribed as part of a larger effort to "domesticate" Native Americans.[8] The lack of food composition information on local and traditional foods also limited culturally appropriate foods from being integrated into any kind of nutrition and health education programming. It is thus somewhat ironic that Atwater received his doctorate in 1869 in agricultural chemistry with a thesis titled "The Proximate Composition of Several Types of American Maize."

MARGINALIZATION AND TRAUMATIC LOSSES OF FOODWAYS

The overall historical and ongoing process of marginalizing Native American indigenous foodways by institutions such as the USDA, BIA, and eventually Indian Health Services, however well meaning, sought to modernize and homogenize their dietary traditions under the public health pretext of disease prevention and control. It is difficult to separate this type of dietary assimilation from the parallel strategies used to suppress expressions of their language, religion, and culture. For example, in the case of Native American languages, the erasure of Native tongues has been clearly documented through the government boarding school education experience. Children were physically punished for speaking anything other than English.[9] The historical trauma resulting from the systematic attempt to disrupt the foodways of hundreds of indigenous nations cannot be separated from the classification of those traditions as being cults embedded in larger ideological systems in need of conversion. While the term *cults* may not have been used explicitly, the tone was one that often implied unclean, unsanitary, unbalanced, restricted, or monotonous diets. Of course, such descriptors were tagged as a result of stubborn old traditions that died hard, rather than revealing them as a result of intentional disruptions of their traditional food systems as a calculated plan to force treaties and a reservation lifestyle that established Native communities as wards of the state. Nor did it recognize the arts of resistance and agency being utilized by indigenous communities themselves. Defining and redefining authenticity, in either a culture or its foodways, is a dynamic process where voices of diversity and memory must be given as much, if not greater, credence over merely the posturing of authority.

A case in point can be to look at the impact of the forces of assimilation that ultimately led to the distribution of commodities such as wheat flour, lard, and sugar—the stuff of fry bread—and canned meats as a means to address the high levels of malnutrition and food insecurity associated with reservation life. These programs ushered in a new low-quality and insufficient food system with federal aid programs that failed to incorporate or support traditional foods and thus became the foundation of chronic diseases such as diabetes. However, there is no denying that the pan-Indian and pantribal identity of the culinary consequence of the commodities programs has resulted in fry bread being seen as a "traditional" Indian food. The clearly unhealthy fat content of fry bread[10] has become part of a discourse over authenticity, wherein fry bread has become a traditional food that is nontraditional.[11] From this perspective, fry bread can be viewed as the ultimate indigenous "cult food." However, perhaps the more important question is linked to the memories of how it became a traditional food as part of a larger process of identity building and maintenance in the face of historical trauma and assimilation. Beyond fry bread, food is defined as part of a homogenized American diet and can be labeled with an even deeper meaning when it is used in the contexts surrounding culturally centered events.

RITUALIZED ACTS OF EATING

While fry bread has become the singular symbolic "traditional" Native American food among non–Native Americans, it remains a food that has been actively incorporated into traditional ceremonies such as drum birthing rituals in the Upper Midwest and offered as the foundation of Indian tacos at powwows across the United States. There is as much variability in fry bread as there is heterogeneity among American Indian communities, a little-known truth among non-Native populations. For instance, fry bread takes many forms, from soft flatbreads to harder, doughnut-like dense breads. Following a five-hour-long drum birthing ceremony in a traditional wigwam, I was offered fry bread with black coffee for breakfast along with other attendees. Fry bread, in this case, has replaced the quintessential doughnut as the American breakfast for those in a hurry. More than that, having fry bread with coffee represents a new ritual created by Native Americans and a powerful symbol of adaptation (and a silent response) to the political economic forces of the United States.

In contrast, the single most symbolic food ritual in the United States is arguably Thanksgiving, which cross-cuts multiethnic boundaries and has become a rite of passage for newly arrived immigrants as "being 'Merican." It further conjures stereotypical images such as Louis Gerome Ferris's *The First Thanksgiving* (1915) of the initial fated encounter between the new order of the Pilgrims and the new world of indigenous peoples that continue to marginalize modern Native Americans. In *Food in the USA*, Carole Counihan describes the replacement of the Fourth of July by Thanksgiving Day as the single most celebrated American ritual. She quotes James Robertson, who had written that the "modern celebration of Thanksgiving is a ritual affirmation of what Americans believe was the Pilgrim confronting, settling, adapting to, and civilizing the New World."[12] In addition to reaffirming an idealized (non-Native) American identity, Thanksgiving reaffirms the American family and, annually, resurrects the early American imagination of what it means to be "indigenous" or "Native American" with images that are replete with (idealized and marginalized) conjured images of Pilgrims and Indians standing shoulder to shoulder engaging in a form of mythical, equal dialogue. In history texts, it is claimed that the Pilgrims arrived at Plymouth Rock on December 11, 1620. With a rough first winter, 46 of the 102 pilgrims died. The remaining 56 celebrated their first harvest the following fall of 1621 with a feast with the Natives. The first meal, following the pattern of a more traditional English harvest festival, lasted three days and is believed to have included venison, duck, geese, fish, clams, lobster, and corn. There is no evidence of breads, pies, cranberries, or potatoes. It was much later that President George Washington announced the first Thanksgiving Day in 1789, and in 1863 President Abraham Lincoln made a Thanksgiving Proclamation, closing government offices. Later, in 1941, President Franklin D. Roosevelt signed a bill into law, with Congress making Thanksgiving a national holiday on the fourth Thursday in November. Ironically, the National Turkey Federation in 1947 presented President Harry Truman with a live turkey that labeled it as the main course of a Thanksgiving meal. It is this ritualized non-Native food cult of Thanksgiving and its invented history that suggests the divide between the real and the imagined holiday and, henceforth, the perpetuation and continuous marginalization of the Native identity to date, with the "turkey" symbolizing the Native American "stuffed and served" to the Pilgrims.[13]

The religious cult comparison is not lost on its relevance to understanding the historical framing of indigenous food cults. Religious cults can be defined as ideologically based belief systems that are realized or exhibited through rituals. In the case of food cults, the act of eating is the ritual itself and becomes ritualized. However, in order to understand the ritualized acts of eating, we need to unpack the meanings of "food" in the Anglo context that informed the American ideals. In areas like New England the English yeomen diet brought to the New World by the Puritans consisting of peas porridge, brown bread, boiled meat, dark beer, and fermented cider was still maintained well into the nineteenth century in the former American colonies.[14]

Early nineteenth-century examples of perspectives on diet, food, and health came from a litany of publications, such as medical texts and domestic economy cookbooks. For example, Thomas Graham prescribes in his 1828 treatise on *Sure Methods of Improving Health, and Prolonging Life* healthy meals emphasizing the importance of eating certain foods at specific times: "In case of a late dinner, some *luncheon* is almost always necessary, as it is highly improper to fast from breakfast to a late dinner. It may consist of a little good soup and bread, or an egg and some bread and butter, or a very thin slice of cold meat and bread, with a little malt liquor or half a glass of wine."[15]

With respect to a uniquely American diet, Sarah Josepha Hale, in her 1839 *Good Housekeeper*, calls for dietary proscriptions based on her observation that "foreigners say that our climate is unhealthy; that the Americans have, generally, thin form, sallow complexions and bad teeth. Is it not most likely that these defects are incurred, in part if not wholly, because the diet and modes of living are unsuitable to the climate, and consequently to the health of the people?"[16] Ironically, Hale was also the one who petitioned Lincoln in 1863 to write the Thanksgiving Day celebration proclamation.

Such American meanings of "healthy foods" preceded the widespread industrialization of American foodways and predated the birth of nutritional science as a discipline. As such, these examples of early American notions of "healthy" foods and meals continue to be both prescriptive and proscriptive in indigenous memories today. They also reveal a foundation of contested ethnic foodways that Tompkins has referred to as a form of *racial indigestion.*[17]

Yet some American values and ideals of "healthy eating" in conjunction with the convenient, easy-to-prepare, prepackaged and "unhealthy" foods are embraced alike through the active (re-)imaginations of the Native American communities. In contrast to Thanksgiving, for example, the fall harvest festival in an Upper Midwest community was a more intimate affair reinforcing gendered roles of food preparation. A few Native Americans attended it, and there were many food offerings accompanied by men drumming and children dancing and hula-hooping. Opened with a harvest prayer by the traditional healer, the harvest feast celebrated the fertility and abundance of Mother Earth with prepared "three sisters" from the local community garden and accompanied by corn and an overwhelming array of "American" desserts, including prepackaged, easy-to-prepare, and no-bake blueberry and strawberry cheesecakes, angel food cake, and pies. There was no turkey or chicken as the centerpiece of the table, for turkey is too expensive to purchase on semirural reservations where there are no wild turkeys and (affordable) supermarkets are thirty or more miles away. In another example, a Southwest American Indian woman's involvement in traditional food procurement and processing can range from making the paper-thin blue corn bread piki on a polished stone griddle to providing fry bread or loaves of store-bought white bread for traditional ceremonies. While the woman's preparation of piki would be considered traditional, her purchase of bread would not, a symbol of the complex (re-)construction of meaning used by Native Americans such as the Hopi. In this manner, we argue that patterns of eating and drinking are products of agentic adaptation and marginalization brought about by the confluence of repeated historical trauma and loss of Native foodways.[18]

FROM A MODERN TO POSTMODERN PUBLIC HEALTH MOVEMENT

As treaties became established between Indian nations and the newly formed United States, the responsibility for overseeing trade and treaty relations and, eventually, Indian health care became assigned to the War Department. By 1849 the BIA, along with its Indian medical service, was transferred from military to civilian control within the Department of the Interior. The move to assimilate Indian nations and end federal treaty responsibilities was seen through Christian missions, boarding schools, and legislation that sought to break up the reservation system in the late nineteenth century and provide Indian citizenship by the turn of the twentieth century.

Reports on Indian health during this time were focused on problems arising from poor living conditions, diet, inadequate sanitation, and infectious disease control, particularly against tuberculosis. Rates of child and maternal mortality were the highest for any group in the United States. The Meriam report released in 1928[19] provided a scathing analysis of the inadequate and incompetent administration of Indian affairs. It called for both public health and preventive medicine measures to be taken to address the poor state of Indian health.

Depression-era New Deal legislation led to the Indian Reorganization Act of 1934, which promoted Indian self-governance, and the Social Security Act and began providing block grants to states to address Indian health issues. By the 1950s policies began to be implemented to terminate Indian reservations and federal responsibility for Indian health care. In 1955 the Indian Health Services (IHS) was finally transferred from the BIA to the U.S. Public Health Service.

The fight against termination and raising awareness about Indian rights, health, and welfare became a central focus during the Civil Rights era of the 1950s and 1960s and the war against poverty. Federal policies eventually changed course with the passage of the 1975 Indian Self-Determination Act, which began to shift administrative responsibilities from the BIA and IHS to tribal governments. The Indian Health Care Improvement Act of 1976 and subsequent amendments in the 1980s and 1990s reaffirmed the federal government's legal responsibility for assuring the highest level of health care.[20] This act was made permanent in 2010 as part of the Patient Protection and Affordable Care Act.

Over the past fifty years the shift from a focus on sanitation and infectious disease to chronic disease has been the most substantial marker of change in Indian health. Clearly dietary change has been central to nutritional and consequently epidemiologic transitions.[21] Today, in an age of Indian gaming and casinos and congressional budget cuts and inaction, and the ongoing shifting of responsibilities of federal programs to states, the effectiveness of Indian health care and public health preventative measures vary widely from one Indian community to the next. The one commonality is that in comparison to the average U.S. population, American Indians have, on average, higher overall mortality disparity rates for the combined category of all causes. Health and social disparities ratios are disproportionately higher among American Indians as compared to the average U.S. population for conditions such as liver disease (4.7 times higher), diabetes (2.8 higher), accidents (2.4 higher), homicide (1.9 higher), and suicide (1.6 higher).[22]

Yet the notion and term *research* is itself considered "one of the dirtiest words in the Indigenous world's vocabulary," with many roadblocks to participation and ethical concerns about research led by non-Natives,[23] and, consequently, there are many barriers to holistically understanding community perceptions on many health- and food-related topics. Among many topics, what largely remains unpublished in health sciences is the perception among Native Americans that historical trauma[24] is the single most influential social determinant of health that is embodied in household structures, foodways, interpersonal relationships, and diets, and that gets translated downstream into individual physical, mental, and emotional health behaviors.[25] This issue reared its beastly head early in our respective dissertation fieldwork experiences. As the first author, I witnessed the elderly, parents, and even some adolescents who spoke of the critical need to address historical trauma through social programs for all physical and mental health programs using a holistic approach for all conditions, chronic diseases, infectious diseases, injuries, and substance abuse. They spoke of this embodiment of intergenerational historical trauma early among young children, as they are experiencing this wave of premature disease and disability, including being overweight and obese.

It is in the postmodern public health movement for indigenous health that there is an increased focus upon Native American community-driven collaborative partnerships between non-Native and Native American communities, researchers, and practitioners for culturally tailored, sensitive, and relevant public health interventions. There are numerous examples, including works done by the first author's dissertation advisor's team, of academic researchers, for instance, who have been collaborating with Native American communities for years and outlined information in a review article previously published,[26] highlighting several culturally sensitive and relevant collaborative research projects, including Pathways,[27] OPREVENT,[28] and Zhinwaapenewin Akin'maagewin (ZA),[29] as well as other health researchers. Moreover, such cross-cultural partnerships have focused on a variety of health topics, including health care systems strengthening,[30] mental health and substance abuse/alcohol abuse,[31] and women's health,[32] among others, in countries such as Canada, New Zealand, and Australia, from which the United States can learn and apply best practices for future interventions.[33]

CONCLUSIONS

While the overall trend of continued federal policies of assimilation, termination, and removal that contributed to the erasure of indigenous food memories and meaning is still active, we cannot understate the resiliency of communities in response to these forces of historical trauma. Indigenous foodways are dynamic processes in the larger context of defining indigeneity. As community-based researchers, we have a duty to take great care in how we navigate public health interventional spaces within indigenous communities. When we find ourselves at the cross-cultural nexus of food symbolism, health, and well-being, we must (re-)emphasize the importance of recognizing and valuing the cultural context of acts of eating for healthy outcomes, be they physical, emotional, social, or spiritual. This minimally begins with a process of valuation and validating traditional foodways as the focus rather than the limiting American prescriptions of "healthy eating" established by the dominant food system. Where we must head, in the future, is toward building the collaborative anthropology models for research and practice between non-Native and Native Americans to develop sensitive and relevant strategies for improving the well-being of such indigenous communities.

NOTES

1. U.S. Department of the Interior, Bureau of Indian Affairs, "Services Overview," accessed February 22, 2016, http://www.bia.gov/.

2. U.S. Department of the Interior, Bureau of Indian Affairs, "Status of Acknowledgement Cases," accessed February 22, 2016, http://www.bia.gov/cs/groups/xraca/documents/text/idc1-023074.pdf.

3. William T. Jarvis, "Food Faddism, Cultism, and Quackery," *Annual Review of Nutrition* 3 (1983): 35–52; Brian Wansink, "Position of the American Dietetic Association: Food and Nutrition Misinformation," *Journal of the American Dietetic Association* 106 (2006): 601–7.

4. Wilbur O. Atwater, *Principles of Nutrition and Nutritive Value of Food*, Farmer's Bulletin 142 (Washington, DC: U.S. Department of Agriculture, 1902).

5. Susan Welsh, "Atwater to the Present: Evolution of Nutrition Education," *Journal of Nutrition* 124 (1994): 1799S–1807S.

6. Gyorgy Scrinis, *Nutritionism: The Science and Politics of Dietary Advice* (New York: Columbia University Press, 2013).

7. Michael Pollan, *In Defense of Food: An Eater's Manifesto* (New York: Penguin, 2008).

8. Jane E. Simonsen, *Making Home Work: Domesticity and Native American Assimilation in the American West, 1860–1919* (Chapel Hill: University of North Carolina Press, 2006).

9. Jon Reyhner and Jeanne Eder, *American Indian Education: A History* (Norman: University of Oklahoma Press, 2006).

10. Janell Smith and Dennis Wiedman, "Fat Content of South Florida Indian Frybread: Health Implications for a Pervasive Native-American Food," *Journal of the Academy of Nutrition and Dietetics* 101 (2001): 582–85.

11. Devon A. Mihesuah, *Recovering Our Ancestors' Gardens: Indigenous Recipes and Guide to Diet and Fitness* (Lincoln: University of Nebraska Press, 2005).

12. Mihesuah, *Recovering Our Ancestors' Gardens*; James O. Robertson, *American Myth, American Reality* (New York: Hill and Wang, 1980), 15.

13. Carole M. Counihan, ed., *Food in the USA: A Reader* (New York: Routledge, 2002).

14. Susan Williams, *Food in the United States, 1820s–1890* (Westport, CT: Greenwood Press, 2006), 103.

15. Thomas J. Graham, *Sure Methods of Improving Health, and Prolonging Life; or, A Treatise on the Art of Living Long and Comfortably, by Regulating the Diet and Regimen* (Philadelphia: Carey, Lea and Carey, 1828), 77.

16. S. J. Hale, *Good Housekeeper, or The Way to Live Well and to Be Well While We Live* (Boston: Weeks, Jordan and Company, 1839), vii.

17. Kyla Wazana Tompkins, *Racial Indigestion: Eating Bodies in the 19th Century* (New York: New York University Press, 2012).

18. While the focus of this chapter is on food products, we feel the need to mention briefly the ritualized act of drinking alcoholic beverages among indigenous Native Americans. This becomes specifically relevant and critical because of the historical trauma associated with food, drink, tobacco, and other substances during the initial encounter between Native peoples and

colonizers. However, a normative discussion on food focuses only upon eating; therefore, we will save a dialogue on drinking for a future publication.

19. Lewis Meriam et al., *The Problem of Indian Administration: Institute for Government Research Studies in Administration* (Baltimore: Johns Hopkins Press, 1928).

20. Betty Pfefferbaum, Rennard Strickland, Everett R. Rhoades, and Rose L. Pfefferbaum, "Learning How to Heal: An Analysis of the History, Policy, and Framework of Indian Health Care," *American Indian Law Review* 20 (1995–1996): 365–91.

21. Charlene W. Compher, "The Nutrition Transition in American Indians," *Journal of Transcultural Nursing* 17 (2006): 217–23.

22. Indian Health Services (IHS), *Trends in Indian Health 2014 Edition* (Washington, DC: U.S. Department of Health and Human Services, Indian Health Services, 2014).

23. K. Humphrey, "Dirty Questions: Indigenous Health and 'Western Research,'" *Australian and New Zealand Journal of Public Health* 25 (2001): 197–202.

24. Historical trauma from colonialization results from the action of being subjugated through the act of subjugation (cf. Edwin N. Wilmsen, ed., *We Are Here: Politics of Aboriginal Land Tenure* [Berkeley: University of California Press, 1989]).

25. Pertice M. Moffitt, "Colonization: A Health Determinant for Pregnant Dogrib Women," *Journal of Transcultural Nursing* 15 (2004): 323–30.

26. Joel Gittelsohn, Megan Rowan, and Preety Gadhoke, "Interventions in Small Food Stores to Change the Food Environment, Improve Diet, and Reduce Risk of Chronic Disease," *Preventing Chronic Disease* 9 (2012): 1–15.

27. J. Stevens, M. Story, K. Ring, D. M. Murray, et al., "The Impact of the Pathways Intervention on Psychosocial Variables Related to Diet and Physical Activity in American Indian Schoolchildren," *Preventive Medicine* (2003): S70–S79; B. Caballero, T. Clay, S. M. Davis, B. Ethelbah, et al., "Pathways: A School-Based, Randomized Controlled Trial for the Prevention of Obesity in American Indian Schoolchildren," *American Journal of Clinical Nutrition* 78 (2003): 1030–38.

28. B. Roberts, S. Fleischhacker, M. Pardilla, M. Treuth, et al., "Self-Reported Physical Activity among American Indian Adults from Two Diverse Regions," *Journal of Rural Health* (2016); Preety Gadhoke, Karina Christiansen, Jackie Schwartz, and Joel Gittelsohn, "'Cause It's Family Talking to You': Children as Change Agents for Adult Nutrition and Physical Activity in Ojibwa and Potawatomi Households in Semi-Rural Upper Midwestern United States," *Childhood* (2014): 1–16; Preety Gadhoke, Karina Christiansen, Maria Pardilla, Kevin Frick, et al., "'We're Changing Our Ways': Women's Coping Strategies for Obesity Risk-Reducing Behaviors in American Indian Households," *Ecology of Food and Nutrition* 56 (2014): 1–20.

29. L. S. Ho, J. Gittelsohn, S. B. Harris, and E. Ford, "Development of an Integrated Diabetes Prevention Program with First Nations in Canada," *Health Promotion International* 21 (2006): 88–97.

30. R. Bailie, D. Si, C. Shannon, J. Semmens, et al., "Study Protocol: Native Research Partnership to Improve Primary Health Care Performance and Outcomes for Indigenous Peoples," *BMC Health Services Research* 10 (2010): 129–41.

31. James Allen, Gerald V. Mohatt, Sarah Beehler, and Hillary L. Rowe, "People Awakening: Collaborative Research to Develop Cultural Strategies for Prevention in Community Intervention," *American Journal of Community Psychology* 54 (2014): 100–111.

32. Janelle F. Palacios and Carmen J. Portillo, "Understanding Native Women's Health: Historical Legacies," *Journal of Transcultural Nursing* 20 (2009): 15–27.

33. We argue that indigenous health research is better developed outside the United States, in countries such as Canada, Australia, and New Zealand. A comparative discussion is beyond the scope of this chapter.

BIBLIOGRAPHY

Allen, James, Gerald V. Mohatt, Sarah Beehler, and Hillary L. Rowe. "People Awakening: Collaborative Research to Develop Cultural Strategies for Prevention in Community Intervention." *American Journal of Community Psychology* 54 (2014): 100–111.

Atwater, Wilbur O. *Principles of Nutrition and Nutritive Value of Food*. Farmer's Bulletin 142. Washington, DC: U.S. Department of Agriculture, 1902.

Bailie, R., D. Si, C. Shannon, J. Semmens, et al. "Study Protocol: Native Research Partnership to Improve Primary Health Care Performance and Outcomes for Indigenous Peoples." *BMC Health Services Research* 10 (2010): 129–41.

Caballero, B., T. Clay, S. M. Davis, B. Ethelbah, et al. "Pathways: A School-Based, Randomized Controlled Trial for the Prevention of Obesity in American Indian Schoolchildren." *American Journal of Clinical Nutrition* 78 (2003): 1030–38.

Compher, Charlene W. "The Nutrition Transition in American Indians." *Journal of Transcultural Nursing* 17 (2006): 217–23.

Counihan, Carole M., ed. *Food in the USA: A Reader*. New York: Routledge, 2002.

Gadhoke, Pretty, Karina Christiansen, Maria Pardilla, Kevin Frick, et al. "'We're Changing Our Ways': Women's Coping Strategies for Obesity Risk-Reducing Behaviors in American Indian Households." *Ecology of Food and Nutrition* 56 (2014): 1–20.

Gadhoke, Preety, Karina Christiansen, Jackie Schwartz, and Joel Gittelsohn. "'Cause It's Family Talking to You': Children as Change Agents for Adult Nutrition and Physical Activity in Ojibwa and Potawatomi Households in Semi-Rural Upper Midwestern United States." *Childhood* (2014): 1–16.

Gittelsohn, Joel, Megan Rowan, and Preety Gadhoke. "Interventions in Small Food Stores to Change the Food Environment, Improve Diet, and Reduce Risk of Chronic Disease." *Preventing Chronic Disease* 9 (2012): 1–15.

Graham, Thomas J. *Sure Methods of Improving Health, and Prolonging Life; or, A Treatise on the Art of Living Long and Comfortably, by Regulating the Diet and Regimen*. Philadelphia: Carey, Lea and Carey, 1828.

Hale, S. J. *Good Housekeeper, or The Way to Live Well and to Be Well While We Live*. Boston: Weeks, Jordan and Company, 1839.

Ho, L. S., J. Gittelsohn, S. B. Harris, and E. Ford. "Development of an Integrated Diabetes Prevention Program with First Nations in Canada." *Health Promotion International* 21 (2006): 88–97.

Humphrey, K. "Dirty Questions: Indigenous Health and 'Western Research.'" *Australian and New Zealand Journal of Public Health* 25 (2001): 197–202.

Indian Health Services (IHS). *Trends in Indian Health 2014 Edition*. Washington, DC: U.S. Department of Health and Human Services, Indian Health Services, 2014.

Jarvis, William T. "Food Faddism, Cultism, and Quackery." *Annual Review of Nutrition* 3 (1983): 35–52.

Meriam, Lewis, et al. *The Problem of Indian Administration: Institute for Government Research Studies in Administration*. Baltimore: Johns Hopkins Press, 1928.

Mihesuah, Devon A. *Recovering Our Ancestors' Gardens: Indigenous Recipes and Guide to Diet and Fitness*. Lincoln: University of Nebraska Press, 2005.

Moffitt, Pertice M. "Colonization: A Health Determinant for Pregnant Dogrib Women." *Journal of Transcultural Nursing* 15 (2004): 323–30.

Palacios, Janelle F., and Carmen J. Portillo. "Understanding Native Women's Health: Historical Legacies." *Journal of Transcultural Nursing* 20 (2009): 15–27.

Pfefferbaum, Betty, Rennard Strickland, Everett R. Rhoades, and Rose L. Pfefferbaum. "Learning How to Heal: An Analysis of the History, Policy, and Framework of Indian Health Care." *American Indian Law Review* 20 (1995–1996): 365–91.

Pollan, Michael. *In Defense of Food: An Eater's Manifesto*. New York: Penguin, 2008.

Reyhner, Jon, and Jeanne Eder. *American Indian Education: A History*. Norman: University of Oklahoma Press, 2006.

Roberts, E. B., S. Fleischhacker, M. Pardilla, M. Treuth, et al. "Self-Reported Physical Activity among American Indian Adults from Two Diverse Regions. *Journal of Rural Health* (2016).

Robertson, James O. *American Myth, American Reality*. New York: Hill and Wang, 1980.

Scrinis, Gyorgy. *Nutritionism: The Science and Politics of Dietary Advice*. New York: Columbia University Press, 2013.

Simonsen, Jane E. *Making Home Work: Domesticity and Native American Assimilation in the American West, 1860–1919*. Chapel Hill: University of North Carolina Press, 2006.

Smith, Janell, and Dennis Wiedman. "Fat Content of South Florida Indian Frybread: Health Implications for a Pervasive Native-American Food." *Journal of the Academy of Nutrition and Dietetics* 101 (2001): 582–85.

Stevens, J., M. Story, K. Ring, D. M. Murray, et al. "The Impact of the Pathways Intervention on Psychosocial Variables Related to Diet and Physical Activity in American Indian Schoolchildren." *Preventive Medicine* (2003): S70–S79.

Tompkins, Kyla Wazana. *Racial Indigestion: Eating Bodies in the 19th Century*. New York: New York University Press, 2012.

U.S. Department of the Interior, Bureau of Indian Affairs. "Services Overview." Accessed February 22, 2016. http://www.bia.gov/.

U.S. Department of the Interior, Bureau of Indian Affairs. "Status of Acknowledgement Cases." Accessed February 22, 2016. http://www.bia.gov/cs/groups/xraca/documents/text/idc1-023074.pdf.

Wansink, Brian. "Position of the American Dietetic Association: Food and Nutrition Misinformation." *Journal of the American Dietetic Association* 106 (2006): 601–7.

Welsh, Susan. "Atwater to the Present: Evolution of Nutrition Education." *Journal of Nutrition* 124 (1994): 1799S–1807S.

Williams, Susan. *Food in the United States, 1820s–1890*. Westport, CT: Greenwood Press, 2006.

Wilmsen, Edwin N., ed. *We Are Here: Politics of Aboriginal Land Tenure*. Berkeley: University of California Press, 1989.

Chapter Fourteen

"Herb Is for the Healing of the Nation!"

Marijuana as a Consumable Vegetable among Ghetto Muslim Youth of Maamobi in Accra, Ghana

De-Valera N. Y. M. Botchway and Charles Prempeh

The consumption and use of marijuana (*Cannabis sativa*) are as ancient as the origin of humankind. The making of it as part of the human diet, as medicine, as an industrial and recreational substance, and as a religious object stems from antiquity. Yet, despite its significance over millennia, the vegetable is a subject of controversy in the discourses of scholars, legal experts, and the general public today.

Negative testimonies about its inhalation or ingestion or topical application have increased calls from anti-marijuana campaigners for it to be criminalized. They produce "data" and different reasons to discredit its usage in whatever context. Pro-marijuana people have endeavored to prove it is harmless. Some writers, such as Grinspoon and Bakalar[1] and Zimmer and Morgan,[2] deem it a plant with beneficial chemical and nutritional assets and want it decriminalized. Conversely, detractors such as Nahas and Latour[3] and Walters[4] think otherwise. In Ghana, many persons, reflecting popular knowledge installed by the police that marijuana is often found on hardcore criminals, identify marijuana with social misdemeanour and violence. Nevertheless, the herb enjoys widespread cultivation, production, consumption, and use globally.[5] In 2012, about 227 million people were estimated to have used cannabis, corresponding to between 2.7 and 4.9 percent of the population aged fifteen to sixty-four years.[6] The vagueness about the perceived harm or benefits of marijuana has largely resulted in a universal criminalization of it by governments, even though the United States, United Kingdom, and some few countries have taken steps to declassify it as a Class A drug and accepted it in their pharmacopoeia, and prescriptions of it for therapeutic purposes are limited to special physicians or psychiatrists. Holland and Canada permits its use for specific medicinal and recreational purposes.

In Ghana, the cultivation, possession, use, or sale of marijuana is a felony. The Provisional National Defence Council (PNDC) Law 236 and the Narcotic Drug Law (1990) state, "No person should undertake any activity for the purpose of establishing or promoting any enterprise relating to narcotic drugs." Marijuana is considered a narcotic; hence, using marijuana, which in the legal lexicon refers to all parts of the herb (seeds, resin, every compound, manufacture, salt, derivative, mixture, or preparation of the plant),[7] for any purpose, is illegal under Ghana's laws. It is ironic, though, that Ghana's market imports marijuana-derived items such as hair creams, fabrics, and ropes.

Despite Ghana's legal position, the cultivation of marijuana for a domestic market and export is a major business for a number of farmers in the least accessible areas of Ghana's forest.[8] The tropical climatic conditions of the countryside favor its growth. It is eaten, smoked, infused in water and drunk as bitters, and mixed with local gin and drunk as a beverage,[9] and its consumption is trans age, trans gender, trans social class, and trans locality in Ghana. Many secondary school and university students patronize it.[10] Daniel Akwasi Amankwah of the Narcotics Control Board disclosed on national media in October 2014 that, in terms of marijuana consumption, Ghana tops the list in Africa and places third in the world.

In Maamobi, a suburb in Accra, Ghana's capital, the consumption of marijuana, which has acquired currency among many of the youth, especially in established "ghettos"—special places where marijuana is sold and consumed—goes back to the 1950s. Maamobi has a large Muslim community, and many of the youth (male and female) who consume marijuana profess Islam. Information we obtained from the police stations of Maamobi and the adjoining community of Nima indicated that many of the youth who were prosecuted for consuming marijuana claimed to be Muslims. Marijuana is illegal in Ghana; it is also considered *haram* by many leaders in Ghana's *ummah* (Islamic community). So what sociocultural structural forces in the history of marijuana use in Maamobi and Ghana predispose some Muslim youth to consume marijuana? How do they rationalize their consumption of the herb and conceptualize its effects on their lives?

PROFILE OF THE MAAMOBI COMMUNITY

The Maamobi land originally belonged to the Ga ethnic group of Accra. However, it has largely become a migrant community that evolved from the settling of early Fulani and Hausa traders in the urbanized space of Accra in the 1940s. Hence only a few Ga people live there today. Ex-servicemen of the British West African Frontier Force, mainly Muslims from northern Ghana, and Hausa soldiers from Nigeria and other Anglophone West African countries also settled there after World War II. By the mid-1960s the community was multiethnic in character. Different West African ethnicities live there today. The early settlers were mostly Muslim, so Islam is dominant in the region. The majority of the population share the commonwealth of the faith. Hausa, which was largely used by the early Muslim traders and missionaries to propagate Islam, is the lingua franca of that multiethnic community. This migrant community, encased in the pressures of urbanization in Accra, suffers from the problems of overcrowding, squalor, and paucity of social amenities. Many children are thus exposed to different economic activities to make a livelihood for self and family. Some work alongside schooling. The advent of *Sakawa* (online cyber scam) has induced some of the youth to discontinue schooling and go into the practice with the hope of making quick money to meet different needs.

The ghetto has been one space where a lifestyle of friendship and sharing, revolving around a common cult(ure) of marijuana use, persists. This character attracts many of the youth whose poor backgrounds are unable to give them a sense of social security to go to the ghetto in search of comradeship and social security among the ghetto commune of marijuana users who experience the herb as a euphoric and crucial mystical sacrament capable of enlightenment and alleviating sufferings from the reality of social insecurity, alienation, and poverty.

HISTORY OF MARIJUANA USE IN GHANA

Marijuana is commonly known as *wee* in Ghana, but some people also refer to it as *ganja*, *tampe/ntampi*, *sundu*, *obonsam tawa*, *apopo*, *taba*, and *wee bitters*. Oral tradition avers that it was used as a psychotropic substance or depressant or stimulant because of indigenous knowledge about its chemical properties in the precolonial era.[11] Some indigenous ritual specialists must have chewed marijuana leaves and/or other more potent hallucinatory leaves before they initiated themselves into the psychic realm and trances. Many priests and priestesses of popular indigenous shrines and mystery cults in Ghana still use some hallucinatory substances to alter or heighten their state of consciousness during initiation rites and incantations.[12] Some indigenous warriors also used hallucinogens from the vegetable world to remove fear and give them psychological strength for the rigors of fighting. Among the Akan this practice was expressed as *Ye ko noa asa* ("We are going to cook war"). This secret activity was usually done in the thickest forest.[13] Some traditional priests and priestesses and herbalists still use marijuana for rituals and explore its properties for medicinal purposes.[14]

Next to the view of local traditions that the herb is indigenous to Ghana is the opinion that ex-servicemen who returned from India and Burma after World War II were responsible for the prevalence of the plant in postcolonial Ghana. Even though an ex-serviceman in Maamobi, who pleaded anonymity, stated that some ex-servicemen brought marijuana to Ghana, Yussif Iddris Konate, an imam of Accra and the chief imam of Maamobi, argued that the ex-servicemen were not known for smoking marijuana, although they did smoke tobacco that the colonial administrators supplied to them. Two of the earliest settlers and assemblymen of the Maamobi community, Alhaji Haruna Bukari Dabre and Abdul Godwin Baba Ali, corroborated the imam's information. Vincent Adjei, a World War II veteran, did not accept or deny the allegation that veterans brought the herb back and used it in the country. Cautioning that the possibility should not be overruled, nor the allegation generalized, he opined that the bravery of some of the ex-servicemen, which, it was alleged, was induced by their use of marijuana, gave currency to the claim that they brought marijuana into the country.[15] The Krio from Sierra Leone who worked as stevedores along West Africa's coast may have also introduced cannabis to the country during the colonial period.[16] Marijuana's medicinal and nonmedicinal value was popular in Sierra Leone, and in the 1930s some Sierra Leoneans began to explore a market for cannabis within British West Africa. They capitalized on Freetown's importance as a major port, the presence of Sierra Leonean sailors on steamships, and a Sierra Leonean diaspora in port towns in West Africa, where many worked as stevedores, and spread cannabis in other West African countries, including Ghana.[17] Despite this multivocality about the genesis of marijuana in Ghana, the colonial regime's law classified its cultivation, use, and possession as criminal.[18] The steady flux of governments that have come and gone have never up to this date legalized the herb. Despite the law, marijuana's popularity soared in the late 1950s because "[w]ith the decline in world market price for cocoa from 1958, cocoa farmers may have been encouraged to diversify into cannabis cultivation"[19] to satisfy an existing local clientele, which included some Muslim youth in Maamobi.

THE BACKGROUND OF SMOKING MARIJUANA IN MAAMOBI

The consumption of marijuana, especially smoking, in Maamobi became noticeable in the 1950s. Imam Yussif Iddris Konate of Maamobi avers that Krio stevedores who occasionally worked at the Light House Port in Accra introduced marijuana smoking to the community through the youth. The early consignments were allegedly sourced from Congo, so marijuana became popularly known as "Congo tobacco" in Maamobi in the early days.[20] America House, a unit in the community, became a popular ghetto. Apart from America House, the area of Avenor also supplied marijuana to users in Maamobi. The early "pushers" (sellers) in the ghetto then included Mahma Issaka, Awolah, Medicine, and Mamare. They obtained marijuana from different parts of Ghana for sale in Maamobi. The prevalence of social vices and criminal activities such as armed robbery came to be associated with smokers of marijuana.[21] It was alleged that robbers were involved in the sale of marijuana and the glamorization of smoking it among the youth. Armed robbery, accompanied by the Hausa expression *Kawokudi* ("Bring money"), was so rife that this scenario gave a section of the community the name *Kawokudi.* Consequently, Maamobi became a major target of the country's security agencies when the Armed Forces Revolutionary Council (AFRC), a military government that claimed that it wanted to rid the country of crime and corruption, came to power in 1979. This focus on Maamobi by the police and soldiers contributed to the collapse of America House. Barracks and later Four Junction emerged as major alternative ghettos. They are still popular and major ghettos that different consumers, including some Muslim youth, frequent. In the view of these Muslims, their ghetto marijuana smoking cult(ure) is spiritually, psychologically, and socially functional to their existence in an economically hard and squalid space like Maamobi, and not at variance or illegal or to be deemed un-Islamic.

MARIJUANA CONSUMPTION IN EARLY ISLAM AND VIEWS OF THE SCHOOLS OF THOUGHT ABOUT IT IN ISLAM

The legality or illegality of marijuana has been debated in the post-Muhammed era of Islam for centuries. The contention basically evolves from the multiple definitions of *khamr*. No particular definition is sacrosanct, because it is the Qur'an that is infallible and not the interpreters.[22] The definition of khamr can be contextualized in a specific geocultural milieu and time and it is difficult to wholly apply it to all Muslim communities, because in some areas in Africa staple foods contain some traces of intoxicants. For example, Muslims of the Savanna belt of West Africa continue to take fermented millet, corn, and sorghum without deeming them un-Islamic.

The consumption of marijuana found some currency in the culture of the Muslim world in the ninth century. Muslims from the Arabian world contacted marijuana-consuming societies in places such as Syria, Persia, and parts of Asia Minor through jihads after the Prophet's demise. The Islamic culture assimilated some of the eating norms, including marijuana consumption, of these places. Furthermore, the translations of Greek literature on medicine into Arabic by Islamic scholars exposed marijuana's therapeutic value. Consequently, some Muslim physicians cautiously experimented and recommended the therapeutic values of marijuana in the early part of the history of Islam. The physician al-Rhazes (c. 854/865–925) prescribed it for ear infections, dandruff, flatulence, and epileptic cases.[23] Some people used it to treat asthma, gonorrhea, constipation, and poisoning;[24] to stimulate the appetite and aid concentration and hearing;[25] and to reduce libido. However, the abuse of it as a drug emerged in Muslim societies.

> The spread of political unrest in various parts of the Muslim domain and the rise of many religious schools of thought, mysticism, sufism and sectarianism helped further the need for ways of escape from hard realities for many, and led to the wide spread [abuse of cannabis and] drug addiction.[26]

Some Sufis used cannabis to endure the long hours of fasting, prayers, and solitary meditation.[27] Allegedly some members of the Hashishiyya, from which the word *assassin* evolved, which was a Sufi group reportedly founded around 1090, killed their opponents under the influence of marijuana. The marijuana connection to Hashishiyya violence partly provided a political motivation for the criminalization of marijuana in the Western world.[28] Shaikh Haidar, founder of the Haidari Sufi order in Kharasan (northwest Iran and Afghanistan), who lived around AD 1200, reportedly used it and told his disciples, "Almighty God has bestowed upon you by a special favour the virtues of this plant, which will dissipate the shadows that cloud your souls and will brighten your spirits."[29] Other Sufis do not use marijuana because they deem it a bad psychoactive substance.[30]

Arab Muslim traders may have also picked up the marijuana consumption norm from China and India and popularized it in the Arabian and Islamic world.[31] Ibn Batuta reported that people ate marijuana, even in the mosques sometimes,[32] during his travel through parts of the Islamic world in the fourteenth century. In Morocco, marijuana ("kaif" or "kif") featured in the religious ceremonies of the Sunusis sect.[33] The authorities prohibited it because of abuse in the thirteenth century.[34] Muslim jurists, historians, theologians, poets, and storytellers who were confronted by the silence of the Qur'an about marijuana and, more important, the multiple definitions of khamr discussed the "merits" and "evils" of the herb for centuries.[35] Some legal scholars interpreted khamr, often cited as wine, to include any intoxicant that befogs the mind. According to Dixon (1972),[36] khamr is derived from the verb *khamara* (to cover, or conceal) and could be extended to denote any substance that covers up the mind. However, some interpreters equated khamr with wine only.[37] Notwithstanding the semantic confusion, Maliki, Shafi'i, and Hanbali schools of law broadly defined khamr and consequently classified marijuana as an intoxicant, hence outlawed in Islam.[38] Consequently, Sheikh ibn Taymiyyah opined:

> Sinful people smoke hashish because . . . it produces rapture and delight . . . to drunkenness. . . . [I]t promotes dullness and lethargy . . . disturbs the mind and temperament, excites sexual desire, and leads to shameless promiscuity.[39]

Shak-al-Harin, a thirteenth-century jurist, also argued, "All the destructive effects of wine are found in hashish many times over."[40]

The Hanafi school of law's restricted definition of khamr allows moderate therapeutic use of marijuana. In the light of that outlook, a Shafute legal scholar, az-Zarkashi, opined in 1360 that "any use of wine is forbidden because it is unclean, unlike hashish which is permitted but not for intoxication." Another jurist, Agfashi, also declared in 1390, "Contrary to wine, hashish is used as medicine. It is not subject to punishment, and eating a small quantity of it is not forbidden as long as it does not influence the mind or senses."[41] The outright rejection of marijuana by schools of thought apart from Hanafi is a kneejerk response to a challenge in society—abuse—and not essentially a demonization of a plant, which is part of God's creation, a creation that Islam deems good.

MARIJUANA CONSUMPTION CULT(URE) OF THE GHETTO

The conscious consumption of marijuana as a vegetable "food" in Maamobi's ghettos, mainly animated by the deprived suffering masses, is considered by the Muslim youth who partake in it as a way of life that upholds a "special food." Whether they ingest it by chewing or drinking a concoction of it or inhaling smoke from the leaves, they regard the herb as food. Food here is construed as any substance that is consciously put into the human body to nourish and sustain its physiological, biological, spiritual, and psychic parts. The intention of consuming marijuana, within the context of this ghetto-based feeding lifestyle, a cult(ure), is to assist the holistic human composition to derive certain spiritual and health benefits and not to befog the mind. Hence they do not deem the herb, which they perceive as a visionary plant, as khamr. This ghetto-based lifestyle provides partakers with a certain sense of group distinctiveness and moral judgment.

As a supplier of social and moral identity, food generally transcends mere nourishment and fitness for humans. Some people rally around a particular diet or food item in their efforts to acquire a unique identity and/or a worldview in their pursuit of satisfaction in life. This is a direction that produces diet or food cults. For example, the ancient Hebrews derived an unusual sense of a unique group identity and a conviction of moral superiority over adherents of nonkosher dietary regulations. Those who deemed themselves true Hebrews therefore had to adhere to the kosher cult(ure). They disapproved of others who did not share their food preference. Similar is the African Hebrew Israelites community's obsession with a vegan diet. This community, which was started in the 1960s in the United States by African Americans but has now raised branches internationally, believes that a vegan diet is the healthiest and original food requirement that Yah (God) gave to humans (Genesis 1:29), the first blacks (Hebrews) of which they are descendants. Members of the group strictly adhere to a plant-based diet because it signifies a return to their true identity and obeisance to Yah, who chose them over others.

Food cults provide unique names to a particular food or dietary style that they draw their special identity from. For example, kosher as against nonkosher, plant-based diet as against non-plant-based diet. They usually find scientific (pseudoscientific) and at times religious explanations and scriptural hermeneutics to justify their special food/diet as "best," superior, and healthy—physical, spiritual, and mental health—than others, or as a *conditio sine qua non* for health, even if one takes other foods. Followers tend to be emotionally attached to the food, not rationally per se, because of the sense of identity that they and the community that enfolds their membership derive from the diet. Such groups commonly advocate nutritional "musts." Consequently, their demonization of certain "foods" helps them to define their culture as distinct from the others whose dietary culture or foods they criticize as unhealthy to the human constitution. Their forceful rhetoric about their "hallowed" dietary preference helps them to attract followers who desire to move away from what the group criticizes as toxic and addictive.

The rhetoric of the culture of marijuana consumption in the ghetto advances certain fantastic scientific and religious and economic ideas about why the herb is a necessary food despite the opposing views of some Islamic scholars and Ghana's laws. In the ghetto opinion, many nonusers labor in trepidation before the mass media's adverse publicity of oppositions and hysteria, which has accompanied the reality of the herb. One of the realities of the ghettos about marijuana is the perceived supernatural powers of the herb to protect the consumer from evil. The second is its power to bring the user closer to God (Allah), the third is the silence of the Qu'ran about it, and the fourth is that their consumption of marijuana negotiates a form of nationalist resistance to the conspiracy of Western economic imperialists to kill its economic benefits to Ghana.

The consumption of marijuana has a unique way of fomenting group solidarity among smokers in the ghetto. The sharing of "joints," similar to the Rastafari practice of "Reasoning" and the Christian practice of the Eucharist, has a way of establishing a sense of we-feeling among smokers in the ghetto. In the ghettos, many smokers have a different hermeneutical meaning for *wee*. In the logic of the ghetto, the word *wee* means "all of us." The ghetto members have some degree of emotional attachment to each other due to the sharing of marijuana. It is the understanding of the communalism of the smoking cult(ure) that has over the years frustrated every attempt by nonsmoking members of the community to eradicate all ghettos. The sense of we-feeling among smokers finds expression in the assistance that is extended to members in need. A number of the smokers have acquired vocational skills such as block molding, driving, and auto mechanics because of their association with the ghetto. Also, the cultic nature of the marijuana culture is exemplified in the fact that members deem it their responsibility to unite in defense of another member who finds himself in trouble outside of the ghetto. The ghetto philosophy of solidarity is similar to the pre-Islamic Arabic philosophy that enjoined the Arabs to stand by their brother whether he is being oppressed or is the oppressor. In the Maamobi community, any attack on a marijuana smoker by a nonsmoker is often interpreted by smokers to mean an attack on all marijuana smokers. Thus, until quite recently, feuds have been a major feature of the Maamobi community. As part of the orientation into ghetto life, neophytes learn to see themselves as having a responsibility to protect other members of the ghetto.

Similarly, because marijuana smokers consider marijuana to be a type of food that has spiritual significance, smokers claim to possess some esoteric knowledge that is unavailable to nonsmokers. For example, another name for Four Junction, one of the oldest ghettos in the community, is the University of Four Junction. Members in the ghetto believe that the smoking of marijuana predisposes them to a kind of knowledge that helps them to offer cultic attention to Allah, the Ultimate Reality. Smokers consider nonsmokers absolutely ignorant about the ethos of social life, since the kind of knowledge that marijuana exposes them (marijuana smokers) to is unavailable to them (nonsmokers). It is also widely believed in the ghettos that marijuana has a way of stimulating critical and analytical thinking among smokers. That marijuana is able to stimulate critical thinking has encouraged some smokers to dabble in cyber scams, since they believe that, with the aid of marijuana, they are able to stay behind the computer for longer hours and also stupefy their clients. Proceeds from *Sakawa* are used to support members during marriage ceremonies (*awure*) and naming ceremonies (*Suuna*). Also, the belief that marijuana is a cultic food with spiritual significance has informed the decision by ghetto leaders to not encourage the sale of cigarettes and alcohol in the ghettos. While some ghetto members consume cigarettes and alcohol, albeit very moderately, the general understanding in the ghetto is that these other substances could undermine the inherent spiritual potency of marijuana. The prescribed practice in the ghetto is, therefore, that members "must" consume marijuana.

The cultogenic nature of the marijuana culture dovetails with the politics of the sale of marijuana. In the ghettos, marijuana is not sold to nonmembers. The substance is sold only to members of the ghetto and close friends of members of the ghetto. Much as this practice is well carved to outwit the police, who often organize swoops (known in the ghetto as "scatter"), it is believed that nonmembers may not be able to identify with the kind of common episteme that is shared by all ghetto members.

Finally, the cult(ure) of marijuana has gender implications in terms of membership. It is believed that marijuana consumption predisposes smokers to a kind of knowledge that must be kept secret within the smoking fraternity. For example, it is believed that when one smokes, the jinns inhabiting the substance are able to lead one into venturing on business enterprises that could be very rewarding. Females, according to the philosophy of the ghetto, are ontologically unable to keep secrets. So the ghettos do not admit females as members. The cult(ure) of marijuana has been a magnetic force that attracts nonsmokers to the ghettos. Thus, over the years, state-sponsored negative testimonies, which filter through the media—print and electronic—have not been able to discourage new members from being initiated into the marijuana cult(ure). The cultogenic nature of marijuana has likewise been demonstrated in rituals that have evolved around the substance.

SMOKING OUT THE WITCH FROM THE SLUMS: MARIJUANA TO THE RESCUE

Marijuana's importance in the ghettos of Maamobi stems from the seemingly cultic belief of users that it has an inherent divine ability to make a positive impact on them. The most common way of consumption is smoking, which is a form of feeding/eating according to the smokers. Thus the herb is food, whether it is smoked or cooked and ingested. The herb is believed to be disliked by malevolent spirits. Smoke from it repels such spirits, especially those that support witchcraft. The marijuana users in the ghetto uphold a belief in witchcraft because such a notion is part of the cosmology of their indigenous society. Belief in the force of witchcraft as mostly antilife is very ubiquitous in African societies. The belief that witches use negative energy to retard the progress of people is a prevalent idea in Maamobi. The activities of witches are believed to be mainly nocturnal, and they are superhuman and cannot be understood by material investigation. Witches operate with their astral bodies to cause harm, especially diseases, death, and poverty to people. Thus, they cannot be confronted physically. Targets of witches experience the effect of a witchcraft attack not immediately but later, after the event. According to the cult(ure) lore of the ghetto, marijuana is an antidote to the metaphysical operations of witches who cause harm to their relatives and nonrelatives. Muslim youth in Maamobi are wary of the activities of witches.

Because of this fear, many resort to different spiritual means; they wear charms, rings, and amulets and inject into their bodies anti-witchcraft substances prepared by some Muslim ritual experts to protect themselves from witchcraft activities. It is this same mindset of finding security, and also a burgeoning mistrust in the commercialization of the anti-witchcraft services of many ritual experts, that has made some Muslim youth resort to feeding on marijuana, the ghetto-prescribed anti-witchcraft food. According to ghetto lore the spirit of a person is what witchcraft attacks; however, when people feed on marijuana the anti-witchcraft divine essence of the herb establishes with their spirit and protects it. Thus, the Muslim youth in the ghetto believe that the smoke of the herb undermines witchcraft and protects the smoker.

This conviction is a rationalized outlet for marijuana smokers in the ghetto to find a causative explanation for the existential challenges of life. Interestingly, witches are blamed for insanity and other psychotic cases in the ghetto community and not on marijuana, as most psychiatry books and experts will do. Witches are perpetually at work to mischievously interfere in people's lives and even cause them harm, such as insanity or death as they smoke. Thus, within the cult(ure) of marijuana use among Muslim youth in the ghetto, a ritual invocation of God's presence and security is performed before the herb is consumed. Most smokers recite the Fatiha, the first chapter of the Qur'an, and this is believed to also heighten the spiritual potency of marijuana. MacDanji[42] explained this rite as follows:

> I always recite the Fatiha before I smoke taba. I do this because taba has its own power and to activate that power, one must first plead with Allah, the creator of all things, including taba, to enjoy the spiritual benefits of taba. It is the activation of the inherent spirit in marijuana that drives away the spirit of witchcraft. Witches do not like the smoke of taba, because the smoke of taba is charged with the spirit of Allah. As researchers, you might have heard that every plant has a spirit inhabiting it. That explains why herbalists perform special rituals before they make use of any herb. In the ghettoes, we also believe that taba as an herb has its own powers, and its powers are best invoked to counter evil spirits.

This practice is similar to what most herbalists do in Ghana. Herbalists perform rituals before taking parts of certain plants for medicine because they believe that permission must be sought from the spirits in the plant, which would also make the therapeutic components of the plant potent. Many of the Muslim youth in the ghetto believe that it is a benevolent spirit;

many deem it jinn, in or attached to marijuana, and that gives the vegetable an anti-witchcraft ability.

The belief in jinns is prevalent among Muslims in Ghana. The Qur'an expressly justifies the existence of jinns, whom it is reported share certain attributes with humans. For example, they worship and depend on God (Qur'an 51:56); they are social, and they can learn and listen (Qur'an 46:29–30); and they can work (Qur'an 34:13). Nevertheless, they are not human; they are invisible, fiery in composition, and can perform miracles. The belief about the jinns-marijuana nexus is part of a unique marijuana food cult(ure) carried by ghetto Muslim youth, which is not universally shared by all Muslims. The general understanding among the ghetto community is that a symbiotic relationship is between the vegetable and spiritual worlds, hence the one between marijuana and jinns, and humans can exploit that alliance to fight evils spirits, especially witchcraft in the human world. In line with this thought, an older Muslim mystic, locally known as a Mallam, who consumes marijuana even though he is not a member of the marijuana culinary cult(ure) of the ghetto, shared his experience:

> [J]inns can be ordered to work [for] human beings . . . for negative things, [and] for constructive purposes. Those of us who use marijuana are able to implore the jinns to protect us from witches. And this we believe works for us. [J]inns are more powerful than witches.

WORSHIPPING GOD IN SILENCE: THE GRACE OF MARIJUANA

Marijuana has a tranquillizing chemical compound. The ghetto Muslim youth claim that since marijuana keeps one in a relaxed mood it is able to induce a high level of concentration in them, and also helps them in their spirituality because it allows them to "stay cool" in deep thought and meditate on Allah and the Qu'ran when they "feed" on it. The popular out-of-the-ghetto assumption that marijuana induces aggressiveness and violence does not hold legitimacy in the psyche of the Muslim youth in the ghetto. They believe that aggression is produced by synthetic drugs and not the natural herb of marijuana. Masud apologetically contended:

> Taba alone cannot let anyone go wild . . . to be violent. Anyone who smokes taba and misbehaves should be checked properly. Such a person uses other substances. Such a person is likely to quaff alcohol . . . or . . . uses heroin and cocaine in addition to taba. I have been smoking taba for so many years and I

> have lots of experience . . . concerning this precious herb. . . . [M]arijuana rather helps one to concentrate on Allah and meditate upon His word. Whenever I smoke taba in the company of my friends, [I] am able to think deeply about Allah and . . . about my life.

The view that marijuana alone will not predispose anyone to violence until another drug or chemical is consumed alongside it, because the herb is a tranquilizer that can also aid the spiritual exercise of meditating on Allah and by extension life, is common to many youth in the ghetto. Because of the perceived ability of marijuana to connect the consumers to the divine, the Muslim youth circle of the ghetto deem the herb a "sacred" vegetable food that "must" be taken and venerated as a natural conduit to spiritual experience despite the fact that several Muslim scholars have proscribed it because of the unsettled controversy about the herb's propriety in the wider space of Islam and the risk of being prosecuted if caught using or possessing marijuana in Ghana.

THE SILENCE OF THE QUR'AN: A JUSTIFICATION FOR THE CONSUMPTION OF MARIJUANA

It is curious that this circle of youth will risk their freedom to pursue a foodway fixated on the consumption of marijuana even though one can be shunned by other Muslims and can be imprisoned for a minimum of five years if one is caught experimenting with marijuana. What justification do they give? The first is that the Qur'an and Hadith are silent about the herb and the consumption and smoking of it. Nevertheless, jurists who criticized the post-Mohammed social issue of the consumption of marijuana broaden the definition of khamr to include marijuana and use the injunctions against alcohol to incriminate the consumption of marijuana. Even though marijuana and alcohol are both intoxicants, the two are not the same. Also, according to knowledge from the ghettos, consumers of this medicinal plant are capable of performing religious rituals, while alcohol-intoxicated persons can hardly perform them. One of Muslim youth respondents who sought a defense from the Bible, a book that Muslims are enjoined to respect, and the Qur'an to justify marijuana consumption revealed in his ghetto hermeneutics of the books that

> the silence of the Qur'an is not for nothing. Allah knew that the smoking [consumption] of marijuana is not haram. Granted that it is bad, Allah would

> have revealed it to the Prophet even if it was unknown during the time of the Prophet. [L]ogically . . . Allah is all knowing and He knew . . . that today marijuana would be smoked. [I]f Allah did not want marijuana, He would have revealed its prohibition to the Prophet. There are . . . issues that the Qur'an talks about that were unknown during the Prophet's time. If marijuana were bad, Allah would not have also created it. But since the Qur'an and the Hadith are silent about hemp, we should go to the Bible, because . . . the two religious books are all from the same one God, who gave the same message to all the prophets, but only at different times. Psalm 87 and Numbers 6 . . . come to the same conclusion with me that God, after all, is not against the smoking of hemp. If you agree with me on this principle then we can refer to all those who criminalize hemp as hypocrites and blind . . . about God's creation. People who condemn the smoking of hemp do so out of ignorance and religious bigotry—they are forever blind . . . and they will never know anything about its potency until God opens their eyes one day. Out of ignorance when I go to the mosque to pray as a Muslim, some people tend to look down on me as someone who is practicing a syncretism of religion—Islam and Rastafarianism,[43] because of my dreadlock. I know that no man other than God can judge me and so I am not worried about their ignorance.

The silence of the Qur'an and Hadith is a justification leeway for the peculiar feeding habit in the ghetto, so despite the contention of some Muslim scholars that alcohol befogs the mind and so does marijuana so the ban on alcohol should be extended to the use of the plant, the ghetto marijuana smokers deem alcohol and marijuana as two different things in terms of composition and the effects they have on humans. All the marijuana smokers that we conversed with in the ghettos were of the opinion that if marijuana were inherently bad, God would have revealed that to the Prophet. Claiming that there are harmful things that have not been criminalized, such as cigarettes, whose boxes commonly bear the inscription that it is harmful to health, yet their precious vegetable has been demonized, they remain steadfast in believing that marijuana is harmless.

WHY MARIJUANA AND NOT TOBACCO?

Marijuana, according to ghetto knowledge, has no negative effect and should not be criminalized, unlike other legalized substances like cigarettes and alcohol that should rather be criminalized because they commonly cause cancer and dipsomania. With a contrived Afrocentric view, the lore contends that the criminalization of marijuana is part of a grand plan that is politically and economically motivated by some Western capitalist powers to keep Ghana, and by extension Africa, a puppet of the West. The criminalization of the herb during the colonial period is linked to the assumption that marijuana, which was comparatively cheap and readily available, especially in the forest areas, competed with the sale of cigarettes, which was introduced by the colonizer's economy. As a result, the colonial regime's commercial interests in the sale of cigarettes had to be protected with the purposeful criminalization of marijuana. Thus, the criminalization of marijuana's cultivation, sale, and use is a neocolonial plan to deprive Ghana, and many African countries, of a huge source of revenue. Consequently, its proscription by the government in the postcolonial moment today is a neocolonialist appeasement. The above view was articulated by a ghetto member as follows:

> They will criminalize everything African. Why would they criminalize taba? Why don't they criminalize cigarettes, which they themselves universally agree is harmful to human health? Why won't they criminalize alcohol since, again, it is believed to be harmful to human health? They always claim they burn taba, when they arrest any pusher with the substance, but have you ever heard them burn cocaine? This white people have an agenda: an agenda to keep Africans continuously poor? If their land were to be good enough to sustain the cultivation of marijuana, do you think they would have criminalized it? You are educated, and it is good you have come to us to seek our opinion on this substance. We will continue to consume taba because we know the benefit we derive from it.

CONCLUSION

Whether marijuana is entirely harmless is contentious. In the ghetto, the herb is taken as each person sees fit, but it is commonly smoked. It can be prepared in the form of a tea or used as condiments to other foods. It is cut and cleaned of excess seeds on a wooden board, sanctified with a few drops of water, and recut and rolled in smoking paper into conical-shaped "rolls" or "spliffs." The act of passing the spliff or the cup of tea from a friend to a friend or around the brethren is considered a reverential and unification practice in the ghetto and an invocation toward powers of the spiritual world. When smoked in a gathering it symbolizes the act of physical, mental, and spiritual association among the assembly. It is accepted as binding the participants together in the fullness of God, thereby creating a concerted flow of mutual meditation and reasoning among those participating in the sacramental feeding. For them, it can reveal the divine and living presence in all humans. It releases an energy flow carrying the revelations of the inner creative source otherwise covered in the grosser reality of the mundane physical body. This experience is a positive act toward God and not a negative end.

Every now and then, some persons are imprisoned for either possessing or cultivating marijuana in Ghana, and yet reports on the consumption of marijuana continue to find space in the newspapers. The ghettos in Maamobi continue to record neophytes who join the ghetto lifestyle to consume marijuana because of the rhetoric of the ghetto lore about the perceived benefits associated with the substance. The users claim that, contrary to outside social rhetoric intended to sway them from their attitude to and belief in the herb, they alone are the sum awareness and reality of their own health, spiritual, and social experience of the herb within their body and spirit and mind. They argue that the ethical and medical reality of the herb resides solely with the individual and his conscience. They choose to see it as fit because they know and for them it is so! Their consumption has not succumbed to the negative testimonies about the substance. Its historical significance in Islam and in the indigenous milieu of Ghana and its assumed ability to ward off witches continue to make the consumption of marijuana current among some Muslim youth in the ghetto. The fact that marijuana continues to enjoy some significant acceptance in Ghana requires a broader discourse on the substance. We need to do a good analysis of this subject to clear doubt about the benefits (or otherwise) of marijuana.

NOTES

1. Lester Grinspoon and James B. Bakalar, *Marihuana, the Forbidden Medicine* (New Haven, CT: Yale University Press, 1993).
2. Lynn Zimmer and John P. Morgan, *Marijuana Myths, Marijuana Facts: A Review of the Scientific Evidence* (New York: Lindesmith Center, 1997).
3. Gabriel Nahas and C. Latour, "The Human Toxicity of Marijuana," *Medical Journal Australian* 156 (1992): 495–97.
4. Elaine Walters, *Marijuana: An Australian Crisis* (Malvern, Australia: E. Walters, 1993).
5. G. E. Woody and W. MacFadden, "Cannabis Related Disorders," in *Comprehensive Textbook of Psychiatry*, 6th ed., edited by H. I. Kaplan and B. Sadock (Baltimore: Williams & Wilkens, 1995), 810–16; United Nations Development Programme, *Human Development Report 2002: Deepening Democracy in a Fragmented World* (Oxford: Oxford University Press, 2002); United Nations Office on Drugs and Crime (UNODC), *World Drug Report 2009* (New York: United Nations, 2009); United Nations Office on Drugs and Crime (UNODC), *World Drug Report 2010* (New York: United Nations, 2010).

6. United Nations Office on Drugs and Crime (UNODC), *World Drug Report 2014* (New York: United Nations, 2014), 41.

7. Gary J. Miller, *Drugs and the Law: Detection, Recognition & Investigation*, 2nd ed. (Longwood, FL: Gould, 1997), 412.

8. Henry Bernstein, "Ghana's Drug Economy: Some Preliminary Data," *Review of African Political Economy* 26, no. 79 (1999): 13–32.

9. Joseph B. Asare, *The Problems of Drug Abuse in Ghana* (Accra: Sedco Publishing Ltd., 2008), 26.

10. N. Joshua Kudadjie and Robert Kwasi Aboagye-Mensah, *Christian Social Ethics* (Accra: Asempa, 2004), 159.

11. Dr. Asiama, a lecturer at the School of Performing Arts, and practitioner of herbal medicine, interview by author, Accra, Ghana, October 4, 2010.

12. Dr. Asiama interview.

13. Dr. Asiama interview.

14. Some of the traditional priests and priestesses interviewed for this study pleaded anonymity because of the legal status of the substance in the country. We are, therefore, unable to mention their names.

15. Vincent Adjei, an ex-serviceman, interview by author, Accra, Ghana, November 13, 2010.

16. Emmanuel Kwaku Akyeampong, "Diaspora and Drug Trafficking in West Africa: A Case Study of Ghana," *African Affairs* 104, no. 416 (2005): 429–47.

17. Akyeampong, "Diaspora and Drug Trafficking in West Africa," 433.

18. Ato Essel, "Ghana's War on Narcotic Drugs," *GhanaWeb*, May 25, 2009, http://209.197.117.98/GhanaHomePage/features/Ghana-s-War-On-Narcotic-Drugs-162563, accessed on October 1, 2015.

19. Akyeampong, "Diaspora and Drug Trafficking in West Africa," 435.

20. The position of the chief imam is supported by other elders of the community, including Baba Moro Issa, chief of Wangara community, and Alhaji Haruna Bukari Dabre, assemblyman for Maamobi East Electoral Area.

21. Anthony Prempeh, interview by author, Accra, Ghana, September 12, 2008.

22. A. Ali Mazrui, *Islam: Between Globalization and Counterterrorism* (Oxford: James Currey, 2006).

23. Gabriel Nahas, "Hashish in Islam: 9th to 18th Century," *Bulletin of the New York Academy of Medicine* 58, no. 9 (1982): 823.

24. Nahas, "Hashish in Islam."

25. Nahas, "Hashish in Islam," 823.

26. Sami Hamarneh, "Pharmacy in Medieval Islam and History of Drug Addiction," *Medical History* 16, no. 3 (1972): 231.

27. Hamarneh, "Pharmacy in Medieval Islam and History of Drug Addiction," 232.

28. Oakley Sten Ray and Charles Ksir, *Drugs, Society & Human Behaviour* (St. Louis: Mosby Year Book, Inc., 1996).

29. Nahas, "Hashish in Islam," 816–17.

30. Nahas, "Hashish in Islam," 817.

31. Nahas, "Hashish in Islam."

32. Nahas, "Hashish in Islam," 820.

33. Hamarneh, "Pharmacy in Medieval Islam."

34. Hamarneh, "Pharmacy in Medieval Islam," 236.

35. Nahas, "Hashish in Islam," 824.

36. Cited in Nahas, "Hashish in Islam."

37. Nahas, "Hashish in Islam."

38. Nahas, "Hashish in Islam," 825.

39. Ruqaiyyah Maqsood, *Islam* (Lincolnwood, IL: NTC, 1994), 160.

40. Nahas, "Hashish in Islam," 826.

41. Nahas, "Hashish in Islam," 825.

42. The real names of our respondents are not used because of security reasons. The statements attributed to the names are accurate, but the names are fictitious.

43. Many followers of Rastafari wear a hairstyle popularly called dreadlocks and consume marijuana as a holy sacrament.

BIBLIOGRAPHY

Akyeampong, Emmanuel Kwaku. "Diaspora and Drug Trafficking in West Africa: A Case Study of Ghana." *African Affairs* 104, no. 416 (2005): 429–47.

Asare, Joseph B. *The Problems of Drug Abuse in Ghana*. Accra: Sedco Publishing Ltd., 2008.

Bernstein, Henry. "Ghana's Drug Economy: Some Preliminary Data." *Review of African Political Economy* 26, no. 79 (1999): 13–32.

Essel, Ato. "Ghana's War on Narcotic Drugs." *GhanaWeb*, May 25, 2009. http://209.197.117.98/GhanaHomePage/features/Ghana-s-War-On-Narcotic-Drugs-162563. Accessed on October 1, 2015.

Grinspoon, Lester, and James B. Bakalar. *Marihuana, the Forbidden Medicine*. New Haven, CT: Yale University Press, 1993.

Hamarneh, Sami. "Pharmacy in Medieval Islam and History of Drug Addiction." *Medical History* 16, no. 3 (1972): 226–37.

Kudadjie, Joshua N., and Robert Kwasi Aboagye-Mensah. *Christian Social Ethics*. Accra: Asempa, 2004.

Maqsood, Ruqaiyyah. *Islam*. Lincolnwood, IL: NTC, 1994.

Mazrui, A. Ali. *Islam: Between Globalization and Counterterrorism*. Oxford: James Currey, 2006.

Miller, Gary J. *Drugs and the Law: Detection, Recognition & Investigation*, 2nd ed. Longwood, FL: Gould, 1997.

Nahas, Gabriel. "Hashish in Islam: 9th to 18th Century." *Bulletin of the New York Academy of Medicine* 58, no. 9 (1982): 814–31.

Nahas, Gabriel, and C. Latour. "The Human Toxicity of Marijuana." *Medical Journal of Australia* 156 (1992): 495–97.

Ray, Oakley Sten, and Charles Ksir. *Drugs, Society & Human Behavior*. St. Louis: Mosby Year Book, Inc., 1996.

United Nations Development Programme. *Human Development Report 2002: Deepening Democracy in a Fragmented World*. Oxford: Oxford University Press, 2002.

United Nations Office on Drugs and Crime (UNODC). *World Drug Report 2009*. New York: United Nations, 2009.

United Nations Office on Drugs and Crime (UNODC). *World Drug Report 2010*. New York: United Nations, 2010.

United Nations Office on Drugs and Crime (UNODC). *World Drug Report 2014*. New York: United Nations, 2014.

"US State Dept on Ghana's Narcotics Trade: International Narcotics Control Strategy Report on Ghana—2006." *GhanaWeb*, March 2006. http://www.ghanaweb.com/GhanaHomePage/economy/artikel.php?ID=103459.

Woody, G. E., and W. McFadden. "Cannabis Related Disorders." In *Comprehensive Textbook of Psychiatry*, 6th ed., edited by H. I. Kaplan and B. Sadock, 810–16. Baltimore: Williams & Wilken, 1995.

Walters, Elaine. *Marijuana: An Australian Crisis*. Malvern, Australia: E. Walters, 1993.

Zimmer, Lynn, and John P. Morgan. *Marijuana Myths, Marijuana Facts: A Review of the Scientific Evidence*. New York: Lindesmith Center, 1997.

Chapter Fifteen

What Makes a Good Mother?

Mother's Conceptions of Good Food

Liora Gvion and Irit Sharir

The formation of social groups that revolve around food ideologies and practices are limited in Israel. However, with the growing concern for healthy eating and the mounting popularity of vegetarianism, veganism, and consumption of organic foods, there has been an increase in individual agencies formed around food consumption. These agencies often seek support from individuals who uphold similar food beliefs. This chapter focuses on a group of mothers of young children (pre-K through sixth grade). Each of these mothers applies strict food practices, aiming to provide their children with the skills of becoming critical and health-oriented food consumers. Caring for their children's particular food intake is taken as an indication of good motherhood and a means of introducing parental control. However, daily routines require that both the mothers and the children develop strategies for coping with social surroundings in which their food rules are not followed. We point to three major means by which the mothers cope in social environments that are not supportive of their foodways. First, when surrounded by people who eat differently, the mothers loosen up the rules, trusting their children to internalize the principles of correct eating to the extent that they follow them despite the food "temptations" provided. Second, they try shaping their children's food environment by either providing them with homemade foods to be eaten at all times or convincing their children's surroundings to change their food habits. Third, in order to get support, they limit their contacts with people who eat differently by homeschooling their children, affecting the schools' menus, and socializing with peers with similar food beliefs and practices.

FOOD AND GOOD PARENTING

Women often see their domestic kitchens as settings for "doing gender"; for example, engaging in an entirety of socially guided perceptional and interactional activities that cast particular pursuits as expressions of masculine and feminine nature.[1] Feeding, for them, is a pleasurable female labor of love, which is done for specific people whose taste is taken into account[2] and wins the appreciation of their family members.[3]

However, industrial and technological developments have reduced the amount of the domestic food labor. As convenient as it is to use ready-made foods, a growing number of parents, and mothers particularly, claim feeding their families healthily is their primary concern. They worry about the safety of the foods they feed their children and often do not trust the government to guarantee the food is appropriate for human consumption.[4] Since children grow to like foods to which they have been exposed, the greater their exposure to a healthy form of eating, the more they develop healthy eating habits.[5] When parents understand that they set an example for their children's eating habits, it is also easier for them to stick to the nutritional codes they have set.[6] These healthy eating habits, they claim, will guide the children throughout their lives.[7]

Various factors prevent mothers from following the food rules they wish their offspring to respect. First, their children spend a great deal of their time out of the home where they are exposed to foods that contradict the house rules. Consequently, in order for their children to have a social life when in the company of friends, the mothers often ease their restrictions, trusting their children to have internalized the house food rules and to follow them at all times. Second, as strict as the women are about their food practices, they still prioritize their good relationships with their children. The decision to let the children deviate from the food rules is, therefore, a means of expressing respect and trust in their children and ensuring that the children develop their own taste. Some parents even distinguish between weekday and weekend foods, claiming that when the entire family eats together the food is interpreted in social and emotional terms rather than in its health-related terms.[8]

Parents usually employ one out of two strategies to ensure their children eat healthily. They either limit the consumption of unhealthy foodstuffs or apply pressure to consume healthy food only. Both practices may limit the children's freedom of choosing and controlling their diet. For example, Brown and Ogden[9] found that the greater the parents' attempt to control their offspring's food intake, the stronger the need to negotiate their children's consumption of both healthy and nonhealthy food items and the greater their difficulties of instilling parental authority in general. Children who are denied the freedom of choice often develop a liking for the types of foods of which they have been denied.[10] Allowing children to have their own say about their diet and providing them with information about the consequences of consuming both healthy and nonhealthy food, rather than just following their parents' orders, enables parents to limit the consumption of junk food. Food does not become a subject against which the children revolt because they are equipped with all the necessary means of selecting healthy foodstuffs even when not supervised.[11]

In light of the above, this chapter suggests looking at a unique group of professional women, all of whom live in a small town an hour north of Tel Aviv. Following the birth of their first child, they either stopped working out of the home or switched to careers that allowed flexible working hours and could mostly be done from home. They embedded their perception of good motherhood with food practices that called for the consumption of whole foods, organic vegetables and fruits, as well as abstention from dairy products, sweets, and mass-produced food items. They were all between thirty and forty-three years of age at the time of the interview and had at least one child. We reached them via a forum they had established on Facebook with the aim of getting information about healthy food and making friends with mothers with similar food beliefs. They make a good case study for examining the connection between motherhood and thinking about food and for looking at the way in which they later bring people together.

We stipulate that in light of lacking a yardstick against which motherhood is estimated, the participants used their food rules and the extent to which their children followed them as a means of reinforcing their self-perception as mothers. They developed strategies for their children to follow a healthy diet, claiming that ensuring appropriate eating was part of their maternal duties.

FOOD AND PARENTAL RESPONSIBILITY

Healthy eating for our interviewees was a means by which the women reassured themselves they were good mothers who equipped their offspring with the necessary skills to be critical food consumers, assume responsibility for their health, and prevent future illnesses. However, their inability to control their children's food intake at all times obliged them to make certain compromises and adjustments. Some trusted their children to eat properly even at settings in which unhealthy food was served. Others tried to manipulate the environments where their children spent time and to change the menu so it matched their dietary rules. Nevertheless, in order to minimize their children's exposure to foods they did not approve of, all of them constructed their social lives around people who followed similar food practices so their children were not isolated.

Upon the birth of their first child, our interviewees realized how little they knew about the food they themselves ate and fed others with. Hence, they started reading about nutrition and changing their diets accordingly. Feeding their child "correctly" became a manifestation of parental authority and responsibility. Anna, a thirty-nine-year-old mother of three and an economist who became a dietary consultant, says:

> My oldest didn't gain enough weight. I started consulting pediatricians and clinical dietitians and became obsessive with it. So I started asking myself questions and realized I was a thirty-year-old mother who knew nothing about the food her family ate.

Motherhood made Anna interrelate parental responsibility with "correct" eating, seeing feeding as a manifestation of good motherhood. One of her ways of making sure she was providing her baby with good food was to select the sources she relied on for information.

Meirav, a thirty-four-year-old dance therapist and a four-month pregnant mother of a two-year-old, also assessed her maternal performance by the control she exerted over her child's diet:

> I had this need to be the perfect mother. I started reading about nutrition and gradually making changes. All of a sudden it wasn't only me I was responsible for but another human being as well.

It was the responsibility for another human being that caused the women to reconstruct their knowledge of food in connection with their maternal feelings and to deconstruct their new knowledge into a set of food practices that would ensure correct feeding. Nevertheless, it was while attending to their children's needs that they realized their offspring might wish to eat food items they did not approve of. Yael, a thirty-nine-year-old mother of four and a lactation consultant, tells us:

> We were vegetarians. Once, we had dinner at our friends' house and my daughter grabbed a chicken leg and ate it with great pleasure. I understood that I was depriving her of food items she was entitled to have. I was worried that she'd eat meat out of the home and I'd lose control over her eating. So I started preparing meat and eating it with them.

Her daughter's behavior compelled Yael to adjust domestic food practices to meet her particular needs even if they challenged the home food rules. With the aim of gaining control over her daughter's eating, exercising parental authority, and supporting her daughter's right to develop her own taste, Yael integrated meat into the family's diet.

The dietary principles the women introduced to their families also required the cooperation of their spouses. However, the latter were often reluctant to give up their old eating habits. Some of them ate healthy at home but kept eating whatever they wished when out of the house. Most of the men, like Anna's husband, made some compromises:

> My husband used to live on junk food, coke, and lots of coffee. It took me a while to change his diet. Today he eats healthy with the exception of coffee with cow milk.

By running the domestic kitchen according to their food beliefs, claiming their particular diet provides them with the necessary means to lead a healthy life, mothers gain control over members of their household. However, spouses may disagree about the centrality of food in the family's life and the proportion of the family's budget spent on food. Women negotiate with their husbands over the amount of money spent on health food and claim the latter is as important as the children's education. Yael says:

> We decided to spend money on food and schooling for the children because we believe they constitute an investment in their future. These are things the kids will use for the rest of their lives.

Setting food rules does not necessarily imply they are followed by the children and at all times. Our interviewees realize the limitation of maternal control, especially when exposing their children to social settings in which different food rules apply. This turns social and familial gatherings into opportunities for testing the extent to which children have internalized the food rules to which they have been socialized so they can be trusted to follow them. Yael says:

> I have a duty to set them on the right track so they can go on without me. I won't be there forever to tell them what they can and can't eat. My inner voice will always be with them.

Trusting one's children, according to Yael, is an ongoing process. It is by correct upbringing she hopes her children are going to internalize her food rules and follow them distinctly. Anna, conversely, believes in being stricter with her children in order to set them on the right path:

> Will you let your child ride his bike without a helmet? The same goes for food. A mother has to set her limits. Children will always challenge them. If I let them have junk food I'll poison them.

In addition to trusting their children to eat properly, eating out of the house requires that the mothers decide on the degree of freedom given to their children in choosing their food. Chen, a forty-three-year-old stay-at-home mother, has ongoing conflicts with her parents over food:

> At first my parents deliberately went against me. They prepared cake, frozen meat, and candy saying my kids needed to be spoiled because they were deprived of the good things of life. At a certain point I put an end to it and said: if you want to spoil them bring them food we consider as a treat. Sometimes they still bring cookies.

Miri, a thirty-eight-year-old stay-at-home mother of four who is expecting her fifth child, decided not to turn against her parents and lets them "spoil" the children:

> They have a need to feed them junk. It has its benefits. My kids know that they eat enough junk at their grandparent's house. I set a limit to the quantities. My parents babysit and love them dearly. So letting them feed my kids on junk is a price I pay.

Yael, conversely, uses her children's exposure to unhealthy foods as an opportunity to teach them how to eat healthy in an "unhealthy" environment:

> We spent the weekend in a big hotel. The first time we went into the dining room they were amazed by the food choices. We said: You can choose whatever you want but only after you eat what one should eat. They didn't object because by now they can feel what their bodies need.

The fact that Yael trusts her children to feel the needs of their bodies and eat accordingly is based on their socialization. A meal, according to her, must include certain food items, and once one follows them she or he is not tempted into deviating from their diet. Miri, by contrast, stresses the importance of emotional gestures via food that sustain familial relations even at the price of deviating from domestic food rules. By limiting the quantities of junk food her children eat, she exercises parental control and also shows her children she respects her parents by letting them set their own food rules.

In addition to compromising and showing the children how important it is to be flexible when the circumstances require it, the women also try to minimize future rebellions against their food rules. Anna says:

> They have three possibilities: rebelling and eating junk food, following my way because they understand how important it is, or be somewhere in the middle. All I can do is give them my knowledge and hope they use it.

Meirav agrees:

> I can give them the means to choose the right foods. One day they'll choose their own ways of eating and may even go against all I've taught them.

One of the ways of minimizing future rebellions of their children and contemporary conflicts is to let them choose part of the food they eat even if it is "unhealthy." Shira, a forty-one-year-old beautician, says:

> They each planned their favorite menu so that we could prepare the dishes they liked. I let them have ketchup and mayonnaise because they don't eat a lot of it. But I prepare pastrami at home and never buy it.

Another way of minimizing conflicts is by disguising health food items. Shira, who feeds her children on brown rice and whole-wheat pasta without mentioning it, says:

> I don't talk to my kids about rice. I just serve it. I talk about junk food because it's bad for them. Rice and pasta are common in every household, just as soap is. Why talk about it?

By serving healthy food items in a form of "regular" items yet different in their content and nutritional value, without referring to the actual nature of the dish, Shira wins her children's cooperation and controls their eating. But the older the children are, the harder it gets to manipulate them into eating healthy. They are influenced by peers, and the women have to believe that, although their children vocalize their protest, they still eat healthy, as Anna does:

> My older kids are aware of the difference between the way we eat and the way their friends eat. They often challenge me, but I know that when they're out of the house they follow the house rules and even try to convince their friends to eat differently. As long as they eat healthy I don't mind their protest.

Some of the children, according to our interviewees, already realize the long-term rewards of healthy eating. Shira tells us:

> The dentist said she could see that they drink water and not sodas. On our way back my son said, thanks mom for teaching us to drink water. I said to myself: It worked because I never forced anything on them.

Chen adds:

> My kids never visited a pediatrician because eating healthy minimizes one's chance and probability of getting sick.

Tal, a thirty-nine-year-old stay-at-home mother of a two-year-old girl, adds:

> I explain everything. Yesterday, we were at a health store. She took a bottle of preserved lemon juice and I told her we use fresh lemons only. She said "not healthy." That's what happens when you explain everything.

On the one hand, the expectation to follow a healthy diet requires women to negotiate with their children over their food intake and to set limits on the consumption of unhealthy food items. Simultaneously, eating healthy obliges the children to assume responsibility for their eating in addition to developing their own tastes. Being able to equip the children with the principle of correct eating and allowing them a certain freedom to choose what to eat reassures and reinforces the women's self-perception as good mothers.

Just as social gatherings embody challenges to parental control, schools, where different food rules apply, also require that the mothers make certain decisions. For instance, should they single their children out by sending them homemade food, or should they let them eat what the rest of the children eat? Some prioritize food to an extent that they choose schools that either follow the same diet or let children bring their own food, regardless of the school philosophy or curriculum. Most of the mothers enroll their children in the public or private school system, whose menus consist of items they do not approve of. This implies that certain compromises need to be made. Yael, for instance, sends her children to an anthroposophical school because their menu is the closest to the home menu:

> Most of the parents don't choose a school for their children by its menu. They start thinking about it upon realizing their child is willing to eat only a limited variety of foods. They give up because they want to minimize familial arguments. For me the menu is an integral part of the curriculum. I also make sure there's more in a birthday party than junk food.

By choosing a school with a similar "food philosophy" to her own, Yael minimizes the potential conflicts for her children and integrates their schooling into their daily lives. Most of the women cannot afford to send their children to private schools that serve only health food. Thus, they have to come to terms with losing a certain amount of control over their offspring's foodways. As in the case of social gatherings, they hope their children will choose to eat according to the home food rules. However, it rarely works. Gila, a thirty-four-year-old stay-at-home mother of three, started homeschooling her children after realizing her oldest was not capable of making the right choices:

> At the beginning of the year I packed her lunch and she ate it. With time she started eating the food the rest of the children ate. Every Friday they celebrated someone else's birthday and stuffed the children with junk food. I was the only one who cared.

Another way of ensuring their children do not deviate from the home food rules is to bring to school food items that are similar in form but different in their content from the food served in the school system. The children eat food that resembles what the rest of the children eat, which minimizes the difference between them and their peers and gives the mother a feeling she is still in control of their eating. Meirav says:

> I bring to the kindergarten homemade jam which the teacher spreads over the bread I provide them. This way he doesn't feel different.

But she also realizes the limitations of her control when her child is out of the house:

> I let go because I really like the school in all other aspects but food. Their personnel is wonderful and it's more important than just worrying about the food they serve. So he eats eggs and vegetables that are not organic for breakfast. But he doesn't touch the cheese because he isn't used to eating cheese. I send with him tahini and our own bread. The staff thinks I'm nuts but they let me do it.

In search of support for the way they raise their children and for the children to be part of an environment in which they do not feel different, the women establish social networks that revolve around matters of food. Via their interactions with parents with similar views on nutrition, they are reassured that they are good mothers who raise healthy children. Meirav, for instance, has narrowed her social circles and surrounded herself with people "like me":

> People talk about us as "this group of snobbish mothers who raise their children on tofu." We first met them when my son was a baby and we started meeting regularly and doing things with our children. We talk about food and health. It makes me part of a community. I no longer feel comfortable with my other friends who laugh at me for feeding my child on health food. I hardly see them.

Eating habits generate social bonding among the mothers based on similar food beliefs. Being part of a community makes it easier for them to adhere to their food beliefs and make sure their children follow them as much as the circumstances allow. Being part of a group reassures the women that they are good mothers who have chosen the right path for their children even at the price of being socially isolated and enjoying only a small circle of friends. Anna sums up:

> We are surrounded by people who are highly conscious about their food and understand how essential food is to one's health. It is a great benefit, and it makes our life easier and more pleasant. We are not an exception.

CONCLUSION

This chapter looked at a group of mothers of young children (pre-K through sixth grade) who were brought together due to similar food beliefs and practices and got support and reassurance for their style of parenthood. They were all professionals; yet, upon becoming mothers, they switched to careers that allowed flexible working hours, many of which were done from the home. Some even became stay-at-home mothers in order to devote all their attention to their child. Motherhood, they claimed, generated responsibility for another person's well-being—a duty to equip the dependent ones with the necessary means of eating healthy and preventing future illness.

It is our conclusion that the women surround themselves with people who follow similar foodways in the aim of reassuring themselves they are good mothers who raise healthy children. Food, for them, becomes a means to an end. Lacking a yardstick against which motherhood can be evaluated, the women use food and eating to assess their performance of motherhood. They make inquiries about food and consequently plan a healthy diet. However, the exposure of their children to social settings in which different food rules apply compels the women to trust their children to eat according to the family's food rules, thus assuming responsibility for their own health. Cases in which women are unable to control their children's eating are taken as an expression of the children's entitlement to develop their own taste as well as an opportunity to show respect to other people's foodways. By bonding with other mothers who see food and feeding as major components of their maternal identity, the women are socially acknowledged as being good mothers. They become part of a "superior club" designed for people who are committed to particular forms of eating and see food as an essential component of their parental identity.

NOTES

1. Candance West and Don Zimmerman, "Doing Gender," *Gender and Society* 1, no. 2 (1987): 125–51.
2. Brenda Beagan, Gwen Chapman, Andrea D'Sylva, Raewyn Bassett, et al., "It's Just Easier for Me to Do It: Rationalizing the Family Division of Foodwork," *Sociology* 42, no. 4

(2008): 653–71; Michel De Certeau, Luce Girad, and Pierre Mayol, *The Practice of Everyday Life* (Minneapolis: University of Minnesota Press, 1998); Marjory DeVault, *Feeding the Family* (Chicago: University of Chicago Press, 1991); Arlie Hochschild, *The Second Shift* (New York: Avon Books, 1989); Anne Murcott, "Cooking and the Cooked: A Note on the Domestic Preparation of Meals," in *The Sociology of Food and Eating*, edited by Anne Murcott (Aldershot: Gower, 1983), 78–85; Michelle Szabo, "Men Nurturing through Food: Challenging Gender Dichotomies around Domestic Cooking," *Journal of Gender Studies* 23, no. 1 (2014): 18–31; Helen Vallianatos and Kim Raine, "Consuming Food and Constructing Identities among Arabic and South Asian Immigrant Women," *Food, Culture and Society* 2, no. 3 (2008): 375–400.

3. Liora Gvion, "The Changing Significance of Cooking and Meals for Kibbutz Women," *Food and Foodways* 23 (2015): 163–85; Szabo, "Men Nurturing through Food."

4. Joylin Namie, "Public Displays of Affection: Mothers, Children, and Requests for Junk Food," *Food, Culture and Society* 14, no. 3 (2011): 393–412; Barbro Johansson, Eva Ossiansson, Jessica A. Dreas, and Stafan Marild, "Proper Food and Tight Budget: German and Swedish Parents Reflecting on Children's Food and Health," *Food, Culture and Society* 16, no. 3 (2013): 457–78; Terese Anving and Stine Thorsted, "Feeding Ideals and the Work of Feeding in Swedish Families," *Food, Culture and Society* 10, no. 1 (2010): 29–46; Debbie Kemmer, "Tradition and Change in Domestic Roles and Food Preparation," *Sociology* 34, no. 2 (2000): 323–33.

5. Lucy Cooke, "The Importance of Exposure for Healthy Eating in Childhood," *Journal of Human Nutrition and Dietetics* 20, no. 4 (2007): 294–301.

6. C. A. Vereeckeen, Els Keukelier, and L. Maes, "Influence of Mother's Educational Level on Food Parenting Practices and Food Habits of Young Children," *Appetite* 43, no. 1 (2004): 93–103; Rachael Brown and Jane Ogden, "Children's Eating Attitudes and Behavior: A Study of the Modelling and Control Theories of Parental Influence," *Health Education Research Theory and Practice* 19, no. 3 (2004): 261–71.

7. Johansson et al., "Proper Food and Tight Budget."

8. Johansson et al., "Proper Food and Tight Budget"; Namie, "Public Displays of Affection"; Charlene Elliott, "Parent's Choice: Examining Parent Perspectives on Regulations and Child-Targeted Supermarket Foods," *Food Culture and Society* 16, no. 3 (2013): 437–56.

9. Brown and Ogden, "Children's Eating Attitudes and Behavior."

10. Michelle Szabo, "Foodwork or Foodplay? Men's Domestic Cooking, Privilege and Leisure," *Sociology* 47 (2013): 623–38.

11. Namie, "Public Displays of Affection."

BIBLIOGRAPHY

Anving, Terese, and Stine Thorsted. "Feeding Ideals and the Work of Feeding in Swedish Families." *Food Culture and Society* 10, no. 1 (2010): 29–46.

Beagan, Brenda, Gwen Chapman, Andrea D'Sylva, Raewyn Bassett, et al. "'It's Just Easier for Me to Do It': Rationalizing the Family Division of Foodwork." *Sociology* 42, no. 4 (2008): 653–71.

Brown, Rachael, and Jane Ogden. "Children's Eating Attitudes and Behavior: A Study of the Modelling and Control Theories of Parental Influence." *Health Education Research Theory and Practice* 19, no. 3 (2004): 261–71.

Cooke, Lucy. "The Importance of Exposure for Healthy Eating in Childhood." *Journal of Human Nutrition and Dietetics* 20, no. 4 (2007): 294–301.

De Certeau, Michel, Luce Girad, and Pierre Mayol. *The Practice of Everyday Life*. Minneapolis: University of Minnesota Press, 1998.

DeVault, Marjory. *Feeding the Family*. Chicago: University of Chicago Press, 1991.

Elliott, Charlene. "Parent's Choice: Examining Parent Perspectives on Regulation and Child-Targeted Supermarket Foods." *Food, Culture and Society* 16, no. 3 (2013): 437–56.

Gvion, Liora. "The Changing Significance of Cooking and Meals for Kibbutz Women." *Food and Foodways* 23 (2015): 163–85.

Hochschild, Arlie. *The Second Shift*. New York: Avon Books, 1989.

Johansson, Barbro, Eva Ossiansson, Jessica A. Dreas, and Stafan Marild. "Proper Food and Tight Budget: German and Swedish Parents Reflecting on Children Food and Health." *Food, Culture and Society* 16, no. 3 (2013): 457–78.

Kemmer, Debbie. "Tradition and Change in Domestic Roles and Food Preparation." *Sociology* 34, no. 2 (2000): 323–33.

Murcott, Anne. "Cooking and the Cooked: A Note on the Domestic Preparation of Meals." In *The Sociology of Food and Eating*, edited by Anne Murcott, 78–85. Aldershot: Gower, 1983.

Namie, Joylin. "Public Displays of Affection: Mothers, Children, and Requests for Junk Food." *Food, Culture and Society* 14, no. 3 (2011): 393–412.

Szabo, Michelle. "Foodwork or Foodplay? Men's Domestic Cooking, Privilege and Leisure." *Sociology* 47 (2013): 623–38.

Szabo, Michelle. "Men Nurturing through Food: Challenging Gender Dichotomies around Domestic Cooking." *Journal of Gender Studies* 23, no. 1 (2014): 18–31.

Vallianatos, Helen, and Kim Raine. "Consuming Food and Constructing Identities among Arabic and South Asian Immigrant Women." *Food, Culture and Society* 11, no. 3 (2008): 375–400.

Vereeckeen, C. A., Els Keukelier, and L. Maes. "Influence of Mother's Educational Level on Food Parenting Practices and Food Habits of Young Children." *Appetite* 43, no. 1 (2004): 93–103.

West, Candace, and Don Zimmerman. "Doing Gender." *Gender and Society* 1, no. 2 (1987): 125–51.

Index

About the Contributors

Ken Albala is professor of history at the University of the Pacific in Stockton, California, where he teaches courses on the Renaissance and Reformation, food history, and the history of medicine. He is the author of many books on food history, including *Eating Right in the Renaissance* (2002), *Food in Early Modern Europe* (2003), *Cooking in Europe 1250–1650* (2005), *The Banquet: Dining in the Great Courts of Late Renaissance Europe* (2007), *Beans: A History* (2007; winner of the 2008 International Association of Culinary Professionals Jane Grigson Award), and *Pancake* (2008). He has coauthored two cookbooks: *The Lost Art of Real Cooking* (2010) and *The Lost Arts of Hearth and Home* (2012). He has also edited the four-volume *Food Cultures of the World Encyclopedia* (2010) and coedits the journal *Food, Culture and Society*.

Lenore Bell received her BA from Amherst College, her MA in English literature from Universiteit Leiden, and her PhD from the University of St. Andrews. Her research interests include the post-traumatic imagination, fitness culture, and Kafka.

De-Valera N. Y. M. Botchway has a PhD and an MPhil in history, which he obtained in 2011 and 2004, respectively. He is a senior lecturer of history and African studies at the University of Cape Coast, Ghana. The focus of his research is a confluence of the social and cultural history of Africa and the African and global historic and cultural exchanges and experiences. His comparative and interdisciplinary research interests are in several fields of

African and African diaspora history and studies. These include the West African history, popular culture and sports (boxing) history in Ghana, African indigenous knowledge systems, world civilizations, and Africans in dispersion. He has had intimate involvements in the scholarship and research enterprises at the University of Cambridge, England, as a fellow of the African Studies Centre from 2006 to 2007; the University of South Florida as a visiting scholar and global academic partner in 2010; and the Grand Valley State University, Michigan, as exchange faculty in 2012. He received an African Humanities Programme Post-Doctoral Fellowship award of 2013–2014 from the American Council of Learned Society and took residence in the University of the Western Cape, Cape Town, South Africa. He edits three journals—*Drumspeak*, *Asemka*, and *Abibisem*—at the University of Cape Coast. He has attended some local and international conferences and authored several works.

Paul A. Brazinski is a fellow in the Department of Church History at the Catholic University of America, where he specializes in the history of Christianity from AD 250 to 1500. His research interests include the formation of Orthodoxy, heresy, and material culture. His book, *Late Antique Pilgrimage and Ampullae*, was published in 2014.

Barrett P. Brenton, PhD, is professor of anthropology and director of the Center for Global Development and Graduate Program in Global Development and Social Justice at St. John's University in Queens, New York. As a specialist on the nutritional anthropology of sustainable food systems, Dr. Brenton's cross-cultural applied fieldwork experience across five continents has ranged from studies of dietary biodiversity, food insecurity, and health in indigenous Native American and Ecuadorian Amazon communities to research on food aid and food sovereignty in Zambia, to community-based urban food systems and health disparities research in New York City.

Kima Cargill is the author of *The Psychology of Overeating: Food and the Culture of Consumerism* and associate professor of psychology at the University of Washington, Tacoma. She studies how the food and pharmaceutical industries use psychology to trick us into consuming more by distorting scientific information, sowing nutritional confusion, and convincing us that the solution to our problems is to consume more.

Leighann R. Chaffee received her master's from Northern Arizona University and currently teaches at the University of Washington, Tacoma. Her research interests focus on food-related attitudes and decision making, as well as the scholarship of teaching and learning.

Corey L. Cook received his PhD from the University of Florida and currently teaches at the University of Washington, Tacoma. His research focuses on the effects of threat perception on social cognition and behavior.

Preety Gadhoke received her PhD from the Johns Hopkins University and her MPH from Emory University. She teaches global health for the Master of Public Health Program at St. John's University, New York. Dr. Gadhoke is a fellow at the Vincentian Center for Church & Society and a mentor for the Ozanam and McNair scholars programs. She engages in community-based research using ethnography, visual anthropology, and mixed methodology to inform culturally tailored public health programs and policies for marginalized populations. Her research experiences include social network analysis for vaccines in Nigeria, health assessment for artisanal small-scale gold miners in Mozambique, childhood obesity prevention in Baltimore, youth empowerment and women's coping strategies for food security and health in New York City homeless populations, and community health and food security in indigenous Native American and Ecuadorian Amazon Shuar communities.

Liona Gibbs-Bravo studies anthropology and linguistics at McGill University. Her research focuses on the intersections between food, self-perception, and the linguistic mediation of self-image and food behaviors.

L. Sasha Gora studied art history and museum studies in Montreal, Canada; Copenhagen, Denmark; and Gothenburg, Sweden. She is a doctoral candidate at the Rachel Carson Center for Environment and Society. Her research charts connections between the New Nordic food movement and contemporary Canadian cuisine and reimaginations of First Nations food cultures. She writes about art and food and has contributed to publications such as *Gather*, *MUNCHIES: Food by VICE*, *Chickpea*, and *C Magazine*.

Carlnita P. Greene is visiting assistant professor in the media studies program at the University of Oregon's School of Journalism and Communication. Her research broadly operates at the intersections of food, rhetoric, media, and popular culture. Previously published on subjects as diverse as identity, style, and nostalgia, she is the author of *Gourmands and Gluttons: The Rhetoric of Food Excess* (2015) and coeditor of *Food as Communication/Communication as Food* (2011). Dr. Greene obtained her PhD in communication studies from the University of Texas at Austin, where she also earned a doctoral portfolio from the Amèrcio Paredes Center for Cultural Studies.

Liora Gvion is professor of sociology at the Kibbutzim College of Education in Tel Aviv, Israel. Her work mostly focuses on the sociology of food and the sociology of the body. She conducted a big study on Palestinian food in Israel, which matured into two books and several articles. Her current research centers on food and reality television and on social relationships embedded in the production of the human voice.

Jennifer Martin is a PhD candidate and presidential teaching fellow in social advocacy and ethical life at the University of South Carolina. Her book, coedited with Cammie M. Sublette, *Devouring Cultures: Perspectives on Food, Power, and Identity from the Zombie Apocalypse to Downton Abbey* (2016), examines food as a means to define cultural identity.

Amanda Maxfield is a doctoral candidate in biological anthropology at Emory University in Atlanta, Georgia. Her research interests include nutrition, social status, and health inequalities. Her dissertation focuses on the links between food insecurity, the nutrition transition, and mental health in India.

Charles Prempeh obtained a first-degree education at the University of Cape Coast, Ghana, where he graduated with first-class honors and a BA in African studies in 2008. Later in 2009, he enrolled at the Institute of African Studies, University of Ghana, for his MPhil degree and completed it in 2011. He is currently a third-year PhD student at the Makerere Institute of Social Research, Makerere University. His research interests are in contemporary Islamic practices in Ghana.

Andrea Rissing is a doctoral candidate in cultural anthropology at Emory University in Atlanta, Georgia. Her research interests include sustainable food systems, entrepreneurship, and the political history of U.S. agriculture. Her dissertation is focused on beginning farmer livelihoods in Iowa's alternative agriculture.

Michele Scott is a PhD student at North Carolina State University in the Department of Sociology and Anthropology. She currently holds a master of arts in sociology and is the author of *Barbecue Tofu and the Most Southern Food on Earth*.

Irit Sharir is a puppeteer and theatrical producer. Her BA thesis laid the foundations of her chapter.

Tina Sikka is currently a lecturer in media and cultural studies at the University of Newcastle in Australia. In addition to her work in the area of consumption, food, and identity, Dr. Sikka has published extensively on the importance of democratizing technology as it relates to sustainable energy and climate-mitigating technologies in such noted journals as *Technology in Society*, *Communication Review*, and *Critical Discourse Studies*. In these pieces, she focuses specifically on finding ways to build sustainable communities through citizen science projects that rely on empowered local decision making. Tina has also done work in the area of genetically modified foods, indigenous rights, and corn in Oaxaca, Mexico.

Samuel Veissière, PhD, is a cultural and cognitive anthropologist and visiting professor in the Division of Social and Transcultural Psychiatry, the Department of Anthropology, and the Raz Lab in Cognitive Neuroscience at McGill University. His work seeks to bridge gaps and foster dialogues between anthropological, philosophical, neurocognitive, and poetic traditions in the study of the human experience—an approach he terms *contemplative*. In addition to applied work in community education and public health with indigenous populations in Canada and Brazil, Veissière has conducted ethnographic fieldwork on street livelihoods, emergent modes of sociality, and social suffering in Brazil, the Amazon, and transnational contexts. He is presently involved in a series of studies on the social contexts of placebo and the comparative development of social cognition, personhood, and body consciousness across cultures.

www.ingramcontent.com/pod-product-compliance
Lightning Source LLC
LaVergne TN
LVHW101446200926
848483LV00001B/58